Office-Based Laryngeal Surgery

Abdul-latif Hamdan • Robert Thayer Sataloff
Mary J. Hawkshaw

Office-Based Laryngeal Surgery

Springer

Abdul-latif Hamdan
Otolaryngology, Head & Neck Surgery
American University of Beirut Medical Center
Beirut, Lebanon

Robert Thayer Sataloff
Otolaryngology – Head and Neck Surgery
Drexel University
Philadelphia, PA, USA

Mary J. Hawkshaw
Otolaryngology – Head and Neck Surgery
Drexel University
Philadelphia, PA, USA

ISBN 978-3-030-91935-1 ISBN 978-3-030-91936-8 (eBook)
https://doi.org/10.1007/978-3-030-91936-8

This Springer imprint is published by the registered company Springer Nature Switzerland AG
The registered company address is: Gewerbestrasse 11, 6330 Cham, Switzerland

To Sawsan, Aya, Adam, and Jad Hamdan

To Dahlia, Ben, and John
Sataloff, and Shyam Akula

To Luke James Kilcur

Preface

Advances in technology and instrumentation during the last few decades have improved the precision, case, and popularity of office-based laryngeal surgery. In-office surgery of the larynx has been performed with increasing frequency throughout the world. In patients who have been selected correctly, office-based surgery may provide several advantages over MicroDirect laryngoscopy in the operating room. These include eliminating the risks of general anesthesia, hastening the time from diagnosis to receipt of biopsy results, decreasing health care costs, and other benefits. However, in-office surgery requires expertise, informed patient selection, adequate instrumentation, patient education, and office staff training in order to be performed safely and effectively.

This book is intended to provide otolaryngologists with the information necessary to perform office-based surgery of the larynx appropriately. Much of the information may be known to laryngologists who already perform such procedures; however, many other otolaryngologists could add office-based laryngeal surgery to their practices, thereby offering a valuable option for selected patients. The authors discuss core knowledge essential to laryngeal surgeons, administration of topical anesthesia in an office setting, patient counseling and selection, techniques of various procedures, and other topics that we believe will be helpful for physicians who perform office-based laryngeal surgery.

The first four chapters provide core knowledge helpful in understanding voice disorders and are essential for accurate diagnosis, surgical patient selection, and understanding modern surgical techniques. They are modified with permission from prior publications by the author (RTS). This core information also has been included in the authors' prior books published by Springer for the convenience of our readers, and because mastery of these topics is critical to understanding voice and other laryngeal disorders and to providing optimal treatment. Chapter 1 provides a focused, brief review of the anatomy and physiology of phonation. This information is essential not only in helping to understand and establish diagnoses of laryngeal disorders but also to understand the precision required to achieve optimal outcomes with laryngeal surgery, whether it is performed in the operating room or in the office. Chapters 2 and 3 review the comprehensive medical evaluation (history and physical examination) performed for patients with voice complaints. Chapter 4, written in collaboration with Johnathan Sataloff, MD, offers an overview of many medical conditions that may affect the voice and of their treatments. In a majority of patients, nonsurgical treatment including voice therapy is appropriate before decisions are made regarding the need for laryngeal surgery, and prior to decisions about the venue in which laryngeal surgery should be performed.

Chapters 5, 6, 7, 8, 9, 10, 11, and 12 provide background information (including literature review) needed for various office-based surgical procedures, details of surgical techniques, illustrations, and videos. Chapter 5 discusses basic principles of in-office surgery, patient selection, safety, and patient tolerance. Much of the material in this chapter is new, but portions of the chapter are modified with permission from prior publications by the author (RTS). Chapter 6 on topical anesthesia discusses appropriate anesthetic agents, modes of administration, effects of topical anesthesia on the larynx and pharynx, and potential systemic complications of topical anesthesia. Chapter 7 discusses basics in surgical techniques and operative approaches for office-based laryngeal surgery including transnasal, percutaneous, and transoral approaches. Chapter 8 reviews office-based injection laryngoplasty. This chapter reviews important anatomical and surgical considerations, sites and force of injection, short-term and long-term outcomes of office-based injection laryngoplasty, and potential complications. The chapter includes case and video examples to assist the reader in understanding the principles put forth. Chapter 9 on office-based laryngeal injection of botulinum toxin discusses the various indications and techniques. Videos provide examples of injection through a flexible endoscope, and external injection using laryngeal electromyographic guidance. Chapter 10, "Office-Based Laryngeal Laser Therapy," provides information on various kinds of lasers, lesions appropriate for office-based laser management, techniques, limitations and complications of in-office laser surgery, and clinical case discussion. Chapter 11 reviews office-based injection of steroids and other substances including cidofovir, 5-fluorouracil, saline, growth factors, and other materials. Special considerations and clinical examples are included. Chapter 12, "Office-Based Laryngeal Biopsy, Excision of Masses and Dilation," presents information on biopsy, precise resection of vocal fold masses, the little-known procedure of in-office laryngeal dilation for laryngeal stenosis, and other topics.

As the popularity of office-based laryngeal surgery continues to increase, it is important for laryngologists, otolaryngologists, nurses and medical assistants, physician assistants, nurse practitioners, speech-language pathologists, singing voice specialists, acting voice specialists, and others involved in the care of patients with voice disorders to understand the principles, precautions, and limitations of office-based laryngeal surgery. While office-based surgery seems intrinsically safer than general anesthesia, monitoring and access to emergency care usually is better in an operating room than in an office, especially if that office is not close to a hospital. For some patients, surgery in an operating room is safer. Patients undergoing surgery in the office require medical evaluation and clearance, informed consent, and other procedures similar to those required for patients undergoing surgery in an operating room and under anesthesia, in many cases. A thorough understanding of the strengths and limitations of office-based laryngeal surgery allows safe and effective application of this in a valuable option for patient care. The authors hope that this book proves helpful to collect interest in understanding and/or mastering the techniques and judgments required for optimal office-based laryngeal surgery.

Beirut, Lebanon
Philadelphia, PA, USA

Abdul-latif Hamdan
Robert Thayer Sataloff
Mary J. Hawkshaw

Contents

Part II In-Office Surgery

Editors and Contributors

About the Authors

Abdul-latif Hamdan MD, EMBA, MPH, FACS, is currently Professor of Otolaryngology—Head and Neck Surgery, head of the Division of Laryngology, and director of "Hamdan Voice Unit" at the American University of Beirut Medical Center AUBMC. He is also Adjunct Professor of Otolaryngology—Head and Neck Surgery at Drexel University College of Medicine. Dr. Hamdan completed his medical education and residency training in otolaryngology—head and neck surgery at AUBMC, following which he completed a fellowship in laryngology at Vanderbilt University Medical Center. He has also earned a master's degree in health science, a master's degree in hospital administration, and an executive master's degree in business administration from AUB, in addition to a diploma in strategy and innovation from Oxford University. He is the founder of the "Hamdan Voice Unit" at AUBMC, the "Lebanese Voice Association" in Lebanon, the "Hamdan International Award" at the Voice Foundation, and the Voice Foundation Lebanon Chapter. He is a member of the Voice Foundation Board of Directors and Advisory Board, a fellow of the American College of Surgeons, corresponding fellow of the American Laryngological Association, in addition to being a member of International Association of Phonosurgeons.

Dr. Hamdan is a faculty member in the Department of Otolaryngology Head and Neck Surgery at AUBMC providing clinical care in the field of voice and laryngology, performing the full spectrum of phonosurgical procedures with special emphasis on office-based laryngeal surgery. He has authored and co-authored 160 publications in peer-reviewed and indexed journals. His research covers mainly the laryngeal manifestations of systemic diseases in addition to unsedated office-based laser therapy. He has assumed the position of medical director of strategy and innovation at AUBMC for 3 years following his position as the chairperson of the Faculty Development Committee for 2 years. During his tenure, he had organized several workshops to promote the business aspect of medicine among faculty members. He is the author of seven books, among which are *Strategic Thinking in a Hospital*

Setting, Laryngeal Manifestations of Systemic Diseases , *Obesity and Voice*, *Non-Laryngeal Cancer and Voice*, and *Voice Disorders in Athletes, Coaches and other Sports Professionals.* Dr. Hamdan is also a member of the Lebanese Syndicate of Professional Artists and member of Societe des Auteurs, Compositeurs et Editeurs de Musique. He has composed 36 musical tracks and has released four musical CDs.

Robert Thayer Sataloff MD, DMA, FACS, is professor and chairman of the Department of Otolaryngology—Head and Neck Surgery and senior associate dean for clinical academic specialties, Drexel University College of Medicine. Dr. Sataloff is Director of Otolaryngology and Communication Sciences Research at the Lankenau Institute for Medical Research, and Director of Otolaryngology Education at Lankenau Medical Center. He also holds adjunct professorships in the Departments of Otolaryngology—Head and Neck Surgery at Thomas Jefferson University, Temple University, and the Philadelphia College of Osteopathic Medicine, and he is a faculty of the Academy of Vocal Arts. He serves as conductor of the Thomas Jefferson University Choir. Dr. Sataloff is also a professional singer and singing teacher. He holds an undergraduate degree from Haverford College in music theory and composition; graduated from Jefferson Medical College, Thomas Jefferson University; received a Doctor of Musical Arts in Voice Performance from Combs College of Music; and completed residency in otolaryngology – head and neck surgery and a fellowship in otology, neurotology, and skull base surgery at the University of Michigan. Dr. Sataloff is chairman of the board of directors of the Voice Foundation and of the American Institute for Voice and Ear Research. He also has served as chairman of the board of governors of Graduate Hospital; president of the American Laryngological Association, the International Association of Phonosurgery, the Pennsylvania Academy of Otolaryngology—Head and Neck Surgery, and the American Society of Geriatric Otolaryngology; and numerous other leadership positions. Dr. Sataloff is editor-in-chief of the *Journal of Voice*, editor emeritus of *Ear, Nose and Throat Journal*, associate editor of the *Journal of Singing*, editorial board member of *Medical Problems of Performing Artists*, and editorial reviewer for numerous otolaryngology journals. He has written over 1,000 publications including 69 books, and he has been awarded more than $5 million in research funding. His H-index is 43 (as of May 2022). He has invented more than 75 laryngeal microsurgical instruments distributed currently by Integra Medical, ossicular replacement prostheses produced by Grace Medical, and a novel laryngeal prosthesis (patent pending). He holds a patent on a unique thyroplasty implant. His medical practice is limited to care of the professional voice and to otology/neurotology/skull base surgery. Dr. Sataloff has developed numerous novel surgical procedures including total temporal bone resection for formerly untreatable skull base malignancy, laryngeal microflap and mini-microflap procedures, vocal fold lipoinjection, vocal fold lipoimplantation, and others. Dr. Sataloff is recognized as one of the founders of the field of voice, having written the first modern comprehensive article on care of singers, and the first chapter and book on care of the professional voice, as well as having influenced the evolution of the field through his own efforts and through the Voice Foundation for over four decades. Dr. Sataloff has been recognized by Best Doctors in America (Woodward White Athens) every year since 1992, *Philadelphia Magazine* since 1997, and Castle Connolly's "America's Top Doctors" since 2002.

(*Updated 5/19/2022*)

Mary J. Hawkshaw RN, BSN, CORLN, FCPP, is research professor and vice chair for academic initiatives in the Department of Otolaryngology—Head and Neck Surgery at Drexel University College of Medicine. She has been associated with Dr. Robert Sataloff, Philadelphia Ear, Nose & Throat Associates, and the American Institute for Voice & Ear Research (AIVER) since 1986. Ms. Hawkshaw graduated from Shadyside Hospital School of Nursing in Pittsburgh, Pennsylvania, and received a Bachelor of Science degree in nursing from Thomas Jefferson University in Philadelphia. In addition to her specialized clinical activities, she has been involved extensively in research and teaching. She mentors medical students, residents, and laryngology fellows, and has been involved in teaching research, writing, and editing for over three decades. In collaboration with Dr. Sataloff, she has co-authored more than 183 articles, 102 book chapters, and 20 textbooks. She is on the editorial boards of the *Journal of Voice* and *Ear, Nose and Throat Journal*. She has served as secretary/treasurer of AIVER since 1988 and was named executive director of AIVER in January 000. She has served on the board of directors of the Voice Foundation since 1990. Ms. Hawkshaw has been an active member of the Society of Otorhinolaryngology and Head-Neck Nurses since 1998. She is recognized nationally and internationally for her extensive contributions to care of the professional voice.

(*Updated 4/30/2021*)

Contributors

Johnathan Brandon Sataloff Department of Psychiatry, Beth Israel Deaconess Medical Center, Harvard Medical School, Boston, MA, USA

Ghiath Alnouri Department of Otolaryngology – Head and Neck Surgery, Drexel University College of Medicine, Philadelphia, PA, USA

List of Figures

tion, suggests a second lesion that is hidden from view by the large, easily visible granuloma. (**b**) A transnasal flexible laryngoscopy is performed to visualize the larynx. The laryngoscope is placed initially just beyond the soft palate, at the level of the oropharynx, to allow for ease of transoral placement of indirect laryngoscopy needle, and then the laryngoscope is advanced. (**c**) Four percent lidocaine is applied topically through the indirect laryngoscopy needle under flexible laryngoscopic guidance and is placed directly onto the vocal folds. (**d**) Once the desired anesthetic effect has been established, a subepithelial injection of 1% lidocaine with 1:100,000 epinephrine is injected into the base of the lesion, at the junction of normal and abnormal tissue, for hydrodissection to help separate the mass from normal tissue. ((**a–d**) Republished with permission. Sataloff et al. [35], p. 19). (**e**) In this case, this inflammatory lesion was removed easily after hydrodissection with straight microcup forceps. However, for more delicate lesions without preexisting stiffness at the base, heart-shaped forceps, scissors, and delicate dissection instruments are available and preferable. (**f**) A second, similar granuloma is removed from the right true vocal fold. In this case, Sataloff left-angled cup forceps provided easy, precise resection of the lesion at its base, without the need for excessive traction and without tearing the surrounding normal mucosa. This was possible because this was a small, friable inflammatory lesion. Heart-shaped forceps and scissors are preferable in some cases. The position of these granulomas on the musculomembranous portion of the vocal folds was unusual. ((**e, f**) Republished with permission. Sataloff et al. [35], p. 20). (**g**) Using a 25-gauge Sataloff Indirect Laryngeal Needle, steroid (Decadron 10 mg/ml) is injected into the vocal fold at the site of the base of resection of the granuloma 250

Fig. 12.2 A 62-year-old male, smoker, presenting with a history of dysphonia. On laryngeal examination, the patient had left vocal fold leukoplakia. This figure shows biopsy of the left vocal fold lesion using cup forceps introduced through the working channel of a nasopharyngoscope. (Republished with permission. Sataloff et al. [35], p. 20). 251

Fig. 12.3 Sataloff Indirect Laryngeal Dilator. (Integra LifeSciences, Princeton, NJ, USA) 254

Fig. 12.4 Digital reduction of a dislocated arytenoid can be accomplished in the office occasionally, especially for patients who are edentulous and who have had recent posterior dislocation or redislocation following recent arytenoid reduction. The patient's tongue is retracted by the patient or an assistant,

Part I
Core Knowledge

Chapter 1
Anatomy and Physiology of the Voice

To treat voice patients knowledgeably and responsibly, health care providers must understand the medical aspects of voice disorders and their treatment. This requires core knowledge of the anatomy and physiology of phonation. The human voice consists of much more than simply the vocal folds, popularly known as the vocal cords. State-of-the-art voice diagnosis, nonsurgical therapy, and voice surgery depend on understanding the complex workings of the vocal tract. Physicians and other health care professionals specializing in the care of voice patients, especially voice professionals, should be familiar with at least the basics of the latest concepts in voice function. The physiology of phonation is much more complex than this brief chapter might suggest, and readers interested in acquiring more than a clinically essential introduction are encouraged to consult other literature [1].

1.1 Anatomy

The larynx is essential to normal voice production, but the anatomy of the voice is not limited to the larynx. The vocal mechanism includes the abdominal and back musculature, rib cage, lungs, pharynx, oral cavity, and nose, among other structures. Each component performs an important function in voice production, although it is possible to produce voice even without a larynx—for example, in patients who have undergone laryngectomy. In addition, virtually all parts of the body play some role in voice production and may be responsible for voice dysfunction. Even something as remote as a sprained ankle may alter posture, thereby impairing abdominal, back, and thoracic muscle function and resulting in vocal inefficiency, weakness, and hoarseness.

The larynx is composed of four basic anatomic units: skeleton, intrinsic muscles, extrinsic muscles, and mucosa. The most important components of the laryngeal skeleton are the thyroid cartilage, cricoid cartilage, and two arytenoid cartilages

A.-l. Hamdan et al., *Office-Based Laryngeal Surgery*,
https://doi.org/10.1007/978-3-030-91936-8_1

(Fig. 1.1). Intrinsic muscles of the larynx are connected to these cartilages (Fig. 1.2). One of the intrinsic muscles, the *thyroarytenoid muscle* (its medial belly also is known as the vocalis muscle), extends on each side from the vocal process of the

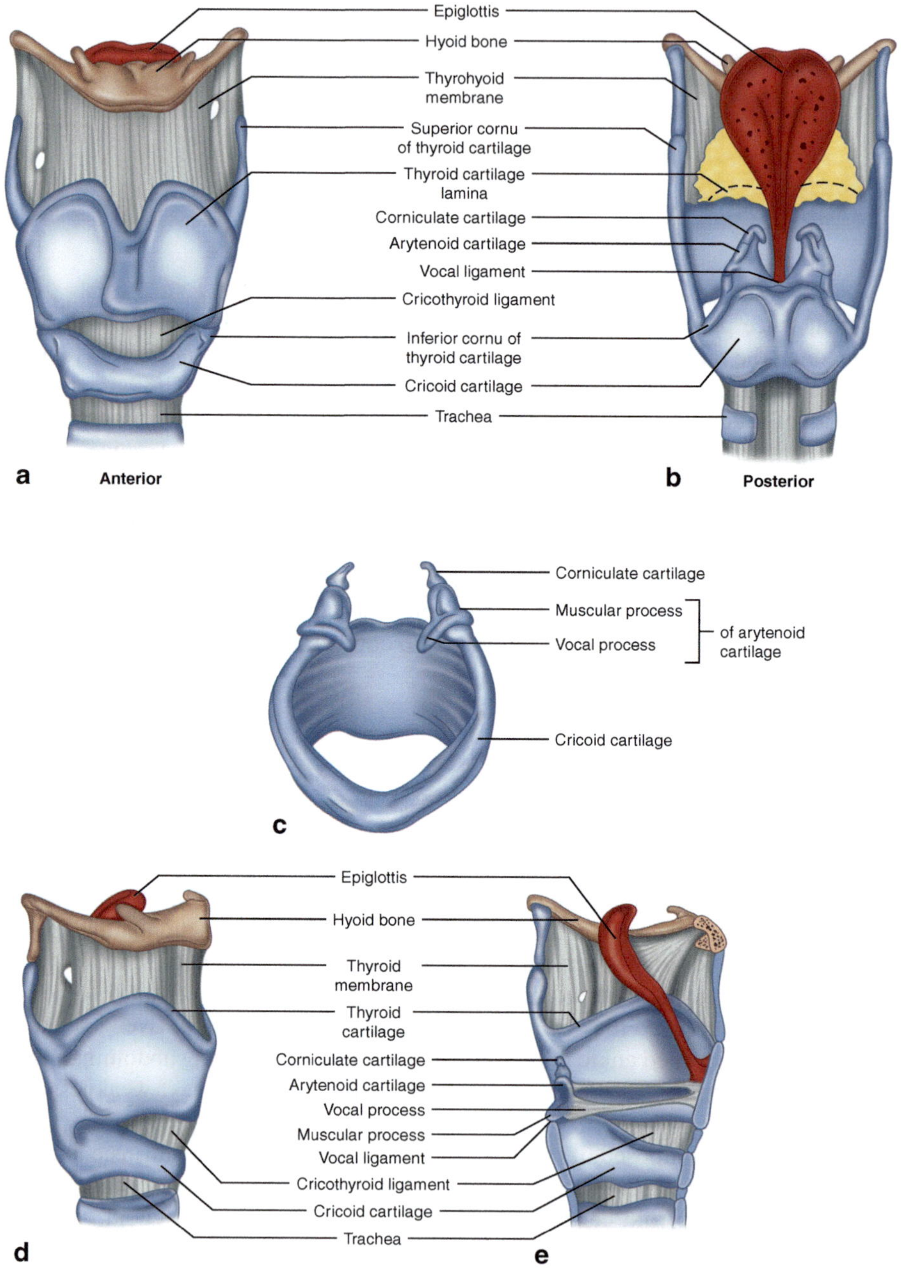

Fig. 1.1 Cartilages of the larynx

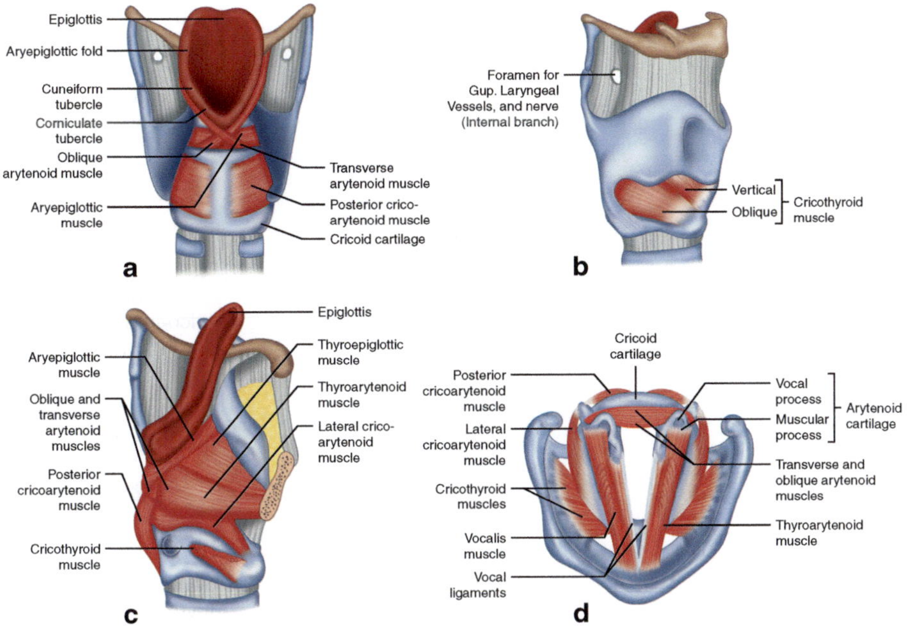

Fig. 1.2 Intrinsic muscles of the larynx

arytenoid cartilage to the inside of the thyroid cartilage just below and behind the thyroid prominence ("Adam's apple"), forming the body of the vocal folds. The vocal folds act as the *oscillator* or *voice source* of the vocal tract. The space between the vocal folds is called the *glottis* and is used as an anatomic reference point. The intrinsic muscles alter the position, shape, and tension of the vocal folds, bringing them together (adduction), moving them apart (abduction), or stretching them by increasing longitudinal tension (Fig. 1.3). They are able to do so because the laryngeal cartilages are connected by soft attachments that allow changes in their relative angles and distances, thereby permitting alteration in the shape and tension of the tissues suspended between them. The arytenoid cartilages on their eliptoid cricoarytenoid joints are capable of motion in multiple planes, permitting complex vocal fold motion and alteration in the shape of the vocal fold edge associated with intrinsic muscle action (Fig. 1.4). All but one of the muscles on each side of the larynx are innervated by one of the two *recurrent laryngeal nerves*. Because this nerve runs in a long course (especially on the left) from the neck down into the chest and then back up to the larynx (hence, the name "recurrent"), it is injured easily by trauma, neck surgery, and chest surgery. Injury may result in vocal fold paresis or paralysis. The remaining muscle (*cricothyroid muscle*) is innervated by the superior laryngeal nerve on each side, which is especially susceptible to viral and traumatic injury. It causes changes in longitudinal tension that are important in voice projection and pitch control. The "false vocal folds" are located above the vocal folds, and unlike

Fig. 1.3 Action of the intrinsic muscles

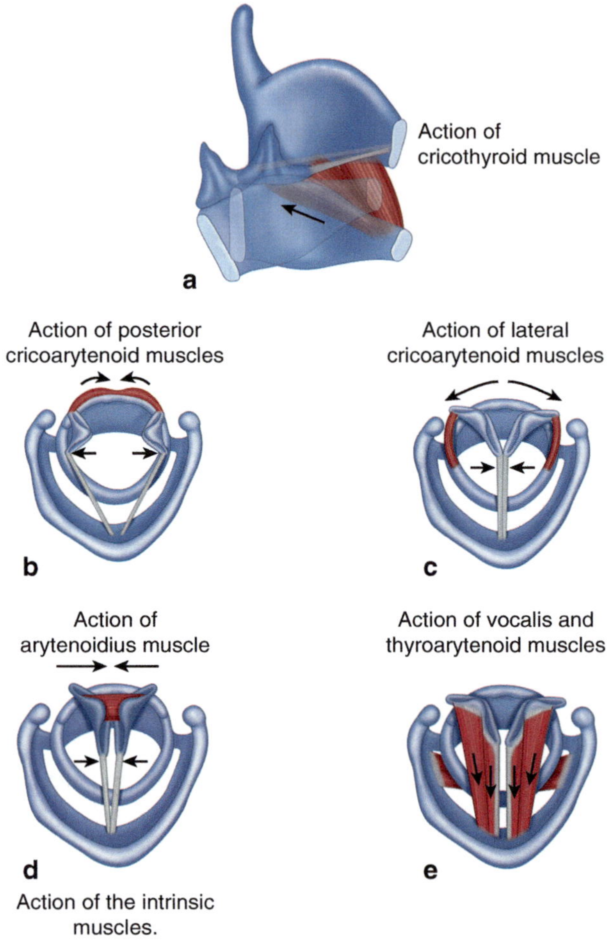

the true vocal folds, usually do not make contact during normal speaking or singing [1]. The neuroanatomy and neurophysiology of phonation are extremely complicated, and only partially understood. As the new field of neurolaryngology advances, a more thorough understanding of the subject is becoming increasingly important to clinicians. Readers interested in acquiring a deeper, scientific understanding of neurolaryngology are encouraged to consult other literature [2] and the publications cited therein.

Because the attachments of the laryngeal cartilages are flexible, the positions of the cartilages with respect to each other change when the laryngeal skeleton is elevated or lowered. Such changes in vertical height are controlled by the extrinsic laryngeal muscles, the strap muscles of the neck. When the angles and distances between cartilages change because of this accordion-like effect, the resting length of the intrinsic muscle changes. Such large adjustments in intrinsic muscle condition interfere with fine control of smooth vocal quality. Classically trained singers

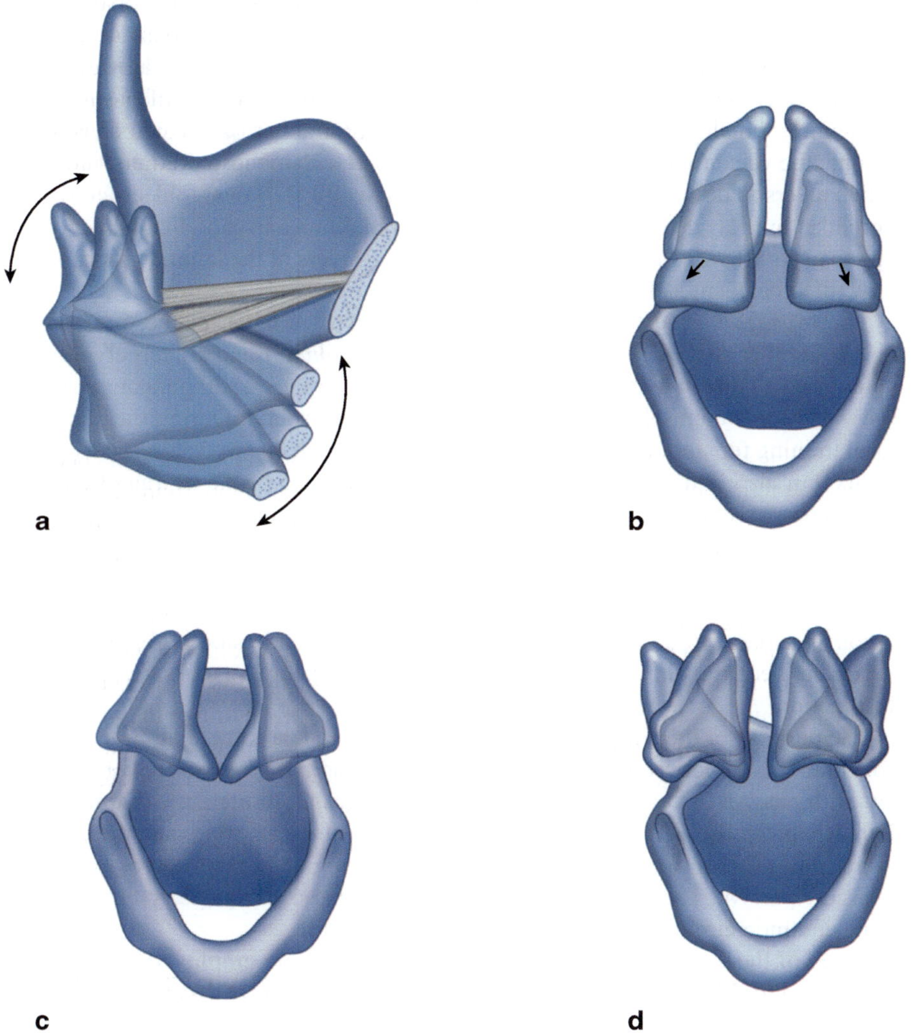

Fig. 1.4 Complex arytenoid motion

generally are taught to use the extrinsic muscles to maintain the laryngeal skeleton at a relatively constant height regardless of pitch. That is, they learn to avoid the natural tendency of the larynx to rise with ascending pitch and fall with descending pitch, thereby enhancing the unity of sound quality throughout the vocal range through effects on both resting muscle condition and supraglottic vocal tract posture.

The soft tissues lining the larynx are much more complex than originally thought. The mucosa forms the thin, lubricated surface of the vocal folds, which makes contact when the two vocal folds are approximated. Laryngeal mucosa might look superficially like the mucosa which lines the inside of the mouth, but it is not.

Throughout most of the larynx, there are goblet cells and pseudo-stratified ciliated columnar epithelial cells designed for producing and handling mucous secretions, similar to mucosal surfaces found throughout the respiratory tract. However, the mucosa overlying the vocal folds is different. First, it is the stratified squamous epithelium, which is better suited to withstand the trauma of vocal fold contact. Second, the vocal fold is not simply muscle covered with mucosa. Rather, it consists of five layers as described by Hirano [3]. Mechanically, the vocal fold structures act more like three layers consisting of the *cover* (epithelium and superficial layer of the lamina propria), *transition* (intermediate and deep layers of the lamina propria), and *body* (the vocalis muscle).

The *supraglottic vocal tract* includes the pharynx, tongue, palate, oral cavity, nose, and other structures. Together, they act as a *resonator* and are largely responsible for vocal quality or timbre and the perceived character of all phonated sounds. The vocal folds themselves produce only a "buzzing" sound. During the course of vocal training for singing, acting, or healthy speaking, changes occur not only in the larynx, but also in the muscle motion, control, and shape of the supraglottic vocal tract, and in aerobic, pulmonary, and bodily muscle function.

The *infraglottic vocal tract* (all anatomical structures below the glottis) serves as the *power source* for the voice. Singers and actors often refer to the entire power source complex as their "support" or "diaphragm." The anatomy of support for phonation is especially complicated and not completely understood. Yet, it is quite important because deficiencies in support frequently are responsible for voice dysfunction.

The purpose of the support mechanism is to generate a force that directs a controlled airstream between the vocal folds. Active respiratory muscles work in concert with passive forces. The principal muscles of inspiration are the diaphragm (a dome-shaped muscle that extends along the bottom of the rib cage) and the external intercostal muscles (located between the ribs). During quiet respiration, expiration is largely passive. The lungs and rib cage generate passive expiratory forces under many common circumstances such as after a full breath.

Many of the muscles used for active expiration also are employed in "support" for phonation. Muscles of active expiration either raise the intra-abdominal pressure, forcing the diaphragm upward, or lower the ribs or sternum to decrease the dimensions of the thorax, or both, thereby compressing air in the chest. The primary muscles of expiration are "the abdominal muscles," but internal intercostals and other chest and back muscles also are involved. Trauma or surgery that alters the structure or function of these muscles or ribs undermines the power source of the voice, as do diseases, such as asthma, that impair expiration. Deficiencies in the support mechanism often result in compensatory efforts that utilize the laryngeal muscles, which are not designed for power functions. Such behavior can result in impaired voice quality, rapid fatigue, pain, and even structural pathology such as vocal fold nodules. Current expert treatment for such vocal problems focuses on the correction of the underlying malfunction rather than surgery whenever possible.

1.2 Physiology

The physiology of voice production is extremely complex. Volitional production of voice begins in the cerebral cortex (Fig. 1.5).

The command for vocalization involves complex interactions among brain centers for speech, as well as other areas. For singing, speech directives must be integrated with information from the centers for musical and artistic expression, which are discussed elsewhere [1]. The "idea" of the planned vocalization is conveyed to

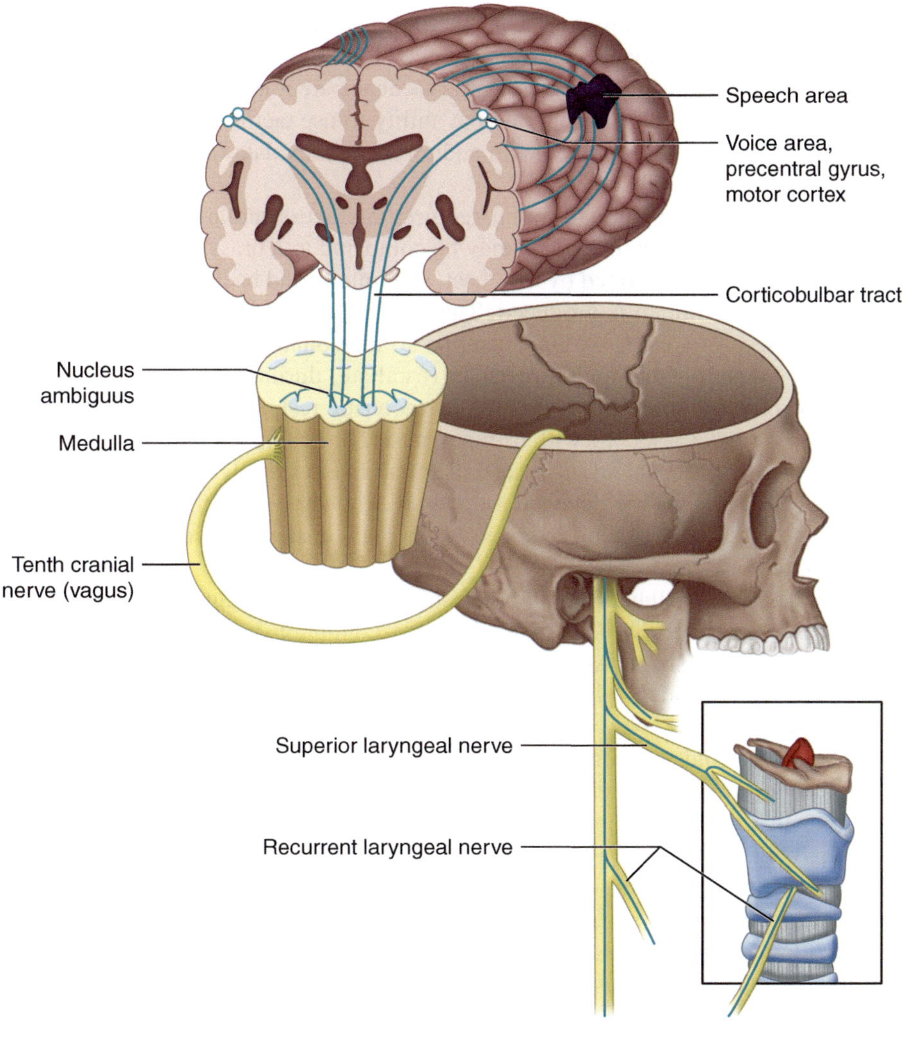

Fig. 1.5 Simplified summary of pathway for volitional phonation

the precentral gyrus in the motor cortex, which transmits another set of instructions to the motor nuclei in the brainstem and spinal cord. These areas send out the complicated messages necessary for the coordinated activity of the larynx, thoracic and abdominal musculature lungs, and vocal tract articulators, among other structures. Additional refinement of motor activity is provided by the extrapyramidal and autonomic nervous systems. These impulses combine to produce a sound that is transmitted not only to the ears of the listener, but also to those of the speaker or singer. Auditory feedback is transmitted from the ear through the brainstem to the cerebral cortex, and adjustments are made within milliseconds that permit the vocalist to match the sound produced with the sound intended, integrating the acoustic properties of the performance environment. Tactile feedback from the throat and other muscles involved in phonation also is believed to help in fine-tuning vocal output, although the mechanism and role of tactile feedback are not understood fully. Many trained singers and speakers cultivate the ability to use tactile feedback effectively because of expected interference with auditory feedback data from ancillary sound such as an orchestra or band.

Phonation, the production of sound, requires interaction among the power source, oscillator, and resonator. The voice may be compared to a brass instrument such as a trumpet. Power is generated by the chest, abdominal, and back musculature, and a high-pressure air stream is produced. The trumpeter's lips open and close against the mouthpiece producing a "buzz" similar to the sound produced by vocal folds when they come together and move apart (oscillate) during phonation. This sound then passes through the trumpet, which has acoustic resonance characteristics that shape the sound we associate with trumpet music. If a trumpet mouthpiece is placed on a French horn, the sound we hear will sound like a French horn, not a trumpet. Quality characteristics are dependent upon the resonator more than on the oscillatory source. The non-mouthpiece portions of a brass instrument are analogous to the supraglottic vocal tract.

During phonation, the infraglottic musculature must make rapid, complex adjustments because the resistance changes almost continuously as the glottis closes, opens, and changes shape. At the beginning of each phonatory cycle, the vocal folds are approximated, and the glottis is obliterated. This permits infraglottic air pressure to build, typically to a level of about 7 cm of water for conversational speech. At that point, the vocal folds are convergent (Fig. 1.6a). Because the vocal folds are closed, there is no airflow. The subglottic pressure then pushes the vocal folds progressively farther apart from the bottom up and from the back forward (Fig. 1.6b) until a space develops (Fig. 1.6c, d) and air begins to flow. Bernoulli force created by the air passing between the vocal folds combines with the mechanical properties of the folds to begin closing the lower portion of the vocal folds almost immediately (Fig. 1.6e–h) even while the upper edges are still separating. The principles and mathematics of Bernoulli force are complex. It is a flow effect more easily understood by familiar examples such as the sensation of pull exerted on a vehicle when passed by a truck at high speed or the inward motion of a shower curtain when the water flows past it.

The upper portion of the vocal folds has elastic properties that also tend to make the vocal folds snap back to the midline. This force becomes more dominant as the

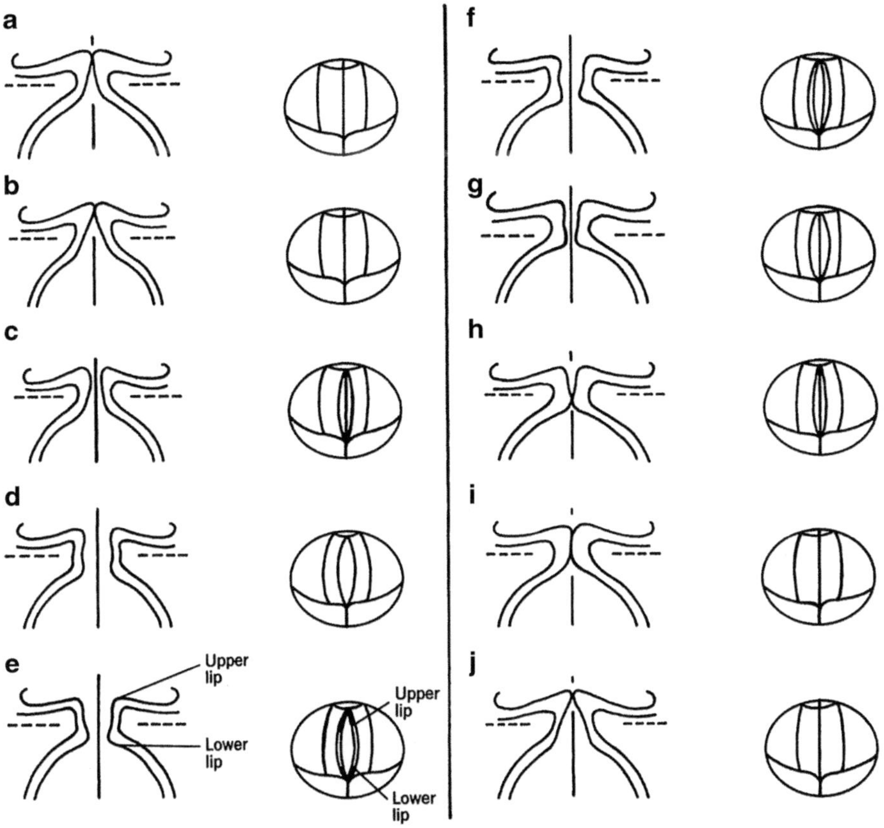

Fig. 1.6 Frontal view (left) and view from above (right) illustrating the normal pattern of vocal fold vibration. The vocal folds close and open from the inferior aspect of the vibratory margin upward, and from posterior to anterior. Vocal folds closed (**a**) opening from the bottom up (**b**), air flowing between the vocal folds (**c**), vocal folds separated (**d**), vocal folds closing from inferior to superior (**e**–**h**), vocal folds adducted (**i**), and vocal folds starting to open again from inferior to superior at the beginning of another cycle (**j**)

upper edges are stretched and the opposing force of the air stream diminishes because of the approximation of the lower edges of the vocal folds. The upper portions of the vocal folds are then returned to the midline (Fig. 1.6i), completing the glottic cycle. Subglottal pressure then builds again (Fig. 1.6j), and the events repeat. Thus, there is a vertical phase difference. That is, the lower portion of the vocal folds begins to open and close before the upper portion. The rippling displacement of the vocal fold cover produces a mucosal wave that can be examined clinically under stroboscopic light. If this complex motion is impaired, hoarseness or other changes in voice quality may cause the patient to seek medical evaluation. The frequency of vibration (number of cycles of openings and closings per second, measured in hertz [Hz]) is dependent on the air pressure and mechanical properties of the vocal folds, which are regulated in part by the laryngeal muscles. Pitch is the perceptual correlate of frequency. Under most circumstances, as the vocal folds are thinned and stretched and air pressure is increased, the frequency of air pulse emissions increases, and pitch goes up. The myoelastic-aerodynamic mechanism of phonation reveals that the vocal folds emit pulses of air, rather than vibrating like strings.

The sound produced by the oscillating vocal folds, called the voice source signal, is a complex tone containing a fundamental frequency and many overtones, or higher harmonic partials. The amplitude of the partials decreases uniformly at approximately 12 dB per octave. Interestingly, the acoustic spectrum of the voice source is about the same in ordinary speakers as it is in trained singers and speakers. Voice quality differences in voice professionals occur as the voice source signal passes through their supraglottic vocal tract resonator system (Fig. 1.7).

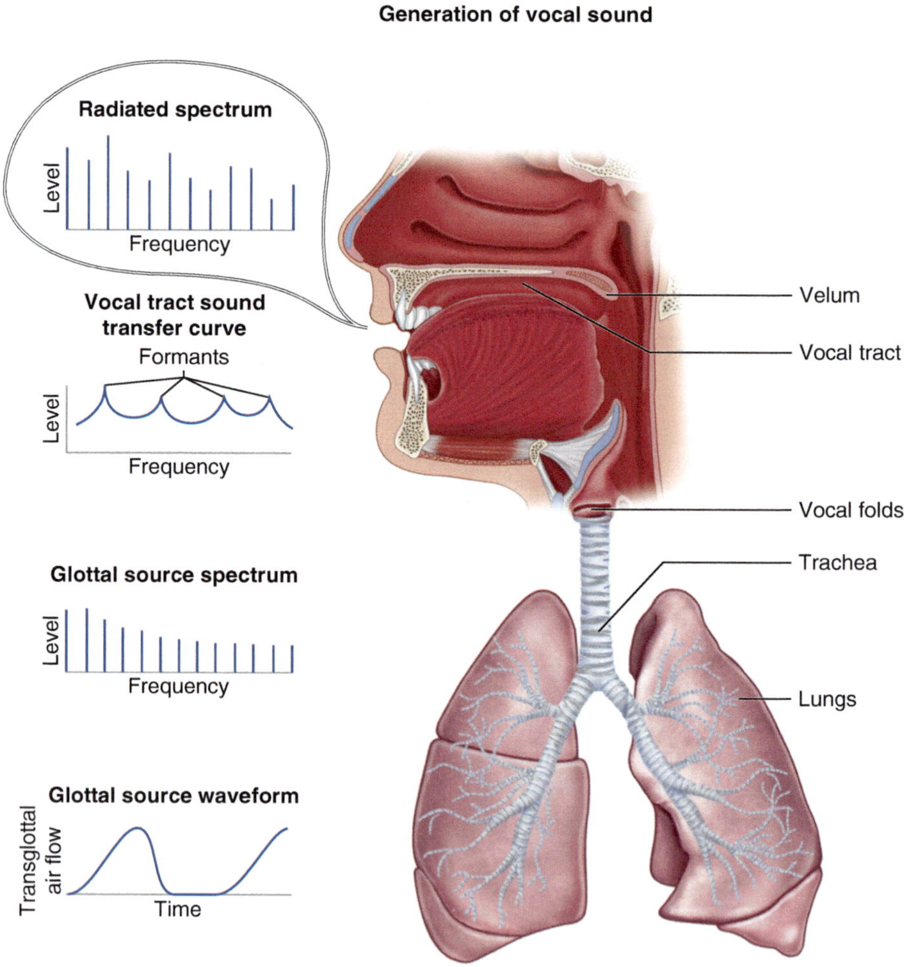

Fig. 1.7 Determinants of the spectrum of a vowel (oral-output signal)

The pharynx, oral cavity, and nasal cavity act as a series of infinitely variable interconnected resonators, which are more complex than that in our trumpet example or other single resonators. As with other resonators, some frequencies are attenuated, others are enhanced. Enhanced frequencies are radiated with higher relative amplitudes or intensities. Sundberg [4] showed long ago that the vocal tract has four or five important resonance frequencies called *formants* and summarized his early findings in a book that has become a classic. The presence of formants alters the uniformly sloping voice source spectrum and creates peaks at formant frequencies. These alterations of the voice source spectral envelope are responsible for distinguishable sounds of speech and song. Formant frequencies are determined by vocal tract shape, which can be altered by the laryngeal, pharyngeal, and oral cavity musculature. Overall vocal tract length and shape are individually fixed and determined by age and sex (females and children have shorter vocal tracts and formant frequencies that are higher than males). Voice training includes conscious physical mastery of the adjustment of vocal tract shape.

Although the formants differ for different vowels, one resonant frequency has received particular attention and is known as the "singer's formant." This formant occurs in the vicinity of 2300 Hz to 3200 Hz for all vowel spectra and appears to be responsible for the "ring" in a singer's or trained speaker's ("speaker's formant") voice. The ability to hear a trained voice clearly even over a loud choir or orchestra is dependent primarily on the presence of the singer's formant [1]. Interestingly, there is little or no significant difference in maximum vocal intensity between trained and untrained singers. The singer's formant also contributes substantially to the differences in fach (voice classification) among voice categories, occurring in basses at about 2400 Hz, baritones at 2600 Hz, tenors at 2800 Hz, mezzo-sopranos at 2900 Hz, and sopranos at 3200 Hz. It is frequently much less prominent in high soprano singing [1].

The mechanisms that control two vocal characteristics are particularly important: fundamental frequency and intensity. Fundamental frequency, which corresponds to pitch, can be altered by changing either air pressure or the mechanical properties of the vocal folds, although the latter is more efficient under most conditions. When the cricothyroid muscle contracts, it makes the thyroid cartilage pivot on the cricothyroid joint and increases the distance between the thyroid and arytenoid cartilages, thus stretching the vocal folds. This increases the surface area exposed to subglottal pressure and makes the air pressure more effective in opening the glottis. In addition, stretching of elastic fibers of the vocal fold makes them more efficient at snapping back together. Hence, the cycles shorten and repeat more frequently, and the fundamental frequency (and pitch) rise. Other muscles, including the thyroarytenoid, also contribute [1]. Raising the pressure of the air stream also tends to increase fundamental frequency, a phenomenon for which singers must learn to compensate. Otherwise, their pitch would go up whenever they tried to sing more loudly.

Voice intensity corresponds to loudness and depends on the degree to which the glottal wave motion excites the air molecules in the vocal tract. Raising the air pressure creates greater amplitude of vocal fold oscillation and therefore increases vocal intensity. However, actually it is not the oscillation of the vocal fold, but rather the sudden cessation of airflow that is responsible for initiating an acoustic signal in the vocal tract and controlling intensity. This is similar to the mechanism of acoustic signal that results from buzzing lips. In the larynx, the sharper the cutoff of airflow, the more intense the sound [1]. In the evaluation of voice disorders, an individual's ability to optimize adjustments of air pressure and glottal resistance is assessed. When high subglottic pressure is combined with high adductory (closing) vocal fold force, glottal airflow and the amplitude of the voice source fundamental frequency are low. This is called *pressed phonation* and can be measured clinically through a technique known as flow glottography. Flow glottogram wave amplitude indicates the type of phonation being used, and the slope (closing rate) provides information about the sound pressure level or loudness. If adductory forces are so weak that the vocal folds do not make contact, the vocal folds become inefficient at resisting air leakage, and the voice source fundamental frequency is low. This is known as *breathy phonation*. *Flow phonation* is characterized by lower subglottic pressure and lower adductory force. These conditions increase the dominance of the fundamental frequency of the voice source in the perceived sound. Sundberg showed that the amplitude of the fundamental frequency can be increased by 15 dB or more when the subject changes from pressed phonation to flow phonation [4]. If a patient habitually uses pressed phonation, considerable effort will be required to achieve loud voicing. The muscle patterns and force that are used to compensate for this laryngeal inefficiency may cause vocal fold damage. Such voice behavior (i.e., pressed voice) can result from laryngeal structural problems, voice technique, psychological abnormalities, and other causes.

Acknowledgments Modified in part from Sataloff RT. *Professional Voice: The Science and Art of Clinical Care, fourth Edition*. San Diego, CA: Plural Publishing; 2017, with permission.

References

1. Sataloff RT. Professional voice: the science and art of clinical care. 4th ed. San Diego: Plural Publishing; 2017.
2. Sataloff RT. Neurolaryngology. San Diego, CA: Plural Publishing; 2017.
3. Hirano M. Phonosurgery: basic and clinical investigations. Otologia (Fukuoka). 1975;21:239–442.
4. Sundberg J. The science of the singing voice. DeKalb: Northern Illinois University Press; 1987.

Chapter 2
Patient History

A comprehensive history and physical examination usually reveal the cause of voice dysfunction. Effective history taking and physical examination depend on a practical understanding of the anatomy and physiology of voice production [1–3]. Because dysfunction in virtually any body system may affect phonation, medical inquiry must be comprehensive. The current standard of care for all voice patients evolved from advances inspired by medical problems of voice professionals such as singers and actors. Even minor problems may be particularly symptomatic in singers and actors, because of the extreme demands they place on their voices. However, a great many other patients are voice professionals. They include teachers, salespeople, attorneys, clergy, physicians, politicians, telephone receptionists, and anyone else whose ability to earn a living is impaired in the presence of voice dysfunction. Because good voice quality is so important in our society, the majority of our patients are voice professionals, and all patients should be treated as such.

The scope of inquiry and examination for most patients is similar to that required for singers and actors, except that performing voice professionals have unique needs, which require additional history and examination. Questions must be added regarding performance commitments, professional status and voice goals, the amount and nature of voice training, the performance environment, rehearsal practices, abusive habits during speech and singing, and many other matters. Such supplementary information is essential to proper treatment selection and patient counseling in singers and actors. However, analogous factors must also be taken into account for stockbrokers, factory shop foremen, elementary school teachers, homemakers with several noisy children, and many others. Physicians familiar with the management of these challenging patients are well equipped to evaluate all patients with voice complaints.

A.-l. Hamdan et al., *Office-Based Laryngeal Surgery*,
https://doi.org/10.1007/978-3-030-91936-8_2

2.1 Patient History

Obtaining extensive historical background information is necessary for a thorough evaluation of the voice patient, and the otolaryngologist who sees voice patients (especially singers) only occasionally cannot reasonably be expected to remember all the pertinent questions. Although some laryngologists consider a lengthy inquisition helpful in establishing rapport, many of us who see a substantial number of voice patients each day within a busy practice need a thorough but less time-consuming alternative. A history questionnaire can be extremely helpful in documenting all the necessary information, helping the patient sort out and articulate his or her problems, and saving the clinician time recording information. The author has developed a questionnaire [4] that has proven helpful. The patient is asked to complete the relevant portions of the form at home prior to his or her office visit or in the waiting room before seeing the doctor. A similar form has been developed for voice patients who are not singers.

No history questionnaire is a substitute for direct, penetrating questioning by the physician. However, the direction of most useful inquiry can be determined from a glance at the questionnaire, obviating the need for extensive writing, which permits the physician greater eye contact with the patient and facilitates rapid establishment of the close rapport and confidence that are so important in treating voice patients. The physician is also able to supplement initial impressions and historical information from the questionnaire with seemingly leisurely conversation during the physical examination. The use of the history questionnaire has added substantially to the efficiency, consistent thoroughness, and ease of managing these delightful, but often complex, patients. A similar set of questions is also used by the speech-language pathologist with new patients and by many enlightened singing teachers when assessing new students.

2.1.1 How Old Are You?

Serious vocal endeavor may start in childhood and continue throughout a lifetime. As the vocal mechanism undergoes normal maturation, the voice changes. The optimal time to begin serious vocal training is controversial. For many years, most singing teachers advocated delay of vocal training and serious singing until near puberty in the female and after puberty and voice stabilization in the male. However, in a child with earnest vocal aspirations and potential, starting specialized training early in childhood is reasonable. Initial instruction should teach the child to vocalize without straining and to avoid all forms of voice abuse. It should not permit premature indulgence in operatic bravado. Most experts agree that taxing voice use and singing during puberty should be minimized or avoided altogether, particularly by the male. Voice maturation (attainment of stable adult vocal quality) may occur at any age from the early teenage years to the fourth decade of life. The dangerous tendency for young singers to attempt to sound older than their vocal years frequently causes vocal dysfunction.

All components of voice production are subject to normal aging. Abdominal and general muscular tone frequently decrease, lungs lose elasticity, the thorax loses its distensibility, the mucosa of the vocal tract atrophies, mucous secretions change character and quantity, nerve endings are reduced in number, and psychoneurologic functions change. Moreover, the larynx itself loses muscle tone and bulk and may show depletion of submucosal ground substance in the vocal folds. The laryngeal cartilages ossify, and the joints may become arthritic and stiff. Hormonal influence is altered. Vocal range, intensity, and quality all may be modified. Vocal fold atrophy may be the most striking alteration. The clinical effects of aging seem more pronounced in female singers, although vocal fold histologic changes may be more prominent in males. Excellent male singers occasionally extend their careers into their 70s or beyond [5, 6]. However, some degree of breathiness, decreased range, and other evidence of aging should be expected in elderly voices. Nevertheless, many of the changes we typically associate with elderly singers (wobble, flat pitch) are due to lack of conditioning, rather than inevitable changes of biological aging. These aesthetically undesirable concomitants of aging can often be reversed.

2.1.2 What Is Your Voice Problem?

Careful questioning as to the onset of vocal problems is needed to separate acute from chronic dysfunction. Often an upper respiratory tract infection will send a patient to the physician's office, but penetrating inquiry, especially in singers and actors, may reveal a chronic vocal problem that is the patient's real concern. Identifying acute and chronic problems before beginning therapy is important so that both patient and physician may have realistic expectations and make optimal therapeutic selections.

The specific nature of the vocal complaint can provide a great deal of information. Just as dizzy patients rarely walk into the physician's office complaining of "rotary vertigo," voice patients may be unable to articulate their symptoms without guidance. They may use the term *hoarseness* to describe a variety of conditions that the physician must separate. Hoarseness is a coarse or scratchy sound that is most often associated with abnormalities of the leading edge of the vocal folds such as laryngitis or mass lesions. Breathiness is a vocal quality characterized by excessive loss of air during vocalization. In some cases, it is due to improper technique. However, any condition that prevents full approximation of the vocal folds can be responsible. Possible causes include vocal fold paralysis, a mass lesion separating the leading edges of the vocal folds, arthritis of the cricoarytenoid joint, arytenoid dislocation, scarring of the vibratory margin, senile vocal fold atrophy (presbyphonia), psychogenic dysphonia, malingering, and other conditions.

Fatigue of the voice is inability to continue to speak or sing for extended periods without a change in vocal quality and/or control. The voice may show fatigue by becoming hoarse, losing range, changing timbre, breaking into different registers, or exhibiting other uncontrolled aberrations. A well-trained singer should be able to sing for several hours without vocal fatigue.

Voice fatigue may occur through more than one mechanism. Most of the time, it is assumed to be due to muscle fatigue. This is often the case in patients who have voice fatigue associated with muscle tension dysphonia. The mechanism is most likely to be peripheral muscle fatigue and due to chemical changes (or depletion) in the muscle fibers. "Muscle fatigue" may also occur on a central (neurologic) basis. This mechanism is common in certain neuropathic disorders, such as some patients with multiple sclerosis; may occur with myasthenia gravis (actually neuromuscular junction pathology); or may be associated with paresis from various causes. However, the voice may also fatigue due to changes in the vibratory margin of the vocal fold. This phenomenon may be described as "lamina propria" fatigue (our descriptive, not universally used). It, too, may be related to chemical or fluid changes in the lamina propria or cellular damage associated with conditions such as phonotrauma and dehydration. Excessive voice use, suboptimal tissue environment (e.g., dehydration, effects of pollution, etc.), lack of sufficient time of recovery between phonatory stresses, and genetic or structural tissue weaknesses that predispose to injury or delayed recovery from trauma all may be associated with lamina propria fatigue.

Although it has not been proven, this author (RTS) suspects that fatigue may also be related to the linearity of vocal fold vibrations. However, briefly, voices have linear and nonlinear (chaotic) characteristics. As the voice becomes more trained, vibrations become more symmetrical, and the system becomes more linear. In many pathologic voices, the nonlinear components appear to become more prominent. If a voice is highly linear, slight changes in the vibratory margin may have little effect on the output of the system. However, if the system has substantial nonlinearity due to vocal fold pathology, poor tissue environment, or other causes, slight changes in the tissue (slight swelling, drying, surface cell damage) may cause substantial changes in the acoustic output of the system (the butterfly effect), causing vocal quality changes and fatigue much more quickly with much smaller changes in initial condition in more linear vocal systems.

Fatigue is often caused by misuse of abdominal and neck musculature or oversinging, singing too loudly, or too long. However, we must remember that vocal fatigue also may be a sign not only of general tiredness or vocal abuse (sometimes secondary to structural lesions or glottal closure problems) but also of serious illnesses such as myasthenia gravis. So, the importance of this complaint should not be understated.

Volume disturbance may manifest as inability to sing loudly or inability to sing softly. Each voice has its own dynamic range. Within the course of training, singers learn to sing more loudly by singing more efficiently. They also learn to sing softly, a more difficult task, through years of laborious practice. Actors and other trained speakers go through similar training. Most volume problems are secondary to intrinsic limitations of the voice or technical errors in voice use, although hormonal changes, aging, and neurologic disease are other causes. Superior laryngeal nerve paralysis impairs the ability to speak or sing loudly. This is a frequently unrecognized consequence of herpes infection (cold sores) and Lyme disease, and may be precipitated by any viral upper respiratory tract infection.

Most highly trained singers require only about 10 min to half an hour to “warm up the voice.” Prolonged warm-up time, especially in the morning, is most often caused by reflux laryngitis. Tickling or choking during singing is most often a symptom of an abnormality of the vocal fold’s leading edge. The symptom of tickling or choking should contraindicate singing until the vocal folds have been examined. Pain while singing can indicate vocal fold lesions, laryngeal joint arthritis, infection, or gastric acid reflux irritation of the arytenoid region. However, pain is much more commonly caused by voice abuse with excessive muscular activity in the neck rather than an acute abnormality on the leading edge of a vocal fold. In the absence of other symptoms, these patients do not generally require immediate cessation of singing pending medical examination. However, sudden onset of pain (usually sharp pain) while singing may be associated with a mucosal tear or a vocal fold hemorrhage and warrants voice conservation pending laryngeal examination.

2.1.3 Do You Have Any Pressing Voice Commitments?

If a singer or professional speaker (e.g., actor, politician) seeks treatment at the end of a busy performance season and has no pressing engagements, management of the voice problem should be relatively conservative and designed to ensure long-term protection of the larynx, the most delicate part of the vocal mechanism. However, the physician and patient rarely have this luxury. Most often, the voice professional needs treatment within a week of an important engagement and sometimes within less than a day. Younger singers fall ill shortly before performances, not because of hypochondria or coincidence, but rather because of the immense physical and emotional stress of the preperformance period. The singer is frequently working harder and singing longer hours than usual. Moreover, he or she may be under particular pressure to learn new material and to perform well for a new audience. The singer may also be sleeping less than usual because of additional time spent rehearsing or because of the discomforts of a strange city. Seasoned professionals make their living by performing regularly, sometimes several times a week. Consequently, any time they get sick is likely to precede a performance. Caring for voice complaints in these situations requires highly skilled judgment and bold management.

2.1.4 Tell Me About Your Vocal Career, Long-Term Goals, and the Importance of Your Voice Quality and Upcoming Commitments

To choose a treatment program, the physician must understand the importance of the patient's voice and his or her long-term career plans, the importance of the upcoming vocal commitment, and the consequences of canceling the engagement. Injudicious prescription of voice rest can be almost as damaging to a vocal career as injudicious performance. For example, although a singer's voice is usually his or her most important commodity, other factors distinguish the few successful artists from the multitude of less successful singers with equally good voices. These include musicianship, reliability, and "professionalism." Canceling a concert at the last minute may seriously damage a performer's reputation. Reliability is especially critical early in a singer's career. Moreover, an expert singer often can modify a performance to decrease the strain on his or her voice. No singer should be allowed to perform in a manner that will permit serious injury to the vocal folds, but in the frequent borderline cases, the condition of the larynx must be weighed against other factors affecting the singer as an artist.

2.1.5 How Much Voice Training Have You Had?

Establishing how long a singer or actor has been performing seriously is important, especially if his or her active performance career predates the beginning of vocal training. Active untrained singers and actors frequently develop undesirable techniques that are difficult to modify. Extensive voice use without training or premature training with inappropriate repertoire may underlie persistent vocal difficulties later in life. The number of years a performer has been training his or her voice may be a fair index of vocal proficiency. A person who has studied voice for 1 or 2 years is somewhat more likely to have gross technical difficulties than is someone who has been studying for 20 years. However, if training has been intermittent or discontinued, technical problems are common, especially among singers. In addition, methods of technical voice use vary among voice teachers. Hence, a student who has had many teachers in a relatively brief period of time commonly has numerous technical insecurities or deficiencies that may be responsible for vocal dysfunction. This is especially true if the singer has changed to a new teacher within the preceding year. The physician must be careful not to criticize the patient's current voice teacher in such circumstances. It often takes years of expert instruction to correct bad habits.

All people speak more often than they sing, yet most singers report little speech training. Even if a singer uses the voice flawlessly while practicing and performing, voice abuse at other times can cause damage that affects singing.

2.1.6 Under What Kinds of Conditions Do You Use Your Voice?

The Lombard effect is the tendency to increase vocal intensity in response to increased background noise. A well-trained singer learns to compensate for this tendency and to avoid singing at unsafe volumes. Singers of classical music usually have such training and frequently perform with only a piano, a situation in which the balance can be controlled well. However, singers performing in large halls, with orchestras, or in operas early in their careers tend to oversing and strain their voices. Similar problems occur during outdoor concerts because of the lack of auditory feedback. This phenomenon is seen even more among "pop" singers. Pop singers are in a uniquely difficult position; often, despite little vocal training, they enjoy great artistic and financial success and endure extremely stressful demands on their time and voices. They are required to sing in large halls or outdoor arenas not designed for musical performance, amid smoke and other environmental irritants, accompanied by extremely loud background music. One frequently neglected key to survival for these singers is the proper use of monitor speakers. These direct the sound of the singer's voice toward the singer on the stage and provide auditory feedback. Determining whether the pop singer uses monitor speakers and whether they are loud enough for the singer to hear is important.

Amateur singers are often no less serious about their music than are professionals, but generally they have less ability to compensate technically for illness or other physical impairment. Rarely does an amateur suffer a great loss from postponing a performance or permitting someone to sing in his or her place. In most cases, the amateur singer's best interest is served through conservative management directed at long-term maintenance of good vocal health.

A great many of the singers who seek physicians' advice are primarily choral singers. They often are enthusiastic amateurs, untrained but dedicated to their musical recreation. They should be handled as amateur solo singers, educated specifically about the Lombard effect, and cautioned to avoid the excessive volume so common in a choral environment. One good way for a singer to monitor loudness is to cup a hand to his or her ear. This adds about 6 dB [7] to the singer's perception of his or her own voice and can be a very helpful guide in noisy surroundings. Young professional singers are often hired to augment amateur choruses. Feeling that the professional quartet has been hired to "lead" the rest of the choir, they often make the mistake of trying to accomplish that goal by singing louder than others in their sections. These singers should be advised to lead their section by singing each line as if they were soloists giving a voice lesson to the people standing next to them and as if there were a microphone in front of them recording their choral performance for their voice teacher. This approach usually not only preserves the voice but also produces a better choral sound.

2.1.7 How Much Do You Practice and Exercise Your Voice? How, When, and Where Do You Use Your Voice?

Vocal exercise is as essential to the vocalist as exercise and conditioning of other muscle systems is to the athlete. Proper vocal practice incorporates scales and specific exercises designed to maintain and develop the vocal apparatus. Simply acting or singing songs or giving performances without routine studious concentration on vocal technique is not adequate for the vocal performer. The physician should know whether the vocalist practices daily, whether he or she practices at the same time daily, and how long the practice lasts. Actors generally practice and warm up their voices for 10–30 min daily, although more time is recommended. Most serious singers practice for at least 1–2 h per day. If a singer routinely practices in the late afternoon or evening but frequently performs in the morning (religious services, school classes, teaching voice, choir rehearsals, etc.), one should inquire into the warmup procedures preceding such performances as well as cool-down procedures after voice use. Singing "cold," especially early in the morning, may result in the use of minor muscular alterations to compensate for vocal insecurity produced by inadequate preparation. Such crutches can result in voice dysfunction. Similar problems may result from instances of voice use other than formal singing. School teachers, telephone receptionists, salespeople, and others who speak extensively also often derive great benefit from 5 or 10 min of vocalization of scales first thing in the morning. Although singers rarely practice their scales too long, they frequently perform or rehearse excessively. This is especially true immediately before a major concert or audition, when physicians are most likely to see acute problems. When a singer has hoarseness and vocal fatigue and has been practicing a new role for 14 h a day for the last 3 weeks, no simple prescription will solve the problem. However, a treatment regimen can usually be designed to carry the performer safely through his or her musical obligations.

The physician should be aware of common habits and environments that are often associated with abusive voice behavior and should ask about them routinely. Screaming at sports events and at children is among the most common. Extensive voice use in noisy environments also tends to be abusive. These include noisy rooms, cars, airplanes, sports facilities, and other locations where background noise or acoustic design impairs auditory feedback. Dry, dusty surroundings may alter vocal fold secretions through dehydration or contact irritation, altering voice function. Activities such as cheerleading, teaching, choral conducting, amateur singing, and frequent communication with hearing-impaired persons are likely to be associated with voice abuse, as is extensive professional voice use without formal training. The physician should inquire into the patient's routine voice use and should specifically ask about any activities that frequently lead to voice change such as hoarseness or discomfort in the neck or throat. Laryngologists should ask specifically about other activities that may be abusive to the vocal folds such as weight lifting, aerobics, and the playing of some wind instruments.

2.1.8 Are You Aware of Misusing or Abusing Your Voice During Singing?

A detailed discussion of vocal technique in singing is beyond the scope of this chapter. The most common technical errors involve excessive muscle tension in the tongue, neck, and larynx; inadequate abdominal support; and excessive volume. Inadequate preparation can be a devastating source of voice abuse and may result from limited practice, limited rehearsal of a difficult piece, or limited vocal training for a given role. The latter error is common. In some situations, voice teachers are at fault; both the singer and teacher must resist the impulse to "show off" the voice in works that are either too difficult for the singer's level of training or simply not suited to the singer's voice. Singers are habitually unhappy with the limitations of their voices. At some time or another, most baritones wish they were tenors and walk around proving they can sing high Cs in "Vesti la giubba." Singers with other vocal ranges have similar fantasies. Attempts to make the voice something that it is not, or at least that it is not yet, frequently are harmful.

2.1.9 Are You Aware of Misusing or Abusing Your Voice During Speaking?

Common patterns of voice abuse and misuse will not be discussed in detail in this chapter. Voice abuse and/ or misuse should be suspected particularly in patients who complain of voice fatigue associated with voice use, whose voices are worse at the end of a working day or week, and in any patient who is chronically hoarse. Technical errors in voice use may be the primary etiology of a voice complaint, or it may develop secondarily due to a patient's effort to compensate for voice disturbance from another cause.

Dissociation of one's speaking and singing voices is probably the most common cause of voice abuse problems in excellent singers. Too frequently, all the expert training in support, muscle control, and projection is not applied to a singers' speaking voice. Unfortunately, the resultant voice strain affects the singing voice as well as the speaking voice. Such damage is especially likely to occur in noisy rooms and in cars, where the background noise is louder than it seems. Backstage greetings after a lengthy performance can be particularly devastating. The singer usually is exhausted and distracted; the environment is often dusty and dry, and generally a noisy crowd is present. Similar conditions prevail at postperformance parties, where smoking and alcohol worsen matters. These situations should be avoided by any singer with vocal problems and should be controlled through awareness at other times.

Three particularly abusive and potentially damaging vocal activities are worthy of note. *Cheerleading* requires extensive screaming under the worst possible physical and environmental circumstances. It is a highly undesirable activity for anyone considering serious vocal endeavor. This is a common conflict in younger singers because the teenager who is the high school choir soloist often is also student council president, yearbook editor, captain of the cheerleaders, and so on.

Conducting, particularly choral conducting, can also be deleterious. An enthusiastic conductor, especially of an amateur group, frequently sings all 4 parts intermittently, at volumes louder than the entire choir, during lengthy rehearsals. Conducting is a common avocation among singers but must be done with expert technique and special precautions to prevent voice injury. Hoarseness or loss of soft voice control after conducting a rehearsal or concert suggests voice abuse during conducting. The patient should be instructed to record his or her voice throughout the vocal range singing long notes at dynamics from soft to loud to soft. Recordings should be made prior to rehearsal and following rehearsal. If the voice has lost range, control, or quality during the rehearsal, voice abuse has occurred. A similar test can be used for patients who sing in choirs, teach voice, or perform other potentially abusive vocal activities. Such problems in conductors can generally be managed by additional training in conducting techniques and by voice training, including warm-up and cooldown exercises.

Teaching singing may also be hazardous to vocal health. It can be done safely but requires skill and thought. Most teachers teach while seated at the piano. Late in a long, hard day, this posture is not conducive to maintenance of optimal abdominal and back support. Usually, teachers work with students continually positioned to the right or left of the keyboard. This may require the teacher to turn his or her neck at a particularly sharp angle, especially when teaching at an upright piano. Teachers also often demonstrate vocal works in their students' vocal ranges rather than their own, illustrating bad as well as good technique. If a singing teacher is hoarse or has neck discomfort, or his or her soft singing control deteriorates at the end of a teaching day (assuming that the teacher warms up before beginning to teach voice lessons), voice abuse should be suspected. Helpful modifications include teaching with a grand piano, sitting slightly sideways on the piano bench, or alternating student position to the right and left of the piano to facilitate better neck alignment. Retaining an accompanist so that the teacher can stand rather than teach from sitting behind a piano, and many other helpful modifications, are possible.

2.2 Do You Have Pain When You Talk or Sing?

Odynophonia, or pain caused by phonation, can be a disturbing symptom. It is not uncommon, but relatively little has been written or discussed on this subject. A detailed review of odynophonia is beyond the scope of this publication. However, laryngologists should be familiar with the diagnosis and treatment of at least a few of the most common causes, at least, as discussed elsewhere in this book.

2.2.1 *What Kind of Physical Condition Are You In?*

Phonation is an athletic activity that requires good conditioning and coordinated interaction of numerous physical functions. Maladies of any part of the body may be reflected in the voice. Failure to maintain good abdominal muscle tone and respiratory endurance through exercise is particularly harmful because deficiencies in these areas undermine the power source of the voice. Patients generally attempt to compensate for such weaknesses by using inappropriate muscle groups, particularly in the neck, causing vocal dysfunction. Similar problems may occur in the well-conditioned vocalist in states of fatigue. These are compounded by mucosal changes that accompany excessively long hours of hard work. Such problems may be seen even in the best singers shortly before important performances in the height of the concert season.

A popular but untrue myth holds that great opera singers must be obese. However, the vivacious, gregarious personality that often distinguishes the great performer seems to be accompanied frequently by a propensity for excess, especially culinary excess. This excess is as undesirable in the vocalist as it is in most other athletic artists, and it should be prevented from the start of one's vocal career. Appropriate and attractive body weight has always been valued in the pop music world and is becoming particularly important in the opera world as this formerly theater-based art form moves to television and film media. However, attempts at weight reduction in an established speaker or singer are a different matter. The vocal mechanism is a finely tuned, complex instrument and is exquisitely sensitive to minor changes. Substantial fluctuations in weight frequently cause deleterious alterations of the voice, although these are usually temporary. Weight reduction programs for people concerned about their voices must be monitored carefully and designed to reduce weight in small increments over long periods. A history of sudden recent weight change may be responsible for almost any vocal complaint.

2.2.2 *How Is Your Hearing?*

Hearing loss can cause substantial problems for singers and other professional voice users. This may be true especially when the voice patient is unaware that he or she has hearing loss. Consequently, not only should voice patients be asked about hearing loss, tinnitus, vertigo, and family history of hearing loss, but it is also helpful to inquire of spouses, partners, friends, or others who may have accompanied the patient to the office whether they have suspected a hearing impairment in the patient.

2.2.3 Have You Noted Voice or Bodily Weakness, Tremor, Fatigue, or Loss of Control?

Even minor neurologic disorders may be extremely disruptive to vocal function. Specific questions should be asked to rule out neuromuscular and neurologic diseases such as myasthenia gravis, Parkinson's disease, tremors, other movement disorders, spasmodic dysphonia, multiple sclerosis, central nervous system neoplasm, and other serious maladies that may be present with voice complaints.

2.2.4 Do You Have Allergy or Cold Symptoms?

Acute upper respiratory tract infection causes inflammation of the mucosa, alters mucosal secretions, and makes the mucosa more vulnerable to injury. Coughing and throat clearing are particularly traumatic vocal activities and may worsen or provoke hoarseness associated with a cold. Postnasal drip and allergy may produce the same response. Infectious sinusitis is associated with discharge and diffuse mucosal inflammation, resulting in similar problems, and may actually alter the sound of a voice, especially the patient's own perception of his or her voice. Futile attempts to compensate for disease of the supraglottic vocal tract in an effort to return the sound to normal frequently result in laryngeal strain. The expert singer or speaker should compensate by monitoring technique by tactile rather than by auditory feedback, or singing "by feel" rather than "by ear."

2.2.5 Do You Have Breathing Problems, Especially After Exercise?

Voice patients usually volunteer information about upper respiratory tract infections and postnasal drip, but the relevance of other maladies may not be obvious to them. Consequently, the physician must seek out pertinent history.

Respiratory problems are especially important in voice patients. Even mild respiratory dysfunction may adversely affect the power source of the voice [8]. Occult asthma may be particularly troublesome [9]. A complete respiratory history should be obtained in most patients with voice complaints, and pulmonary function testing is often advisable.

2.2.6 Have You Been Exposed to Environmental Irritants?

Any mucosal irritant can disrupt the delicate vocal mechanism. Allergies to dust and mold are aggravated commonly during rehearsals and performances in concert halls, especially older theaters and concert halls, because of numerous curtains, backstage trappings, and dressing room facilities that are rarely cleaned thoroughly. Nasal obstruction and erythematous conjunctivae suggest generalized mucosal irritation. The drying effects of cold air and dry heat may also affect mucosal secretions, leading to decreased lubrication, a “scratchy” voice, and tickling cough. These symptoms may be minimized by nasal breathing, which allows inspired air to be filtered, warmed, and humidified. Nasal breathing, whenever possible, rather than mouth breathing, is a proper vocal technique. While the performer is backstage between appearances or during rehearsals, inhalation of dust and other irritants may be controlled by wearing a protective mask, such as those used by carpenters, or a surgical mask that does not contain fiberglass. This is especially helpful when sets are being constructed in the rehearsal area.

A history of recent travel suggests other sources of mucosal irritation. The air in airplanes is extremely dry, and airplanes are noisy [10]. One must be careful to avoid talking loudly and to maintain good hydration and nasal breathing during air travel. Environmental changes can also be disruptive. Las Vegas is infamous for the mucosal irritation caused by its dry atmosphere and smoke-filled rooms. In fact, the resultant complex of hoarseness, vocal “tickle,” and fatigue is referred to as “Las Vegas voice.” A history of recent travel should also suggest jet lag and generalized fatigue, which may be potent detriments to good vocal function.

Environmental pollution is responsible for the presence of toxic substances and conditions encountered daily. Inhalation of toxic pollutants may affect the voice adversely by direct laryngeal injury, by causing pulmonary dysfunction that results in voice maladies, or through impairments elsewhere in the vocal tract. Ingested substances, especially those that have neurolaryngologic effects, may also adversely affect the voice. Nonchemical environmental pollutants such as noise can cause voice abnormalities, as well. Laryngologists should be familiar with the laryngologic effects of the numerous potentially irritating substances and conditions found in the environment. We must also be familiar with special pollution problems encountered by performers. Numerous materials used by artists to create sculptures, drawings, and theatrical sets are toxic and have adverse voice effects. In addition, performers are exposed routinely to chemicals encountered through stage smoke and pyrotechnic effects. Although it is clear that some of the “special effects” may result in serious laryngologic consequences, much additional study is needed to clarify the nature and scope of these occupational problems.

2.2.7 *Do You Smoke, Live with a Smoker, or Work Around Smoke?*

The effects of smoking on voice performance were reviewed recently in the *Journal of Singing* [11], and that review is recapitulated here. Smoking tobacco is the number one cause of preventable death in the United States as well as the leading cause of heart disease, stroke, emphysema, and cancer. The Centers for Disease Control and Prevention (CDC) attributes approximately 442,000 premature (shortened life expectancy) deaths annually in the United States to smoking, which is more than the combined incidence of deaths caused by highway accidents, fires, murders, illegal drugs, suicides, and AIDS [12]. Approximately four million deaths per year worldwide result from smoking, and if this trend continues, by 2030, this figure will increase to about ten million deaths globally [13]. In addition to causing life-threatening diseases, smoking impairs a great many body systems, including the vocal tract. Harmful consequences of smoking or being exposed to smoke influence voice performance adversely.

Singers need good vocal health to perform well. Smoking tobacco can irritate the mucosal covering of the vocal folds, causing redness and chronic inflammation, and can have the same effect on the mucosal lining of the lungs, trachea, nasopharynx (behind the nose and throat), and mouth. In other words, the components of voice production—the generator, the oscillator, the resonator, and the articulator—all can be compromised by the harmful effects of tobacco use. The onset of effects from smoking may be immediate or delayed.

Individuals who have allergies and/or asthma are usually more sensitive to cigarette smoke with potential for an immediate adverse reaction involving the lungs, larynx, nasal cavities, and/or eyes. Chronic use of tobacco, or exposure to it, causes the toxic chemicals in tobacco to accumulate in the body, damaging the delicate linings of the vocal tract, as well as the lungs, heart, and circulatory system.

The lungs are critical components of the power source of the vocal tract. They help generate an airstream that is directed superiorly through the trachea toward the undersurface of the vocal folds. The vocal folds respond to the increase in subglottic pressure by producing sounds of variable intensities and frequencies. The number of times per second the vocal fold vibrate influences the pitch, and the amplitude of the mucosal wave influences the loudness of the sound. The sound produced by the vibration (oscillation) of the vocal folds passes upward through the oral cavity and nasopharynx where it resonates, giving the voice its richness and timbre, and eventually it is articulated by the mouth, teeth, lips, and tongue into speech or song.

Any condition that adversely affects lung function such as chronic exposure to smoke or uncontrolled asthma can contribute to dysphonia by impairing the strength, endurance, and consistency of the airsteam responsible for establishing vocal fold oscillation. Any lesion that compromises vocal fold vibration and glottic closure can cause hoarseness and breathiness. Inflammation of the cover layer of the vocal folds and/or the mucosal lining of the nose, sinuses, and oral nasopharyngeal cavities can affect the quality and clarity of the voice.

Tobacco smoke can damage the lungs' parenchyma and the exchange of air through respiration. Cigarette manufacturers add hundreds of ingredients to their tobacco products to improve taste, to make smoking seem milder and easier to inhale, and to prolong burning and shelf life [14]. More than 3000 chemical compounds have been identified in tobacco smoke, and more than 60 of these compounds are carcinogens [15]. The tobacco plant, *Nicotiana tabacum*, is grown for its leaves, which can be smoked, chewed, or sniffed with various effects. The nicotine in tobacco is the addictive component and rivals crack cocaine in its ability to enslave its users. Most smokers want to stop, yet only a small percentage are successful in quitting cigarettes; the majority who quit relapse into smoking once again [16]. Tar and carbon monoxide are among the disease-causing components in tobacco products. The tar in cigarettes exposes the individual to a greater risk of bronchitis, emphysema, and lung cancer. These chemicals affect the entire vocal tract as well as the cardiovascular system (Table 2.1).

Cigarette smoke in the lungs can lead also to increased vascularity, edema, and excess mucous production, as well as epithelial tissue and cellular changes. The toxic agents in cigarette smoke have been associated with an increase in the number and severity of asthma attacks, chronic bronchitis, emphysema, and lung cancer, all of which can interfere with the lungs' ability to generate the stream of air needed for voice production.

Table 2.1 Chemical additives found in tobaccos and commercial products

Tobacco chemical additives	Also found in
Acetic acid	Vinegar, hair dye
Acetone	Nail polish remover
Ammonia	Floor cleaner, toilet cleaner
Arsenic	Poison
Benzene	A leukemia-producing agent in rubber cement
Butane	Cigarette lighter fluid
Cadmium	Batteries, some oil paints
Carbon monoxide	Car exhaust
DDT	Insecticides
Ethanol	Alcohol
Formaldehyde	Embalming fluid, fabric, laboratory animals
Hexamine	Barbecue lighter
Hydrazine	Jet fuel, rocket fuel
Hydrogen cyanide	Gas chamber poison
Methane	Swamp gas
Methanol	Rocket fuel
Naphthalene	Explosives, mothballs, paints
Nickel	Electroplating
Nicotine	Insecticides
Nitrobenzene	Gasoline additive
Nitrous oxide phenols	Disinfectant
Phenol	Disinfectants, plastics
Polonium-210	A radioactive substance
Stearic acid	Candle wax
Styrene	Insulation materials
Toluene	Industrial solvent, embalmer's glue
Vinyl chloride	Plastic manufacturing, garbage bags

Chronic bronchitis due to smoking has been associated with an increase in the number of goblet (mucous) cells, an increase in the size (hyperplasia) of the mucosal secreting glands, and a decrease in the number of ciliated cells, the cells used to clean the lungs. Chronic cough and sputum production are also seen more commonly in smokers compared with nonsmokers. Also, the heat and chemicals of unfiltered cigarette and marijuana smoke are especially irritating to the lungs and larynx.

An important component of voice quality is the symmetrical, unencumbered vibration of the true vocal folds. Anything that prevents the epithelium covering the vocal folds from vibrating or affects the loose connective tissue under the epithelium (in the superficial layer of the lamina propria known as the Reinke's space) can cause dysphonia. Cigarette smoking can cause the epithelium of the true vocal folds to become red and swollen, develop whitish discolorations (leukoplakia), undergo chronic inflammatory changes, or develop squamous metaplasia or dysplasia (tissue changes from normal to a potentially malignant state). In chronic smokers, the voice may become husky due to the accumulation of fluid in the Reinke's space (Reinke's edema). These alterations in structure can interfere with voice production by changing the biomechanics of the vocal folds and their vibratory characteristics. In severe cases, cancer can deform and paralyze the vocal folds.

Vocal misuse often follows in an attempt to compensate for dysphonia and an alerted self-perception of one's voice. The voice may feel weak, breathy, raspy, or strained. There may be a loss of range, vocal breaks, long warm-up time, and fatigue. The throat may feel raw, achy, or tight. As the voice becomes unreliable, bad habits increase as the individual struggles harder and harder to compensate vocally. As selected sound waves move upward, from the larynx toward and through the pharynx, nasopharynx, mouth, and nose (the resonators), sounds gain a unique richness and timbre. Exposing the pharynx to cigarette smoke aggravates the linings of the oropharynx, mouth, nasopharynx, sinuses, and nasal cavities. The resulting erythema, swelling, and inflammation predispose one to nasal congestion and impaired mucosal function; there may be predisposition to sinusitis and pharyngitis, in which the voice may become hyponasal, the sinus achy, and the throat painful.

Although relatively rare in the United States, cancer of the nasopharynx has been associated with cigarette smoking [17], and one of the presenting symptoms is unilateral hearing loss due to fluid in the middle ear caused by eustachian tube obstruction from the cancer. Smoking-induced cancers of the oral cavity, pharynx, larynx, and lung are common throughout the world, including in the United States.

The palate, tongue, cheeks, lips, and teeth articulate the sound modified by the resonators into speech. Cigarettes, cigar, or pipe smoking may cause a "black hairy tongue," precancerous oral lesions (leukoplakia), and/or cancer of the tongue and lips [18]. Any irritation that causes burning or inflammation of the oral mucosa can affect phonation, and all tobacco products are capable of causing these effects.

Smokeless "spit" tobacco is highly addictive, and users who dip 8–10 times a day may get the same nicotine exposure as those who smoke 1½ to 2 packs of cigarettes per day [19]. Smokeless tobacco has been associated with gingivitis, cheek carcinoma, and cancer of the larynx and hypopharynx.

Exposure to environmental tobacco smoke (ETS), also called secondhand smoke, sidestream smoke, or passive smoke, accounts for an estimated 3000 lung cancer deaths and approximately 35,000 deaths in the United States from heart disease in nonsmoking adults [20].

Secondhand smoke is the "passive" inhalation of tobacco smoke from environmental sources such as smoke given off by pipes, cigars, cigarettes (side-stream), or the smoke exhaled from the lungs of smokers and inhaled by other people (mainstream). This passive smoke contains a mixture of thousands of chemicals, some of which are known to cause cancer. The National Institutes of Health (NIH) lists ETS as a "known" carcinogen, and the more you are exposed to secondhand smoke, the greater your risk [21].

Infants and young children are affected particularly by secondhand smoke with increased incidences of otitis media (ear infections), bronchitis, and pneumonia. If small children are exposed to secondhand smoke, the child's resulting illness can have a stressful effect on the parent who frequently catches the child's illness. Both the illness and the stress of caring for the sick child may interfere with voice performance. People who are exposed routinely to secondhand smoke are at risk for lung cancer, heart disease, respiratory infection, and an increased number of asthma attacks [22].

There is an intricate relationship between the lungs, larynx, pharynx, nose, and mouth in the production of speech and song. Smoking can have deleterious effects on any part of the vocal tract, causing the respiratory system to lose power, damaging the vibratory margins of the vocal folds, and detracting from the richness and beauty of a voice.

The deleterious effects of tobacco smoke on mucosa are indisputable. Anyone concerned about the health of his or her voice should not smoke. Smoking causes erythema, mild edema, and generalized inflammation throughout the vocal tract. Both smoke itself and the heat of the cigarette appear to be important. Marijuana produces a particularly irritating, unfiltered smoke that is inhaled directly, causing considerable mucosal response. Voice patients who refuse to stop smoking marijuana should at least be advised to use a water pipe to cool and partially filter the smoke. Some vocalists are required to perform in smoke-filled environments and may suffer the same effects as the smokers themselves. In some theaters, it is possible to place fans upstage or direct the ventilation system so as to create a gentle draft toward the audience, clearing the smoke away from the stage. "Smoke eaters" installed in some theaters are also helpful.

2.2.8 *Do Any Foods Seem to Affect Your Voice?*

Various foods are said to affect the voice. Traditionally, singers avoid milk and ice cream before performances. In many people, these foods seem to increase the amount and viscosity of mucosal secretions. Allergy and casein have been implicated, but no satisfactory explanation has been established. In some cases, restriction of these foods from the diet before a voice performance may be helpful. Chocolate may have the same effect and should be viewed similarly. Chocolate also contains caffeine, which may aggravate reflux or cause tremor. Voice patients should be asked about eating nuts. This is important not only because some people experience effects similar to those produced by milk products and chocolate but also because they are extremely irritating if aspirated. The irritation produced by aspiration of even a small organic foreign body may be severe and impossible to correct rapidly enough to permit performance. Highly spiced foods may also cause mucosal irritation. In addition, they seem to aggravate reflux laryngitis. Coffee and other beverages containing caffeine also aggravate gastric reflux and may promote dehydration and/or alter secretions and necessitate frequent throat clearing in some people. Fad diets, especially rapid weight-reducing diets, are notorious for causing voice problems. Eating a full meal before a speaking or singing engagement may interfere with abdominal support or may aggravate upright reflux of gastric juice during abdominal muscle contraction. Lemon juice and herbal teas are considered beneficial to the voice. Both may act as demulcents, thinning secretions, and may very well be helpful.

2.2.9 Do You Have Morning Hoarseness, Bad Breath, Excessive Phlegm, a Lump in Your Throat, or Heartburn?

Reflux laryngitis is especially common among singers and trained speakers because of the high intraabdominal pressure associated with proper support and because of lifestyle. Singers frequently perform at night. Many vocalists refrain from eating before performances because a full stomach can compromise effective abdominal support. They typically compensate by eating heartily at postperformance gatherings late at night and then go to bed with a full stomach.

Chronic irritation of arytenoid and vocal fold mucosa by reflux of gastric secretions may occasionally be associated with dyspepsia or pyrosis. However, the key features of this malady are bitter taste and halitosis on awakening in the morning, a dry or "coated" mouth, often a scratchy sore throat or a feeling of a "lump in the throat," hoarseness, and the need for prolonged vocal warm-up. The physician must be alert to these symptoms and ask about them routinely; otherwise, the diagnosis will often be overlooked, because people who have had this problem for many years or a lifetime do not even realize it is abnormal.

2.2.10 Do You Have Trouble with Your Bowels or Belly?

Any condition that alters abdominal function, such as muscle spasm, constipation, or diarrhea, interferes with support and may result in a voice complaint. These symptoms may accompany infection, anxiety, various gastroenterological diseases, and other maladies.

2.2.11 Are You Under Particular Stress or in Therapy?

The human voice is an exquisitely sensitive messenger of emotion. Highly trained voice professionals learn to control the effects of anxiety and other emotional stress on their voices under ordinary circumstances. However, in some instances, this training may break down or a performer may be inadequately prepared to control the voice under specific stressful conditions. Preperformance anxiety is the most common example, but insecurity, depression, and other emotional disturbances are also generally reflected in the voice. Anxiety reactions are mediated in part through the autonomic nervous system and result in a dry mouth, cold clammy skin, and thick secretions. These reactions are normal, and good vocal training coupled with assurance that no abnormality or disease is present generally overcomes them. However, long-term, poorly compensated emotional stress and exogenous stress (from agents, producers, teachers, parents, etc.) may cause substantial vocal dysfunction and may result in permanent limitations of the vocal apparatus. These conditions must be diagnosed and treated expertly. Hypochondriasis is uncommon among professional singers, despite popular opinion to the contrary.

Recent publications have highlighted the complexity and importance of psychological factors associated with voice disorders [23]. A comprehensive discussion of this subject is also presented elsewhere in this book. It is important for the physician to recognize that psychological problems may not only cause voice disorders but also delay recovery from voice disorders that were entirely organic in etiology. Professional voice users, especially singers, have enormous psychological investment and personality identifications associated with their voices. A condition that causes voice loss or permanent injury often evokes the same powerful psychological responses seen following the death of a loved one. This process may be initiated even when physical recovery is complete if an incident (injury or surgery) has made the vocalist realize that voice loss is possible. Such a "brush with death" can have profound emotional consequences in some patients. It is essential for laryngologists to be aware of these powerful factors and manage them properly if optimal therapeutic results are to be achieved expeditiously.

2.2.12 Do You Have Problems Controlling Your Weight? Are You Excessively Tired? Are You Cold When Other People Are Warm?

Endocrine problems warrant special attention. The human voice is extremely sensitive to endocrinologic changes. Many of these are reflected in alterations of fluid content of the lamina propria just beneath the laryngeal mucosa. This causes alterations in the bulk and shape of the vocal folds and results in voice change. Hypothyroidism [24–28] is a well-recognized cause of such voice disorders, although the mechanism is not fully understood. Hoarseness, vocal fatigue, muffling of the voice, loss of range, and a sensation of a lump in the throat may be present even with mild hypothyroidism. Even when thyroid function tests results are within the low normal range, this diagnosis should be entertained, especially if thyroid-stimulating hormone levels are in the high normal range or are elevated. Thyrotoxicosis may result in similar voice disturbances [25].

2.2.13 Do You Have Menstrual Irregularity, Cyclical Voice Changes Associated with Menses, Recent Menopause, or Other Hormonal Changes or Problems?

Voice changes associated with sex hormones are encountered commonly in clinical practice and have been investigated more thoroughly than have other hormonal changes [29, 30]. Although a correlation appears to exist between sex hormone levels and depth of male voices (higher testosterone and lower estradiol levels in basses than in tenors) [29], the most important hormonal considerations in males occur during or related to puberty [31, 32]. Voice problems related to sex hormones are more common in female singers (C. Carroll, personal communication with Dr. Hans von Leden. Arizona State University at Tempe, 1992) [32–48].

2.2.14 Do You Have Jaw Joint or Other Dental Problems?

Dental disease, especially temporomandibular joint (TMJ) dysfunction, introduces muscle tension in the head and neck, which is transmitted to the larynx directly through the muscular attachments between the mandible and the hyoid bone and indirectly as generalized increased muscle tension. These problems often result in decreased range, vocal fatigue, and change in the quality or placement of a voice. Such tension often is accompanied by excess tongue muscle activity, especially pulling of the tongue posteriorly. This hyperfunctional behavior acts through hyoid attachments to disrupt the balance between the intrinsic and extrinsic laryngeal musculature. TMJ problems are also problematic for wind instrumentalists and some string players, including violinists. In some cases, the problems may actually be caused by instrumental technique. The history should always include information about musical activities, including instruments other than the voice.

2.2.15 Do You or Your Blood Relatives Have Hearing Loss?

Hearing loss is often overlooked as a source of vocal problems. Auditory feedback is fundamental to speaking and singing. Interference with this control mechanism may result in altered vocal production, particularly if the person is unaware of the hearing loss. Distortion, particularly pitch distortion (diplacusis), may also pose serious problems for the singer. This appears to be due not only to aesthetic difficulties in matching pitch but also to vocal strain that accompanies pitch shifts [49].

In addition to determining whether the patient has hearing loss, inquiry should also be made about hearing impairment occurring in family members, roommates, and other close associates. Speaking loudly to people who are hard of hearing can cause substantial, chronic vocal strain. This possibility should be investigated routinely when evaluating voice patients.

2.2.16 Have you Suffered Whiplash or Other Bodily Injury?

Various bodily injuries outside the confines of the vocal tract may have profound effects on the voice. Whiplash, for example, commonly causes changes in technique, with consequent voice fatigue, loss of range, difficulty singing softly, and other problems. These problems derive from the neck muscle spasm, abnormal neck posturing secondary to pain, and consequent hyperfunctional voice use. Lumbar, abdominal, head, chest, supraglottic, and extremity injuries may also affect vocal technique and be responsible for the dysphonia that prompted the voice patient to seek medical attention.

2.2.17 Did You Undergo Any Surgery Prior to the Onset of Your Voice Problems?

A history of laryngeal surgery in a voice patient is a matter of great concern. It is important to establish exactly why the surgery was done, by whom it was done, whether intubation was necessary, and whether voice therapy was instituted pre- or postoperatively if the lesion was associated with voice abuse (vocal nodules). If the vocal dysfunction that sent the patient to the physician's office dates from the immediate postoperative period, surgical trauma must be suspected.

Otolaryngologists frequently are asked about the effects of tonsillectomy on the voice. Singers especially may consult the physician after tonsillectomy and complain of vocal dysfunction. Certainly removal of tonsils can alter the voice [50, 51]. Tonsillectomy changes the configuration of the supraglottic vocal tract. In addition, scarring alters pharyngeal muscle function, which is trained meticulously in the professional singer. Singers must be warned that they may have permanent voice changes after tonsillectomy; however, these can be minimized by dissecting in the proper plane to lessen scarring. The singer's voice generally requires 3–6 months to stabilize or return to normal after surgery, although it is generally safe to begin limited singing within 2–4 weeks following surgery. As with any procedure for which general anesthesia may be needed, the anesthesiologist should be advised preoperatively that the patient is a professional singer. Intubation and extubation should be performed with great care, and the use of nonirritating plastic rather than rubber or ribbed metal endotracheal tubes is preferred. Use of a laryngeal mask may be advisable for selected procedures for mechanical reasons, but this device is often not ideal for tonsillectomy, and it can cause laryngeal injury such as arytenoid dislocation.

Surgery of the neck, such as thyroidectomy, may result in permanent alterations in the vocal mechanism through scarring of the extrinsic laryngeal musculature. The cervical (strap) muscles are important in maintaining laryngeal position and stability of the laryngeal skeleton, and they should be retracted rather than divided whenever possible. A history of recurrent or superior laryngeal nerve injury may explain a hoarse, breathy, or weak voice. However, in rare cases, even a singer can compensate for recurrent laryngeal nerve paralysis and have a nearly normal voice.

Thoracic and abdominal surgery interferes with respiratory and abdominal support. After these procedures, singing and projected speaking should be prohibited until pain has subsided and healing has occurred sufficiently to allow normal support. Abdominal exercises should be instituted before resumption of vocalizing. Singing and speaking without proper support are often worse for the voice than not using the voice for performance at all.

Other surgical procedures may be important factors if they necessitate intubation or if they affect the musculoskeletal system so that the person has to change stance or balance. For example, balancing on 1 foot after leg surgery may decrease the effectiveness of the support mechanism.

2.2.18 What Medications and Other Substances Do You Use?

A history of alcohol abuse suggests the probability of poor vocal technique. Intoxication results in incoordination and decreased awareness, which undermine vocal discipline designed to optimize and protect the voice. The effect of small amounts of alcohol is controversial. Although many experts oppose its use because of its vasodilatory effect and consequent mucosal alteration, many people do not seem to be adversely affected by small amounts of alcohol such as a glass of wine with a meal. However, some people have mild sensitivities to certain wines or beers. Patients who develop nasal congestion and rhinorrhea after drinking beer, for example, should be made aware that they probably have a mild allergy to that particular beverage and should avoid it before voice commitments.

Patients frequently acquire antihistamines to help control "postnasal drip" or other symptoms. The drying effect of antihistamines may result in decreased vocal fold lubrication, increased throat clearing, and irritability leading to frequent coughing. Antihistamines may be helpful to some voice patients, but they must be used with caution.

When a voice patient seeking the attention of a physician is already taking antibiotics, it is important to find out the dose and the prescribing physician, if any, as well as whether the patient frequently treats himself or herself with inadequate courses of antibiotics often supplied by colleagues. Singers, actors, and other speakers sometimes have a "sore throat" shortly before important vocal presentations and start themselves on inappropriate antibiotic therapy, which they generally discontinue after their performance.

Diuretics are also popular among some performers. They are often prescribed by gynecologists at the vocalist's request to help deplete excess water in the premenstrual period. They are not effective in this scenario, because they cannot diurese the protein-bound water in the laryngeal ground substance. Unsupervised use of these drugs may cause dehydration and consequent mucosal dryness.

Hormone use, especially use of oral contraceptives, must be mentioned specifically during the physician's inquiry. Women frequently do not mention them routinely when asked whether they are taking any medication. Vitamins are also frequently not mentioned. Most vitamin therapy seems to have little effect on the voice. However, high-dose vitamin C (5–6 g/day), which some people use to prevent upper respiratory tract infections, seems to act as a mild diuretic and may lead to dehydration and xerophonia [52].

Cocaine use is common, especially among pop musicians. This drug can be extremely irritating to the nasal mucosa, causes marked vasoconstriction, and may alter the sensorium, resulting in decreased voice control and a tendency toward vocal abuse.

Many pain medications (including aspirin and ibuprofen), psychotropic medications, and others may be responsible for a voice complaint. So far, no adverse vocal effects have been reported with selective COX-2 inhibiting anti-inflammatory medications (which do not promote bleeding, as do other nonsteroidal anti-inflammatory medicines and aspirin) such as celecoxib (Celebrex; Pfizer, Inc, New York, New York) and valecoxib (Bextra; Pharmacia Corp, New York, New York). However, this group of drugs has been demonstrated to have other side effects, and should in our view only be taken under the care of a physician [53]. The effects of other new medications such as sildenafil citrate (Viagra; Pfizer, Inc) and medications used to induce abortion remain unstudied and unknown, but it seems plausible that such medication may affect voice function, at least temporarily. Laryngologists should be familiar with the laryngologic effects of the many substances ingested medically and recreationally.

Acknowledgments Modified in part from Sataloff RT. *Professional Voice: The Science and Art of Clinical Care, 4th Edition*. San Diego, CA: Plural Publishing; 2017, with permission.

References

1. Sataloff RT. Professional singers: the science and art of clinical care. Am J Otolaryngol. 1981;2:251–66.
2. Sataloff RT. The human voice. Sci Am. 1992;267:108–15.
3. Sundberg J. The science of the singing voice. DeKalb: Northern Illinois University Press; 1987.
4. Sataloff RT. Efficient history taking in professional singers. Laryngoscope. 1984;94:1111–4.

5. Ackerman R, Pfan W. Gerontology studies on the susceptibility to voice disorders in professional speakers. Folia Phoniatr (Basel). 1974;26:95–9.
6. von Leden H. Speech and hearing problems in the geriatric patient. J Am Geriatr Soc. 1977;25:422–6.
7. Schiff M. Comment. Presented at: seventh symposium on care of the professional voice. New York: The Juilliard School; 15–16 June 1978.
8. Spiegel JR, Cohn JR, Sataloff RT, et al. Respiratory function in singers: medical assessment, diagnoses, treatments. J Voice. 1988;2:40–50.
9. Cohn JR, Sataloff RT, Spiegel JR, et al. Airway reactivity-induced asthma in singers (ARIAS). J Voice. 1991;5:332–7.
10. Feder RJ. The professional voice and airline flight. Otolaryngol Head Neck Surg. 1984;92:251–4.
11. Anticaglia A, Hawkshaw M, Sataloff RT. The effects of smoking on voice performance. J Singing. 2004;60:161–7.
12. Centers for Disease Control and Prevention (CDC). Annual smoking-attributable, mortality, years of potential life lost, and economic costs, United States—1995–1999. MMWR Morb Mortal Wkly Rep. 2002;51(14):300–3.
13. World Health Organization. World health report 1999. Geneva: World Health Organization; 1999.
14. United States Department of Health Services (USDHHS). Tobacco products fact sheet. Washington, DC: Government Printing Office; 2000.
15. National Cancer Institute. Environmental tobacco smoke. Fact sheet 3.9; 1999. http://cis.nci.nih.gov/fact/3_9htm.
16. Centers for Disease Control and Prevention. Cigarette smoking among adults—United States, 1993. MMWR Morb Mortal Wkly Rep. 1994;3:925–9.
17. Chow WH, McLaughlin JK, Hrubec Z, et al. Tobacco use and nasopharyngeal carcinoma in a cohort of US veterans. Int J Cancer. 1993;55(4):538–40.
18. Casiglia J, Woo SB. A comprehensive view of oral cancer. Gen Dent. 2001;49(1):72–82.
19. Centers for Disease Control and Prevention. Determination of nicotine pH and moisture content of six U.S. commercial moist snuff products. MMWR Morb Mortal Wkly Rep. 1999;48(19):398.
20. American Cancer Society. Cancer facts and figures 2002. Atlanta: American Cancer Society; 2002.
21. National Toxicology Program (NTP). Report on carcinogens. 10th ed. Research Triangle Park: U.S. Department Health and Human Services, Public Health Service, National Toxicology Program; 2002. http://ehp.niehs.nih.gov/roc/toc10.html.
22. Academy of Pediatrics, Committee on Environmental Health. Environmental tobacco smoke; a hazard to children. Pediatrics. 1997;99(4):639–42.
23. Rosen DC, Sataloff RT. Psychology of voice disorders. 2nd ed. San Diego: Plural Publishing, Inc.; 2020.
24. Gupta OP, Bhatia PL, Agarwal MK, et al. Nasal pharyngeal and laryngeal manifestations of hypothyroidism. Ear Nose Throat J. 1997;56:10–21.
25. Malinsky M, Chevrie-Muller, Cerceau N. Etude clinique et electrophysiologique des alterations de la voix au cours des thyrotoxioses. Ann Endocrinol (Paris). 1997;38:171–2.
26. Michelsson K, Sirvio P. Cry analysis in congenital hypothyroidism. Folia Phoniatr (Basel). 1976;28:40–7.
27. Ritter FN. The effect of hypothyroidism on the larynx of the rat. Ann Otol Rhinol Laryngol. 1964;67:404–16.
28. Ritter FN. Endocrinology. In: Paparella M, Shumrick D, editors. Otolaryngology, vol. I. Philadelphia: Saunders; 1973. p. 727–34.
29. Meuser W, Nieschlag E. Sex hormones and depth of voice in the male [in German]. Dtsch Med Wochenschr. 1977;102:261–4.

30. Schiff M. The influence of estrogens on connective tissue. In: Asboe-Hansen G, editor. Hormones and connective tissue. Copenhagen: Munksgaard Press; 1967. p. 282–341.
31. Brodnitz F. The age of the castrato voice. J Speech Hear Disord. 1975;40:291–5.
32. Brodnitz F. Hormones and the human voice. Bull N Y Acad Med. 1971;47:183–91.
33. von Gelder L. Psychosomatic aspects of endocrine disorders of the voice. J Commun Disord. 1974;7:257–62.
34. Lacina O. Der Einfluss der Menstruation auf die Stimme der Sangerinnen. Folia Phoniatr (Basel). 1968;20:13–24.
35. Wendler J. The influence of menstruation on the voice of the female singer. Folia Phoniatr (Basel). 1972;24:259–77.
36. Brodnitz F. Medical care preventive therapy (panel). In: Lawrence VL, editor. Transcripts of the seventh annual symposium, care of the professional voice, vol. 3. New York: The Voice Foundation; 1978. p. 86.
37. Dordain M. Etude Statistique de l'influence des contraceptifs hormonaux sur la voix. Folia Phoniatr (Basel). 1972;24:86–96.
38. Pahn J, Goretzlehner G. Voice changes following the use of oral contraceptives [in German]. Zentralbl Gynakol. 1978;100:341–6.
39. Schiff M. "The pill" in otolaryngology. Trans Am Acad Ophthalmol Otolaryngol. 1968;72:76–84.
40. von Deuster CV. Irreversible vocal changes in pregnancy [in German]. HNO. 1977;25:430–2.
41. Flach M, Schwickardi H, Simen R. Welchen Einfluss haben Menstruation and Schwangerschaft auf die augsgebildete Gesangsstimme? Folia Phoniatr (Basel). 1968;21:199–210.
42. Arndt HJ. Stimmstorungen nach Behandlung mit Androgenen und anabolen Hormonen. Munch Med Wochenschr. 1974;116:1715–20.
43. Bourdial J. Les troubles de la voix provoques par la therapeutique hormonale androgene. Ann Otolaryngol Chir Cervicofac. 1970;87:725–34.
44. Damste PH. Virilization of the voice due to anabolic steroids [in Dutch]. Ned Tijdschr Geneeskd. 1963;107:891–2.
45. Damste PH. Voice changes in adult women caused by virilizing agents. J Speech Hear Disord. 1967;32:126–32.
46. Saez S, Francoise S. Recepteurs d'androgenes: mise en evidence dans la fraction cytosolique de muqueuse normale et d'epitheliomas phryngolarynges humains. C R Acad Sci Hebd Seances Acad Sci D. 1975;280:935–8.
47. Vuorenkoski V, Lenko HL, Tjernlund P, et al. Fundamental voice frequency during normal and abnormal growth, and after androgen treatment. Arch Dis Child. 1978;53:201–9.
48. Imre V. Hormonell bedingte Stimmstorungen. Folia Phoniatr (Basel). 1968;20:394–404.
49. Sundberg J, Prame E, Iwarsson J. Replicability and accuracy of pitch patterns in professional singers. In: Davis PJ, Fletcher NH, editors. Vocal fold physiology: controlling chaos and complexity. San Diego: Singular Publishing Group; 1996. p. 291–306.
50. Gould WJ, Alberti PW, Brodnitz F, Hirano M. Medical care preventive therapy (Panel). In: Lawrence VL, editor. Transcripts of the seventh annual symposium, care of the professional voice, vol. 3. New York: The Voice Foundation; 1978. p. 74–6.
51. Wallner LJ, Hill BJ, Waldrop W, Monroe C. Voice changes following adenotonsillectomy. Laryngoscope. 1968;78:1410–8.
52. Lawrence VL. Medical care for professional voice (Panel). In: Lawrence VL, editor. Transcripts from the annual symposium, care of the professional voice, vol. 3. New York: The Voice Foundation; 1978. p. 17–8.
53. Cannon CP. COX-2 inhibitors and cardiovascular risk. Science. 2012;336(6087):1386–7.

Chapter 3
Physical Examination

A detailed history frequently reveals the cause of a voice problem even before a physical examination is performed. However, a comprehensive physical examination, often including objective assessment of voice function, also is essential [1–3].

Physical examination must include a thorough ear, nose, and throat evaluation and assessment of general physical condition. A patient who is extremely obese or appears fatigued, agitated, emotionally stressed, or otherwise generally ill has increased potential for voice dysfunction. This could be due to any number of factors: altered abdominal support, loss of fine motor control of laryngeal muscles, decreased bulk of the submucosal vocal fold ground substance, change in the character of mucosal secretions, or other similar mechanisms. Any physical condition that impairs the normal function of the abdominal musculature is suspected as a cause of dysphonia. Some conditions, such as pregnancy, are obvious; however, a sprained ankle or broken leg that requires the singer to balance in an unaccustomed posture may distract him or her from maintaining good abdominal support and thereby result in voice dysfunction. A tremorous neurologic disorder, endocrine disturbances such as thyroid dysfunction or menopause, the aging process, and other systemic conditions also may alter the voice. The physician must remember that maladies of almost any body system may result in voice dysfunction, and the doctor must remain alert for conditions outside the head and neck. If the patient uses his or her voice professionally for singing, acting, or other vocally demanding professions, physical examination should also include assessment of the patient during typical professional vocal tasks. For example, a singer should be asked to sing. Evaluation techniques for assessing performance are described in greater detail elsewhere in this book.

A.-l. Hamdan et al., *Office-Based Laryngeal Surgery*,
https://doi.org/10.1007/978-3-030-91936-8_3

3.1 Complete Ear, Nose, and Throat Examination

Examination of the ears must include assessment of hearing acuity. Even a relatively slight hearing loss may result in voice strain as a singer tries to balance his or her vocal intensity with that of associate performers. Similar effects are encountered among speakers, but they are less prominent in the early stages of hearing loss. This is especially true of hearing losses acquired after vocal training has been completed. The effect is most pronounced with sensorineural hearing loss. Diplacusis, distortion of pitch perception, makes vocal strain even worse. With conductive hearing loss, singers tend to sing more softly than appropriate rather than too loudly, and this is less harmful.

During an ear, nose, and throat examination, the conjunctivae and sclerae should be observed routinely for erythema that suggests allergy or irritation, for pallor that suggests anemia, and for other abnormalities such as jaundice. These observations may reveal the problem reflected in the vocal tract even before the larynx is visualized. Hearing loss in a spouse may be problematic as well if the voice professional strains vocally to communicate.

The nose should be assessed for patency of the nasal airway, character of the nasal mucosa, and nature of secretions, if any. A patient who is unable to breathe through the nose because of anatomic obstruction is forced to breathe unfiltered, unhumidified air through the mouth. Pale gray allergic mucosa or swollen infected mucosa in the nose suggests abnormal mucosa elsewhere in the respiratory tract.

Examination of the oral cavity should include careful attention to the tonsils and lymphoid tissue in the posterior pharyngeal wall, as well as to the mucosa. Diffuse lymphoid hypertrophy associated with a complaint of "scratchy" voice and irritative cough may indicate infection. The amount and viscosity of mucosal and salivary secretions also should be noted. Xerostomia is particularly important. The presence of scalloping of the lateral aspects of the tongue should be noted. This finding is caused commonly by tongue thrust and may be associated with inappropriate tongue tension and muscle tension dysphonia. Dental examination should focus not only on oral hygiene but also on the presence of wear facets suggestive of bruxism. Bruxism is a clue to excessive tension and may be associated with dysfunction of the temporomandibular joints, which should also be assessed routinely. Thinning of the enamel of the central incisors in a normal or underweight patient may be a clue to bulimia. However, it may also result from excessive ingestion of lemons, which some singers eat to help thin their secretions.

The neck should be examined for masses, restriction of movement, excess muscle tension and/or spasm, and scars from prior neck surgery or trauma. Laryngeal vertical mobility is also important. For example, tilting of the larynx produced by partial fixation of cervical muscles cut during previous surgery may produce voice dysfunction, as may fixation of the trachea to overlying neck skin. Particular attention should be paid to the thyroid gland. Examination of posterior neck muscles and range of motion should not be neglected. The cranial nerves should also be examined. Diminished fifth nerve sensation, diminished gag reflex, palatal deviation, or other mild cranial nerve deficits may indicate cranial polyneuropathy. Postviral, infectious neuropathies may involve the superior laryngeal nerve(s) and cause weakness of the vocal fold muscle secondary to decreased neural input, fatigability, and loss of range and projection in the voice. The recurrent laryngeal nerve is also affected in some cases. The more serious neurologic disease may also be associated with such symptoms and signs.

3.2 Laryngeal Examination

Examination of the larynx begins when the singer or other voice patient enters the physician's office. The range, ease, volume, and quality of the speaking voice should be noted. If the examination is not being conducted in the patient's native language, the physician should be sure to listen to a sample of the patient's mother tongue, as well. Voice use is often different under the strain or habits of foreign language use. Rating scales of the speaking voice may be helpful [4, 5]. The classification proposed by the Japanese Society of Logopedics and Phoniatrics is one of the most widely used. It is known commonly as the GRBAS Voice Rating Scale and is discussed below in the section on psychoacoustic evaluation [6].

Physicians are not usually experts in voice classification. However, the physicians should at least be able to discriminate substantial differences in range and timbre, such as between bass and tenor, or alto and soprano. Although the correlation between speaking and singing voices is not perfect, a speaker with a low, comfortable bass voice who reports that he is a tenor may be misclassified and singing inappropriate roles with consequent voice strain. This judgment should be deferred to an expert, but the observation should lead the physician to make the appropriate referral. Excessive volume or obvious strain during speaking clearly indicates that voice abuse is present and may be contributing to the patient's singing complaint. The speaking voice can be evaluated more consistently and accurately using standardized reading passages, and such assessments are performed routinely by speech-language pathologists, by phoniatricians, and sometimes by laryngologists.

The definition of "register" or "registration" is controversial, and many different terms are used by musicians and scientists. Often, the definitions are unclear. Terms to describe register include chest, creek, falsetto, head, heavy, light, little, low, middle, modal, normal, pulse, upper, vocal fry, voce di petto, voce di mista, voce di testa, and whistle (also called flageolet and flute register). A register is a range of frequencies that has a consistent quality or timbre. The break between registers is an area of instability called the passaggio. During vocal training, singers are taught to integrate qualities of their various registers and to smooth and obscure the transition between registers. Registers occur not only in voices but also in some instruments, notably the organ. Vocal register changes are associated with changes in laryngeal musculature and in vocal fold shape. For example, in chest register, contraction of the thyroarytenoid muscles causes thickening of the vocal folds, with a square-shaped glottis and large vibratory margin contact area. In falsetto in men and head voice in women, cricothyroid muscle contraction is dominant, vocal folds are elongated, and the contact area is much thinner and more triangular than in chest voice. Vertical phase differences are diminished in head voice in comparison with chest voice. Controversy remains on the use of traditional terms in males such as chest, middle, head and falsetto register, or chest and head register in females. Voice scientists commonly prefer terms such as modal register. In any case, health care professionals should understand that there is a difference between the terms *register* and *range*. For example, if a singer complains of inability to sing high notes, this should be described as a loss of upper range, not a loss of upper register. Register and range difficulties should be noted.

Vibrato is a fluctuation of the fundamental frequency of a note. It is produced by the vocal mechanism under neural control and is present naturally in adult voices. The primary components of vibrato include rate (the number of frequency fluctuations per second), extent (number of Hertz of fluctuation above and below the center frequency), regularity (consistency of frequency variations from one cycle to the next), and wave form. Rate and extent have been studied most extensively and are arguably the most important components in determining how the vibrato is perceived. Natural vibrato generally is about 6 Hz. Vibrato rate is slower in males than in females, and vocal pitch and effort do not have a substantial influence on vibrato. However, singers are able to alter vibrato rate and pitch oscillation voluntarily for stylistic purposes. The athletic choice of vibrato rate varies over time. For example, vibrato rates of 6–7 Hz were popular in classical Western (operatic) singing in the early twentieth century, but a vibrato rate of 5.5–6 Hz was considered more attractive by the end of the twentieth century. In general, pitch fluctuation covers about 1 semitone (half a semitone above and half a semitone below the center frequency) at present. A prominent wobble, as may be heard in some elderly singers who are not in ideal physical and vocal condition generally, is referred to as a tremolo. The excessive pitch (and sometimes intensity) fluctuations are caused by muscle activity, sometimes with a respiratory component, and are superimposed on the individual's vibrato in most cases, rather than actually being a widened, distorted vibrato. The true source of natural vibrato is uncertain, although the larynx, pharynx, tongue, and other components of the vocal tract may move in concert with vibrato, as well as with tremolo. Vibrato is thought not to be due primarily to phonatory structural activity rather than to respiratory source. The pressure of vibrato abnormalities or tremolo should be documented.

Any patient with a voice complaint should be examined by indirect laryngoscopy at least. It is not possible to judge voice range, quality, or other vocal attributes by inspection of the vocal folds. However, the presence or absence of nodules, mass lesions, contact ulcers, hemorrhage, erythema, paralysis, arytenoid erythema (reflux), and other anatomic abnormalities must be established. Erythema and edema of the laryngeal surface of the epiglottis are seen often in association with muscle tension dysphonia and with frequent coughing or clearing of the throat. It is caused by direct trauma from the arytenoids during these maneuvers. The mirror or a laryngeal telescope often provides a better view of the posterior portion of the endolarynx than is obtained with flexible endoscopy. Stroboscopic examination

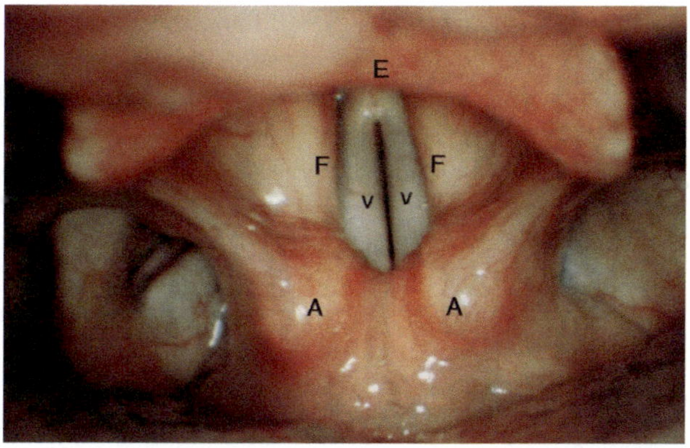

Fig. 3.1 Normal larynx showing the true vocal folds (V), false vocal folds (F), arytenoids (A), and epiglottis (E)

adds substantially to diagnostic abilities (Fig. 3.1), as discussed below. Another occasionally helpful adjunct is the operating microscope. Magnification allows visualization of small mucosal disruptions and hemorrhages that may be significant but overlooked otherwise. This technique also allows photography of the larynx with a microscope camera. Magnification may also be achieved through magnifying laryngeal mirrors or by wearing loupes. Loupes usually provide a clearer image than do most of the magnifying mirrors available.

A laryngeal telescope may be combined with a stroboscope to provide excellent visualization of the vocal folds and related structures. The author usually uses a 70-degree laryngeal telescope, although 90-degree telescopes are required for some patients. The combination of a telescope and stroboscope provides optimal magnification and optical quality for assessment of vocal fold vibration. However, it is generally performed with the tongue in a fixed position, and the nature of the examination does not permit assessment of the larynx during normal phonatory gestures.

Flexible fiberoptic laryngoscopy can be performed as an office procedure and allows inspection of the vocal folds in patients whose vocal folds are difficult to visualize indirectly. In addition, it permits observation of the vocal mechanism in a more natural posture than does indirect laryngoscopy, permitting sophisticated dynamic voice assessment. In the hands of an experienced endoscopist, this method may provide a great deal of information about both speaking and singing techniques. The combination of a fiberoptic laryngoscope with a laryngeal stroboscope may be especially useful. This system permits magnification, photography, and detailed inspection of vocal fold motion. Sophisticated systems that permit flexible or rigid fiberoptic strobovideolaryngoscopy are currently available commercially. They are invaluable assets for routine clinical use. The video system also provides a permanent record, permitting reassessment, comparison over time, and easy consultation. A refinement not currently available commercially is stereoscopic fiberoptic laryngoscopy, accomplished by placing a laryngoscope through each nostril, fastening the two together in the pharynx, and observing the larynx through the eyepieces [7]. This method allows visualization of laryngeal motion in three dimensions. However, it is used primarily in a research setting.

Rigid endoscopy under general anesthesia may be reserved for the rare patient whose vocal folds cannot be assessed adequately by other means or for patients who need surgical procedures to remove or biopsy laryngeal lesions. In some cases, this may be done with local anesthesia, avoiding the need for intubation and the traumatic coughing and vomiting that may occur even after general anesthesia is administered by mask. Coughing after general anesthesia may be minimized by using topical anesthesia in the larynx and trachea. However, topical anesthetics may act as severe mucosal irritants in a small number of patients. They may also predispose the patient to aspiration in the postoperative period. If a patient has had difficulty with a topical anesthetic administered in the office, it should not be used in the operating room. When used in general anesthesia cases, topical anesthetics should usually be applied at the end of the procedure. Thus, if inflammation occurs, it will not interfere with performance of microsurgery. Postoperative duration of anesthesia is also optimized. The author has had the least difficulty with 4% Xylocaine.

3.3 Objective Tests

Reliable, valid, objective analysis of the voice is extremely important and is an essential part of a comprehensive physical examination [2]. It is as valuable to the laryngologist as audiometry is to the otologist [8, 9]. Familiarity with some of the measures and technological advances currently available is helpful. This information is covered in greater detail elsewhere in this book but is included here as a brief overview for the convenience of the reader.

3.3.1 Strobovideolaryngoscopy

Integrity of the vibratory margin of the vocal fold is essential for the complex motion required to produce good vocal quality. Under continuous light, the vocal folds vibrate approximately 250 times per second while phonating at middle C. Naturally, the human eye cannot discern the necessary details during such rapid motion. The vibratory margin may be assessed through high-speed photography, strobovideolaryngoscopy, high-speed video, videokymography, electroglottography (EEG), or photoglottography. Strobovideolaryngoscopy provides the necessary clinical information in a practical fashion. Stroboscopic light allows routine slow-motion evaluation of the mucosal cover layer of the leading edge of the vocal fold. This state-of-the-art physical examination permits detection of vibratory asymmetries, structural abnormalities, small masses, submucosal scars, and other conditions that are invisible under ordinary light [10, 11]. Documentation of the procedure by coupling stroboscopic light with the video camera allows later reevaluation by the laryngologist or other health care providers.

Stroboscopy does not provide a true slow-motion image, as obtained through high-speed photography (Fig. 3.2). The stroboscope actually illuminates different points on consecutive vocal fold waves, each of which is retained on the retina for 0.2 s. The stroboscopically lighted portions of the successive waves are fused visually, and thus the examiner is actually evaluating simulated cycles of phonation. The slow-motion effect is created by having the stroboscopic light desynchronized with the frequency of vocal fold vibration by approximately 2 Hz. When vocal fold vibration and the stroboscope are synchronized exactly, the vocal folds appear to stand still, rather than move in slow motion (Fig. 3.3). In most instances, this approximation of slow motion provides all the clinical information necessary. Our routine stroboscopy protocol is described elsewhere [11]. We use a modification of the standardized method of subjective assessment of strobovideolaryngoscopic images, as proposed by Bless et al. [12] and Hirano [13]. Characteristics evaluated include the fundamental frequency, the symmetry of movements, periodicity, glottic

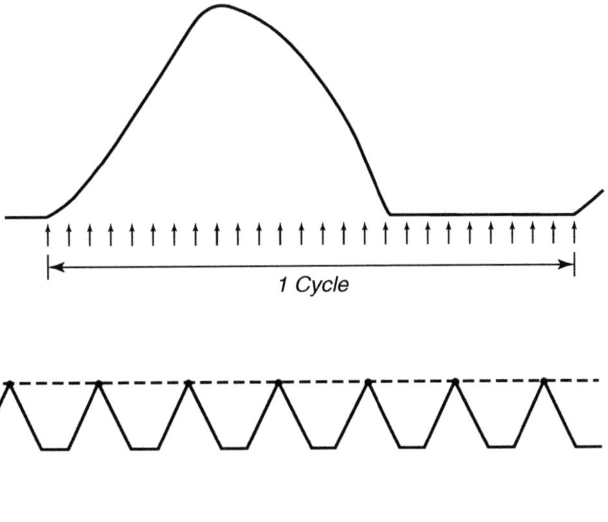

Fig. 3.2 The principle of ultrahigh-speed photography. Numerous images are taken during each vibratory cycle. This technique is a true slow-motion representation of each vocal fold vibration

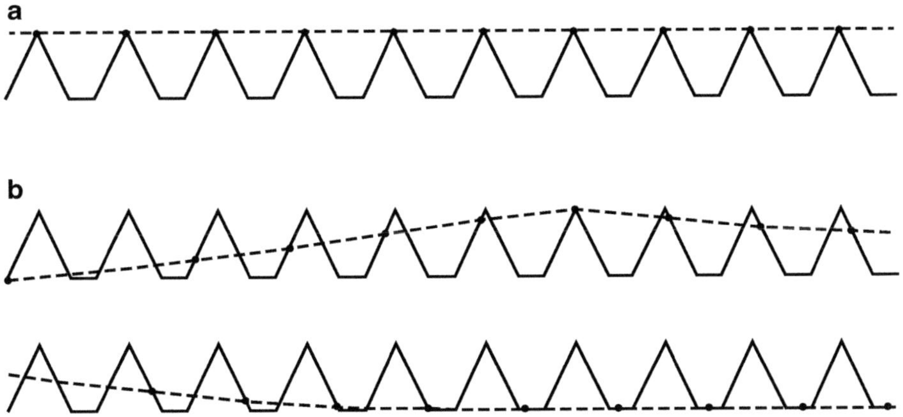

Fig. 3.3 The principle of stroboscopy. The stroboscopic light illuminates portions of successive cycles. The eye fuses the illuminated points into an illusion of slow motion. (**a**) If the stroboscope is synchronized with vocal fold vibration, a similar point is illuminated on each successive cycle and the vocal fold appears to stand still. (**b**) If the stroboscope is slightly desynchronized, each cycle is illuminated at a slightly different point, and the slow-motion effect is created

closure, the amplitude of vibration, the mucosal wave, the presence of nonvibrating portions of the vocal fold, and other unusual findings. With practice, perceptual judgments of stroboscopic images provide a great deal of information. However, it is easy for the inexperienced observer to draw unwarranted conclusions because of normal variations in vibration. Vibrations depend on fundamental frequency, intensity, and vocal register. For example, failure of glottic closure occurs normally in falsetto phonation. Consequently, it is important to note these characteristics and to examine each voice under a variety of conditions.

3.3.2 Other Techniques to Examine Vocal Fold Vibration

Other techniques to examine vocal fold vibration include ultrahigh-speed photography, electroglottography (EGG), photoelectroglottography and ultrasound glottography, and most recently videokymography [14] and high-speed video (digital or analog). Ultrahigh-speed photography provides images that are in true slow motion, rather than simulated. High-speed video offers similar advantages without most of the disadvantages of high-speed motion pictures. Videokymography offers high-speed imaging of a single line along the vocal fold. EGG uses two electrodes placed on the skin of the neck above the thyroid laminae. It traces the opening and closing of the glottis and can be compared with stroboscopic images [15]. EGG allows objective determination of the presence or absence of glottal vibrations and easy determination of the fundamental period of vibration and is reproducible. It reflects the glottal condition more accurately during its closed phase. Photo electroglottography and ultrasound glottography are less useful clinically [16].

3.3.3 Measures of Phonatory Ability

Objective measures of phonatory ability are easy to use, readily available to the laryngologist, helpful in the treatment of professional vocalists with specific voice disorders, and quite useful in assessing the results of surgical therapies. Maximum phonation time is measured with a stopwatch. The patient is instructed to sustain the vowel */a/* for as long as possible after deep inspiration, vocalizing at a comfortable frequency and intensity. The frequency and intensity may be determined and controlled by an inexpensive frequency analyzer and sound level meter. The test is repeated three times, and the greatest value is recorded. Normal values have been determined [16]. Frequency range of phonation is recorded in semitones and documents the vocal range from the lowest note in the modal register (excluding vocal fry) to the highest falsetto note. This is the physiologic frequency range of phonation and disregards quality. The musical frequency range of phonation measures lowest to highest notes of musically acceptable quality. Tests for maximum phonation time, frequency ranges, and many of the other parameters discussed later (including spectrographic analysis) may be preserved on a tape recorder or digitized and stored for analysis at a convenient future time and used for pre- and post-treatment comparisons. Recordings should be made in a standardized, consistent fashion.

Frequency limits of vocal register also may be measured. The registers are (from low to high) vocal fry, chest, mid, head, and falsetto. However, classification of registers is controversial, and many other classifications are used. Although the classification listed above is common among musicians, at present, most voice scientists prefer to classify registers as pulse, modal, and loft. Overlap of frequency among registers occurs routinely.

Testing the speaking fundamental frequency often reveals excessively low pitch, an abnormality associated with chronic voice abuse and development of vocal nodules. This parameter may be followed objectively throughout a course of voice therapy. Intensity range of phonation (IRP) has proven a less useful measure than frequency range. It varies with fundamental frequency (which should be recorded) and is greatest in the middle frequency range. It is recorded in sound pressure level (SPL) (re 0.0002 microbar). For healthy adults who are not professional vocalists, measuring at a single fundamental frequency, IRP averages 54.8 dB for males and 51 dB for females [17]. Alterations of intensity are common in voice disorders, although IRP is not the most sensitive test to detect them. Information from these tests may be combined in a fundamental frequency-intensity profile [16], also called a *phonetogram*.

Glottal efficiency (ratio of the acoustic power at the level of the glottis to subglottal power) provides useful information but is not clinically practical because measuring acoustic power at the level of the glottis is difficult. Subglottic power is the product of subglottal pressure and airflow rate. These can be determined clinically. Various alternative measures of glottic efficiency have been proposed, including the ratio of radiated acoustic power to subglottal power [18], airflow intensity profile [19], and ratio of the root mean square value of the AC component to the mean volume velocity (DC component) [20]. Although glottal efficiency is of great interest, none of these tests is particularly helpful under routine clinical circumstances.

3.3.4 Aerodynamic Measures

Traditional pulmonary function testing provides the most readily accessible measure of respiratory function. The most common parameters measured include (1) tidal volume, the volume of air that enters the lungs during inspiration and leaves during expiration in normal breathing; (2) functional residual capacity, the volume of air remaining in the lungs at the end of inspiration during normal breathing, which can be divided into expiratory reserve volume (maximal additional volume that can be exhaled) and residual volume (the volume of air remaining in the lungs at the end of maximal exhalation); (3) inspiratory capacity, the maximal volume of air that can be inhaled starting at the functional residual capacity; (4) total lung capacity, the volume of air in the lungs following maximal inspiration; (5) vital capacity, the maximal volume of air that can be exhaled from the lungs following maximal inspiration; (6) forced vital capacity, the rate of air flow with rapid, forceful expiration from total lung capacity to residual volume; (7) FEV_1, the forced expiratory volume in 1 s; (8) FEV_3, the forced expiratory volume in 3 s; and (9) maximal mid-expiratory flow, the mean rate of airflow over the middle half of the forced vital capacity (between 25% and 75% of the forced vital capacity). For singers and professional speakers with an abnormality caused by voice abuse, abnormal pulmonary function tests may confirm deficiencies in aerobic conditioning or reveal previously unrecognized asthma [21]. Flow glottography with computer inverse filtering is also a practical and valuable diagnostic for assessing flow at the vocal fold level, evaluating the voice source, and imaging the results of the balance between adductory forces and subglottal pressure [22]. It also has therapeutic value as a biofeedback tool.

The spirometer, readily available for pulmonary function testing, can also be used for measuring airflow during phonation. However, the spirometer does not allow simultaneous display of acoustic signals, and its frequency response is poor. A pneumotachograph consists of a laminar air resistor, a differential pressure transducer, and an amplifying and recording system. It allows measurement of airflow and simultaneous recording of other signals when coupled with a polygraph. A hot-wire anemometer allows determination of airflow velocity by measuring the electrical drop across the hot wire. Modern hot-wire anemometers containing electrical feedback circuitry that maintains the temperature of the hot wire provide a flat response up to 1 kHz and are useful clinically.

The four parameters traditionally measured in the aerodynamic performance of a voice are subglottal pressure (P_{sub}), supraglottal pressure (P_{sup}), glottal impedance, and the volume velocity of airflow at the glottis. These parameters and their rapid variations can be measured under laboratory circumstances. However, clinically their mean value is usually determined as follows:

$$P_{sub} - P_{sup} = \text{MFR} \times \text{GR}$$

where MFR is the mean (root mean square) flow rate and GR is the mean (root mean square) glottal resistance. When vocalizing the open vowel /*a*/, the supraglottic pressure equals the atmospheric pressure, reducing the equation to

$$P_{sub} = \text{MFR} \times \text{GR}$$

The mean flow rate is a useful clinical measure. While the patient vocalizes the vowel /*a*/, the mean flow rate is calculated by dividing the total volume of air used during phonation by the duration of phonation. The subject phonates at a comfortable pitch and loudness either over a determined period of time or for a maximum sustained period of phonation.

Air volume is measured by the use of a mask fitted tightly over the face or by phonating into a mouthpiece while wearing a nose clamp. Measurements may be made using a spirometer, pneumotachograph, or hot-wire anemometer. The normal values for mean flow rate under habitual phonation, with changes in intensity or register, and under various pathologic circumstances, were determined in the 1970s [16]. Normal values are available for both adults and children. Mean flow rate also can be measured and is a clinically useful parameter to follow during treatment for vocal nodules, recurrent laryngeal nerve paralysis, spasmodic dysphonia, and other conditions.

Glottal resistance cannot be measured directly, but it may be calculated from the mean flow rate and mean subglottal pressure. Normal glottal resistance is 20–100 dyne seconds/cm^5 at low and medium pitches and 150 dyne seconds/cm^5 at high pitches [18]. The normal values for subglottal pressure under various healthy and pathologic voice conditions have also been determined by numerous investigators [16]. The phonation quotient is the vital capacity divided by the maximum phonation time. It has been shown to correlate closely with maximum flow rate [23] and is a more convenient measure. Normative data determined by various authors have been published [16]. The phonation quotient provides an objective measure of the effects of treatment and is particularly useful in cases of recurrent laryngeal nerve paralysis and mass lesions of the vocal folds, including nodules.

3.3.5 Acoustic Analysis

Acoustic analysis equipment can determine frequency, intensity, harmonic spectrum, cycle-to-cycle perturbations in frequency (jitter), cycle-to-cycle perturbations in amplitude (shimmer), harmonics/noise ratios, breathiness index, and many other parameters. The DSP Sona-Graph Sound Analyzer Model 5500 (Kay Elemetrics, Lincoln Park, New Jersey) is an integrated voice analysis system. It is equipped for sound spectrography capabilities. Spectrography provides a visual record of the voice. The acoustic signal is depicted using time (x-axis), frequency (y-axis), and intensity (z-axis), shading of light vs dark. Using the bandpass filters, generalizations about quality, pitch, and loudness can be made. These observations are used in formulating the voice therapy treatment plan. Formant structure and strength can be determined using the narrow-band filters, of which a variety of configurations are possible. In clinical settings in which singers and other professional voice users are evaluated and treated routinely, this feature is extremely valuable. A sophisticated voice analysis program (an optional program) may be combined with the Sona-Graph and is an especially valuable addition to the clinical laboratory. The voice analysis program (Computer Speech Lab; Kay Elemetrics) measures speaking fundamental frequency, frequency perturbation (jitter), amplitude perturbation (shimmer), and harmonics-to-noise ratio and provides many other useful values. An electroglottograph may be used in conjunction with the SonaGraph to provide some of these voicing parameters. Examining the EGG waveform alone is possible with this setup, but its clinical usefulness has not yet been established. An important feature of the Sona-Graph is the long-term average (LTA) spectral capability, which permits analysis of longer voice samples (30–90 s). The LTA analyzes only voiced speech segments and may be useful in screening for hoarse or breathy voices. In addition, computer interface capabilities (also an optional program) have solved many data storage and file maintenance problems.

In analyzing acoustic signals, the microphone may be placed at the level of the mouth or positioned in or over the trachea, although intratracheal recordings are used for research purposes only. The position should be standardized in each office or laboratory [24]. Various techniques are being developed to improve the usefulness of acoustic analysis. Because of the enormous amount of information carried in the acoustic signal, further refinements in objective acoustic analysis should prove particularly valuable to the clinician.

3.3.6 Laryngeal Electromyography

Electromyography (EMG) requires an electrode system, an amplifier, an oscilloscope, a loudspeaker, and a recording system [25]. Electrodes are placed transcutaneously into laryngeal muscles. EMG can be extremely valuable in confirming cases of vocal fold paresis, in differentiating paralysis from arytenoid dislocation, distinguishing recurrent laryngeal nerve paralysis from combined recurrent and superior nerve paralysis, diagnosing other more subtle neurolaryngologic pathology, and documenting functional voice disorders and malingering. It is also recommended for needle localization when using botulinum toxin for treatment of spasmodic dysphonia and other conditions.

3.3.7 Psychoacoustic Evaluation

Because the human ear and brain are the most sensitive and complex analyzers of sound currently available, many researchers have tried to standardize and quantify psychoacoustic evaluation. Unfortunately, even definitions of basic terms such as hoarseness and breathiness are still controversial. Psychoacoustic evaluation protocols and interpretations are not standardized. Consequently, although subjective psychoacoustic analysis of voice is of great value to the individual skilled clinician, it remains generally unsatisfactory for comparing research among laboratories or for reporting clinical results.

The GRBAS scale [6] helps standardize perceptual analysis for clinical purposes. It rates the voice from a scale from 0 to 3, with regrading to grade, roughness, breathiness, asthenia, and strain. Grade 0 is normal, 1 is slightly abnormal, 2 is moderately abnormal, and 3 is extremely abnormal. Grade refers to the degree of hoarseness or voice abnormality. Roughness refers to the acoustic/auditory impression of irregularity of vibration and corresponds with gear and shimmer. Breathiness refers to the acoustic/auditory impression of air leakage and corresponds to turbulence. Asthenic evaluation assesses weakness or lack of power and corresponds to vocal intensity and energy in higher harmonics. Strain refers to the acoustic/auditory impression of hyperfunction and may be related to fundamental frequency, noise in the high-frequency range, and energy in higher harmonics. For example, a patient's voice might be graded as G2, R2, B1, A1, and S2.

3.4 Outcomes Assessment

Measuring the impact of a voice disorder has always been challenging. However, recent advances have begun to address this problem. Validated instruments such as the Voice Handicap Index (VHI) [26] are currently in clinical use and are likely to be used widely in future years.

3.5 Voice Impairment and Disability

Quantifying voice impairment and assigning a disability rating (percentage of whole person) remain controversial. This subject is still not addressed comprehensively even in the most recent editions (2008, 6th edition) of the American Medical Association's *Guidelines for the Evaluation of Impairment and Disability* (The Guides). The Guides still do not take into account the person's profession when calculating disability. Alternative approaches have been proposed [27], and advances in this complex arena are anticipated over the next few years.

3.6 Evaluation of the Singing Voice

The physician must be careful not to exceed the limits of his or her expertise, especially in caring for singers. However, if voice abuse or technical error is suspected, or if a difficult judgment must be reached on whether to allow a sick singer to perform, a brief observation of the patient's singing may provide invaluable information. This is accomplished best by asking the singer to stand and sing scales either in the examining room or in the soundproof audiology booth. Similar maneuvers may be used for professional speakers, including actors (who can vocalize and recite lines), clergy and politicians (who can deliver sermons and speeches), and virtually all other voice patients. The singer's stance should be balanced, with the weight slightly forward. The knees should be bent slightly and the shoulders, torso, and neck should be relaxed. The singer should inhale through the nose whenever possible allowing filtration, warming, and humidification of inspired air. In general, the chest should be expanded, but most of the active breathing is abdominal. The chest should not rise substantially with each inspiration, and the supraclavicular

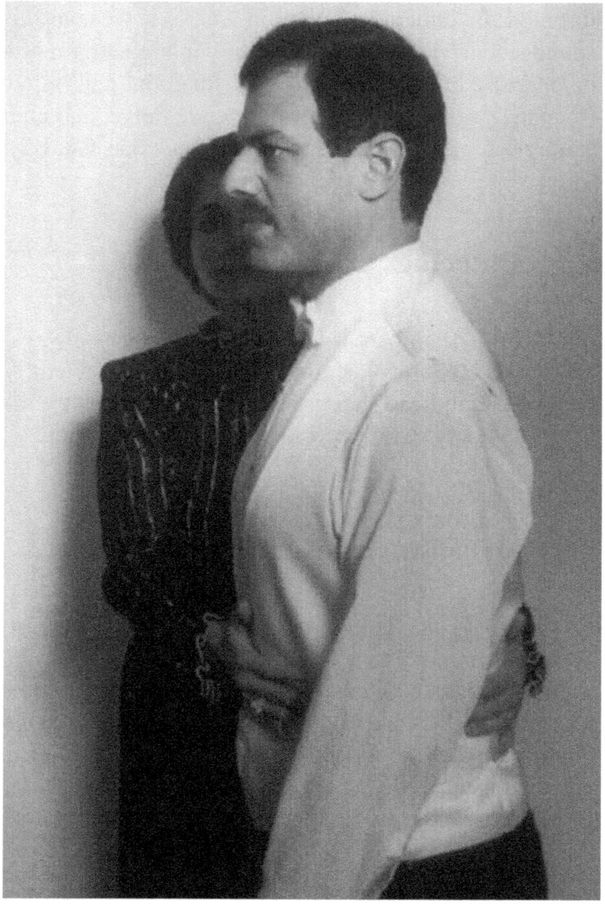

Fig. 3.4 Bimanual palpation of the support mechanism. The singer should expand posteriorly and anteriorly with inspiration. Muscles should tighten prior to onset of sung tone

musculature should not be involved obviously in inspiration. Shoulders and neck muscles should not be tensed even with deep inspiration. Abdominal musculature should be contracted shortly before the initiation of the tone. This may be evaluated visually or by palpation (Fig. 3.4). Muscles of the neck and face should be relaxed. Economy is a basic principle of all art forms. Wasted energy and motion and muscle tension are incorrect and usually deleterious.

The singer should be instructed to sing a scale (a 5-note scale is usually sufficient) on the vowel /a/, beginning on any comfortable note. Technical errors are usually most obvious as contraction of muscles in the neck and chin, retraction of the lower lip, retraction of the tongue, or tightening of the muscles of mastication. The singer's mouth should be open widely but comfortably. When singing /a/, the singer's tongue should rest in a neutral position with the tip of the tongue lying against the back of the singer's mandibular incisors. If the tongue pulls back or demonstrates obvious muscular activity as the singer performs the scales, improper voice use can be confirmed on the basis of positive evidence (Fig. 3.5). The

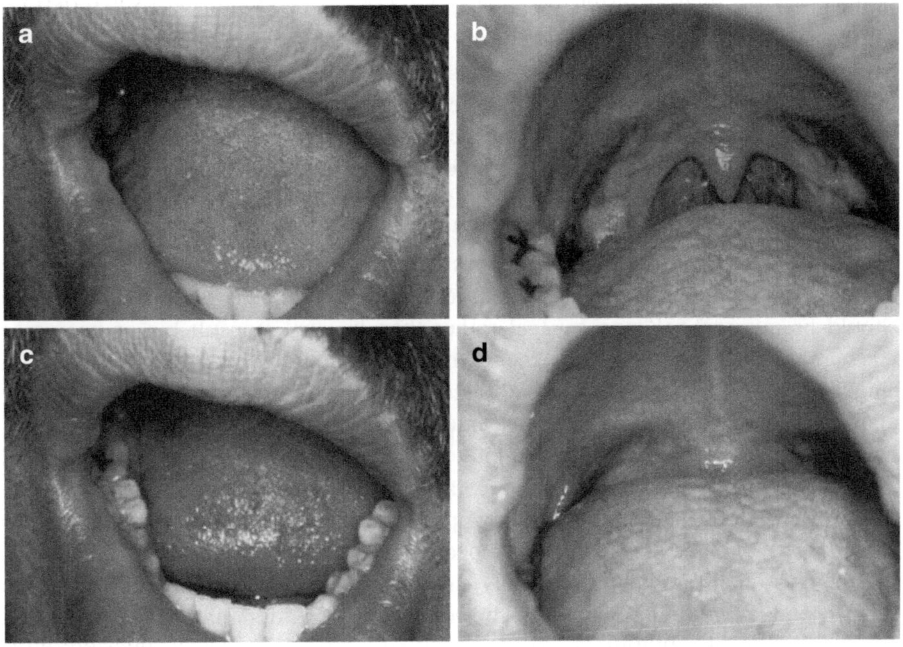

Fig. 3.5 Proper relaxed position of the anterior (**a**) and posterior (**b**) portions of the tongue. Common improper use of the tongue pulled back from the teeth (**c**) and raised posteriorly (**d**)

position of the larynx should not vary substantially with pitch changes. Rising of the larynx with ascending pitch is evidence of technical dysfunction. This examination also gives the physician an opportunity to observe any dramatic differences between the qualities and ranges of the patient's speaking voice and the singing voice. A physical examination summary form has proven helpful in organization and documentation [3].

Remembering the admonition not to exceed his or her expertise, the physician who examines many singers can often glean valuable information from a brief attempt to modify an obvious technical error. For example, deciding whether to allow a singer with mild or moderate laryngitis to perform is often difficult. On one hand, an expert singer has technical skills that allow him or her to compensate safely. On the other hand, if a singer does not sing with correct technique and does not have the discipline to modify volume, technique, and repertoire as necessary, the risk of vocal injury may be increased substantially even by mild inflammation of the vocal folds. In borderline circumstances, observation of the singer's technique may greatly help the physician in making a judgment.

If the singer's technique appears flawless, the physician may feel somewhat more secure in allowing the singer to proceed with performance commitments. More commonly, even good singers demonstrate technical errors when experiencing voice difficulties. In a vain effort to compensate for dysfunction at the vocal fold level, singers often modify their technique in the neck and supraglottic vocal tract.

In the good singer, this usually means going from good technique to bad technique. The most common error involves pulling back the tongue and tightening the cervical muscles. Although this increased muscular activity gives the singer the illusion of making the voice more secure, this technical maladjustment undermines vocal efficiency and increases vocal strain. The physician may ask the singer to hold the top note of a 5-note scale; while the note is being held, the singer may simply be told, “Relax your tongue.” At the same time, the physician points to the singer’s abdominal musculature. Most good singers immediately correct to good technique. If they do, and if upcoming performances are particularly important, the singer may be able to perform with a reminder that meticulous technique is essential. The singer should be advised to “sing by feel rather than by ear,” consult his or her voice teacher, and conserve the voice except when it is absolutely necessary to use it. If a singer is unable to correct from bad technique to good technique promptly, especially if he or she uses excessive muscle tension in the neck and ineffective abdominal support, it is generally safer not to perform with even a mild vocal fold abnormality. With increased experience and training, the laryngologist may make other observations that aid in providing appropriate treatment recommendations for singer patients. Once these skills have been mastered for the care of singers, applying them to other patients is relatively easy, so long as the laryngologist takes the time to understand the demands of the individual’s professional, avocational, and recreational vocal activities.

If treatment is to be instituted, making at least a tape recording of the voice is advisable in most cases and essential before any surgical intervention. The author routinely uses strobovideolaryngoscopy for diagnosis and documentation in virtually all cases as well as many of the objective measures discussed. Pretreatment testing is extremely helpful clinically and medicolegally.

3.7 Additional Examinations

A general physical examination should be performed whenever the patient’s systemic health is questionable. Debilitating conditions such as mononucleosis may be noticed first by the singer as vocal fatigue. A neurologic assessment may be particularly revealing. The physician must be careful not to overlook dysarthrias and dysphonias, which are characteristic of movement disorders and of serious neurologic disease. Dysarthria is a defect in rhythm, enunciation, and articulation that usually results from neuromuscular impairment or weakness such as may occur after a stroke. It may be seen with oral deformities or illness, as well. Dysphonia is an abnormality of vocalization usually caused by problems at the laryngeal level.

Physicians should be familiar with the six types of dysarthria, their symptoms, and their importance [28, 29]. Flaccid dysarthria occurs in lower motor neuron or primary muscle disorders such as myasthenia gravis and tumors or strokes involving the brainstem nuclei. Spastic dysarthria occurs in upper motor neuron disorders (pseudobulbar palsy) such as multiple strokes and cerebral palsy. Ataxic dysarthria is seen with cerebellar disease, alcohol intoxication, and multiple sclerosis. Hypokinetic dysarthria accompanies Parkinson's disease. Hyperkinetic dysarthria may be spasmodic, as in the Gilles de la Tourette disease, or dystonic, as in chorea and cerebral palsy. Mixed dysarthria occurs in amyotrophic lateral sclerosis (ALS) or Lou Gehrig disease. The preceding classification actually combines dysphonic and dysarthric characteristics but is very useful clinically. The value of a comprehensive neurolaryngologic evaluation [30] cannot be overstated. More specific details of voice changes associated with neurologic dysfunction and their localizing value are available elsewhere [2, 31].

It is extremely valuable for the laryngologist to assemble an arts-medicine team that includes not only a speech-language pathologist, singing voice specialist, acting voice specialist, and voice scientist but also medical colleagues in other disciplines. Collaboration with an expert neurologist, pulmonologist, endocrinologist, psychologist, psychiatrist, internist, physiatrist, and others with special knowledge of, and interest in, voice disorders is invaluable in caring for patients with voice disorders. Such interdisciplinary teams have not only changed the standard of care in voice evaluation and treatment but are also largely responsible for the rapid and productive growth of voice as a subspecialty.

Acknowledgments Modified in part from Sataloff RT. Professional Voice: The Science and Art of Clinical Care, 4th Edition. San Diego, CA: Plural Publishing; 2017, with permission.

References

1. Sataloff RT. Professional singers: the science and art of clinical care. Am J Otolaryngol. 1981;2:251–66.
2. Rubin J, Sataloff R, Korovin G. Diagnosis and treatment of voice disorders. 4th ed. San Diego: Plural Publishing; 2014.
3. Sataloff RT. The professional voice: part II, physical examination. J Voice. 1987;1:91–201.
4. Fuazawa T, Blaugrund SM, El-Assuooty A, Gould WJ. Acoustic analysis of hoarse voice: a preliminary report. J Voice. 1988;2(2):127–31.
5. Gelfer M. Perceptual attributes of voice: development and use of rating scales. J Voice. 1988;2(4):320–6.
6. Hirano M. Clinical examination of the voice. New York: Springer-Verlag; 1981. p. 83–4.
7. Fujimura O. Stereo-fiberoptic laryngeal observation. J Acoust Soc Am. 1979;65:70–2.
8. Sataloff RT, Spiegel JR, Carroll LM, Darby KS, Hawkshaw MJ, Rulnick RK. The clinical voice laboratory: practical design and clinical application. J Voice. 1990;4:264–79.
9. Sataloff RT, Heuer RH, Hoover C, Baroody MM. Laboratory assessment of voice. In: Gould WJ, Sataloff RT, Spiegel JR, editors. Voice surgery. St. Louis: Mosby; 1993. p. 203–16.
10. Sataloff RT, Spiegel JR, Carroll LM, Schiebel BR, Darby KS, Rulnick RK. Strobovideolaryngoscopy in professional voice users: results and clinical value. J Voice. 1986;1:359–64.
11. Sataloff RT, Spiegel JR, Hawkshaw MJ. Strobovideolaryngoscopy: results and clinical value. Ann Otol Rhinol Laryngol. 1991;100:725–7.
12. Bless D, Hirano M, Feder RJ. Video stroboscopic evaluation of the larynx. Ear Nose Throat J. 1987;66:289–96.

13. Hirano M. Phonosurgery: basic and clinical investigations. Otologia (Fukuoka). 1975;21:239–442.
14. Svec J, Shutte H. Videokymography: high-speed line scanning of vocal fold vibration. J Voice. 1996;10:201–5.
15. Leclure FLE, Brocaar ME, Verscheeure J. Electroglottography and its relation to glottal activity. Folia Phoniatr (Basel). 1975;27:215–24.
16. Hirano M. Clinical examination of the voice. New York: Springer-Verlag; 1981. p. 25–7, 85–98.
17. Coleman RJ, Mabis JH, Hinson JK. Fundamental frequency sound pressure level profiles of adult male and female voices. J Speech Hear Res. 1977;20:197–204.
18. Isshiki N. Regulatory mechanism of voice intensity variation. J Speech Hear Res. 1964;7:17–29.
19. Saito S. Phonosurgery: basic study on the mechanisms of phonation and endolaryngeal microsurgery. Otologia (Fukuoka). 1977;23:171–384.
20. Isshiki N. Functional surgery of the larynx. In: Report of the 78th annual convention of the Oto-Rhino-Laryngological Society of Japan. Fukuoka: Kyoto University; 1977.
21. Cohn JR, Sataloff RT, Spiegel JR, Fish JE, Kennedy K. Airway reactivity-induced asthma in singers (ARIAS). J Voice. 1991;5:332–7.
22. Sundberg J. The science of the singing voice. Dekalb: Northern Illinois University Press; 1987. p. 11, 66, 77–89.
23. Hirano M, Koike Y, von Leden H. Maximum phonation time and air usage during phonation. Folia Phoniatr (Basel). 1968;20:185–201.
24. Price DB, Sataloff RT. A simple technique for consistent microphone placement in voice recording. J Voice. 1988;2:206–7.
25. Sataloff RT, Mandel S, Heman-Ackah YD, Abaza M. Laryngeal electromyography. 3rd ed. San Diego: Plural Publishing, Inc; 2017.
26. Benninger MS, Syamal MN, Gardner GM, Jacobson BH. New dimensions in measuring voice treatment outcomes and quality of life. In: Sataloff RT, editor. Professional voice: the science and art of clinical care. 4th ed. San Diego: Plural Publishing, Inc; 2017. p. 547–58.
27. Sataloff RT. Voice impairment, disability, handicap, and medical-legal evaluation. In: Sataloff RT, editor. Professional voice: the science and art of clinical care. 4th ed. San Diego: Plural Publishing, Inc; 2017. p. 1741–54.
28. Darley FL, Aronson AE, Brown JR. Differential diagnostic of patterns of dysarthria. J Speech Hear Res. 1969;12(2):246–9.
29. Darley FL, Aronson AE, Brown JR. Clusters of deviant speech dimensions in the dysarthrias. J Speech Hear Res. 1969;12(3):462–96.
30. Rosenfield DB. Neurolaryngology. Ear Nose Throat J. 1987;66:323–6.
31. Raphael BN, Sataloff RT. Increasing vocal effectiveness. In: Sataloff RT, editor. Professional voice: the science and art of clinical care. 4th ed. San Diego: Plural Publishing, Inc; 2017. p. 1201–12.

Chapter 4
Professional Voice Users: An Overview of Medical Disorders and Treatments

Robert Thayer Sataloff, Mary J. Hawkshaw, and Johnathan Brandon Sataloff

Laryngologists specializing in voice devote the majority of their practices to the medical management of benign voice disorders. Although most of us are active surgeons, the good voice specialist takes pride in avoiding the need for laryngeal surgery through expert medical management. Success depends not only on a good laryngologist but also on the availability of a voice team, including a speech-language pathologist, voice scientist, singing voice specialist, and medical consultants who have acquired special knowledge about voice disorders (neurologists, pulmonologists, endocrinologists, internists, allergists, and others). This chapter provides an overview of many of the benign voice problems encountered by health care providers and current nonsurgical management concepts.

Numerous medical conditions affect the voice adversely. Many have their origins primarily outside the head and neck. This chapter is not intended to be all inclusive but rather to highlight some of the more common and important conditions found in professional voice users and wind instrumentalists seeking medical care.

In the 2286 cases of all forms of voice disorders reported by Brodnitz in 1971 [1], 80% were attributed to voice abuse or to psychogenic factors resulting in vocal dysfunction. Of these patients, 20% had organic voice disorders. Of women with organic problems, about 15% had identifiable endocrine causes. A much higher incidence of organic disorders, particularly reflux laryngitis, acute infectious laryngitis, and benign vocal fold masses, is found in the author's (RTS) practice.

R. T. Sataloff (✉) · M. J. Hawkshaw
Otolaryngology – Head and Neck Surgery, Drexel University, Philadelphia, PA, USA
e-mail: rtsataloff@phillyent.com

J. B. Sataloff
Department of Psychiatry, Beth Israel Deaconess Medical Center, Harvard Medical School, Boston, MA, USA

A.-I. Hamdan et al., *Office-Based Laryngeal Surgery*,
https://doi.org/10.1007/978-3-030-91936-8_4

4.1 Voice Abuse

When voice abuse is suspected or observed in a patient with vocal complaints, he or she should be referred to a laryngologist who specializes in voice, preferably a physician affiliated with a voice care team.

Common patterns of voice abuse and misuse will not be discussed in detail in this chapter. They are covered elsewhere in the literature [2]. Voice abuse and/or misuse should be suspected particularly in patients who complain of voice fatigue associated with voice use, whose voices are worse at the end of a working day or week, and in any patient who is chronically hoarse. Technical errors in voice use may be the primary etiology of a voice complaint or may develop secondarily as a result of a patient's efforts to compensate for voice disturbance from another cause.

Speaking in noisy environments such as cars and airplanes is particularly abusive to the voice, as are backstage greetings, post-performance parties, choral conducting, voice teaching, cheerleading, and many other activities. With proper training, all these vocal activities can be done safely. However, most patients, surprisingly even singers, have little or no training for their speaking voice.

If voice abuse is caused by speaking, treatment should be provided by a licensed, certified speech-language pathologist in the United States or by a phoniatrist in many other countries. In many cases, training the speaking voice will benefit singers greatly not only by improving speech but also by indirectly helping singing technique. Physicians should not hesitate to recommend such training, but it should be performed by an expert speech-language pathologist who specializes in voice. Many speech-language pathologists who are well trained in swallowing rehabilitation, articulation therapy, and other techniques are not trained in voice therapy for the speaking voice, and virtually none are trained through their speech and language programs to work with singing unless they are also singing teachers or singing voice specialists.

Specialized singing training also may be helpful to many voice patients who are not singers, and it is invaluable for patients who are singers. Initial singing training teaches relaxation techniques, develops muscle strength, and is symbiotic with standard voice therapy. Abuse of the voice during singing is an even more complex problem, as discussed elsewhere in this book.

4.2 Infection and Inflammation

4.2.1 Upper Respiratory Tract Infection Without Laryngitis

Although mucosal irritation usually is diffuse, patients sometimes have marked nasal obstruction with little or no sore throat and a "normal" voice. If the laryngeal examination showed no abnormality, a singer or professional speaker with a "head cold" should be permitted to use his or her voice and be advised not to try to duplicate his or her usual sound but rather accept the insurmountable alterations in self-perception caused by the change in the supraglottic vocal tract and auditory system. The decision as to whether performing under the circumstances is advisable professionally rests with the voice professional and his or her musical associates. The patient should be cautioned against throat clearing, as it is traumatic and may produce laryngitis. If a cough is present, nonnarcotic medications should be used to suppress it. In addition, the patient should be taught how to "silent cough," which is less traumatic. "Cold sores" or dry, split lips or tongue also may interfere with singing, although they are far more troublesome for wind instrumentalists, as are dental braces which can traumatize mucosal surfaces and affect instrument or voice performance.

4.2.2 Laryngitis With Serious Vocal Fold Injury

Hemorrhage in the vocal folds and mucosal disruption associated with acute laryngitis are contraindications to speaking and singing. When these are observed, treatment includes strict voice rest in addition to correction of any underlying disease. If the patient also plays a wind instrument, laryngoscopy while playing will determine whether there is vocal fold contact during wind performance (there is in many players, but not all). If so, instrument playing should be stopped during the period of voice rest. Vocal fold hemorrhage in voice professionals is most common in premenstrual women who are using aspirin products or nonsteroidal anti-inflammatory drugs (NSAIDS) for dysmenorrhea. Severe hemorrhage or mucosal scarring may result in permanent alternations in vocal fold vibratory function. In rare instances, surgical intervention may be necessary. The potential gravity of these conditions must be stressed, for singers are generally reluctant to cancel an appearance. As von Leden observed, it is a pleasure to work with "people who are determined that the show must go on when everyone else is determined to goof off" [3]. However, patient compliance is essential when serious damage has occurred. At present, acute treatment of vocal fold hemorrhage is controversial. Most laryngologists allow the hematoma to resolve spontaneously. Because this sometimes results in an organized hematoma and scar formation requiring surgery, some physicians advocate incision along the superior edge of the vocal fold and drainage of the hematoma in selected cases. Further study is needed to determine optimal therapy guidelines (Figs. 4.1 and 4.2).

4.2.3 Laryngitis Without Serious Damage

Mild to moderate edema and erythema of the vocal folds may result from infection or from noninfectious causes. In the absence of mucosal disruption or hemorrhage, they are not absolute contraindications to voice use (including wind instrument

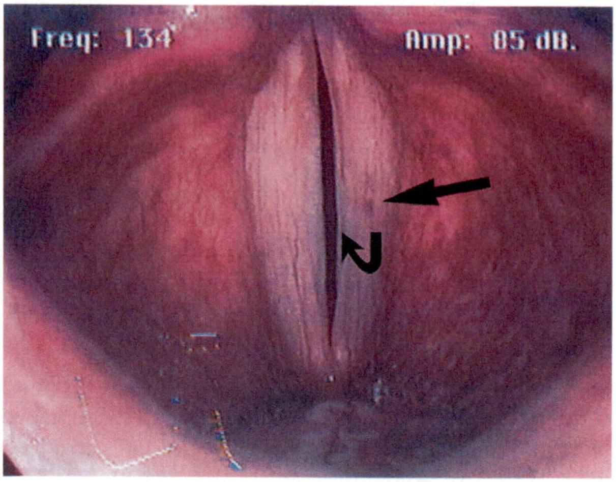

Fig. 4.1 Video print obtained from a strobovideolaryngoscopic examination shows diffuse erythema from acute laryngitis. Additionally, there is a left sulcus vocalis. Also visible is an ecstatic vessel on the superior surface of the left vocal fold (straight arrow). (Figure 40–1 from Sataloff et al. [118]. Republished from Sataloff et al. [118]; with permission)

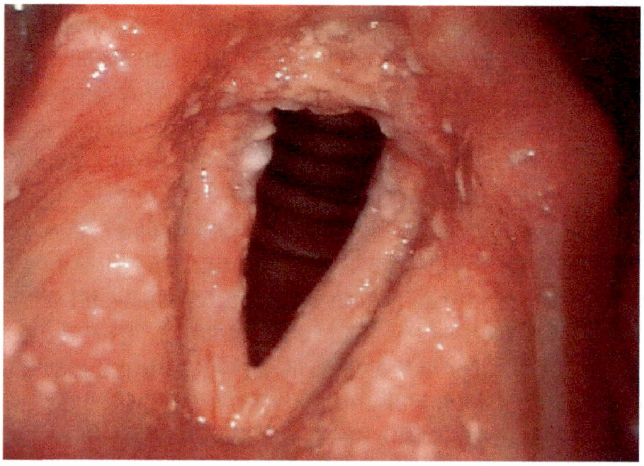

Fig. 4.2 Strobovideolaryngoscopy in this 65-year-old female shows the white, lacy, diffuse plaques embedded in inflamed mucosal surfaces. This appearance is typical of fungal laryngitis, caused most commonly by *Candida albicans*. (Figure 45–1 from Sataloff et al. [118]. Republished from Sataloff et al. [118]; with permission)

performance in selected cases). Noninfectious laryngitis commonly is associated with excessive voice use in pre-performance rehearsals. It also may be caused by other forms of voice abuse and by mucosal irritation produced by allergy, smoke inhalation, and other causes. Mucous stranding between the anterior and middle thirds of the vocal folds is seen commonly in inflammatory laryngitis. Laryngitis sicca (dry voice) is associated with dehydration, dry atmosphere, mouth breathing, and antihistamine therapy (although antihistamines actually cause more mucous thickening than dehydration). Deficiency of mucosal lubrication causes irritation and coughing and results in mild inflammation. If no pressing professional need for performance exists, inflammatory conditions of the larynx are treated best with relative voice rest in addition to other modalities. However, in some instances, speaking and singing may be permitted. The patient should be instructed to avoid all forms of irritation and to rest the voice at all times except during warm-up and performance. Corticosteroids and other medications discussed later may be helpful. If mucosal secretions are copious, low-dose antihistamine therapy may be beneficial, but it must be prescribed with caution and generally should be avoided. Copious, thin secretions are better than scant, thick secretions or excessive dryness. The patient with laryngitis must be kept well hydrated to maintain the desired character of mucosal lubrication. The patient should be instructed to "pee pale," consuming enough water to keep urine diluted. Psychological support is crucial. For example, it is often helpful for the physician to intercede on a singer's behalf and to convey "doctor's orders" directly to agents or theater management. Such mitigation of exogenous stress can be highly therapeutic.

Infectious laryngitis may be caused by bacteria or viruses. Subglottic involvement frequently indicates a more severe infection, which may be difficult to control in a short period of time. Indiscriminate use of antibiotics must be avoided; however, when the physician is in doubt as to the cause and when a major voice commitment is imminent, vigorous antibiotic treatment is warranted. In this circumstance, the damage caused by allowing progression of a curable condition is greater than the damage that might result from a course of therapy for an unproven microorganism while culture results are pending. When a major concert or speech is not imminent, indications for therapy are the same as for the nonsinger or nonprofessional speaker.

Voice rest (absolute or relative) is an important therapeutic consideration in any case of laryngitis. When no professional commitments are pending, a short course of absolute voice rest may be considered, as it is the safest and most conservative therapeutic intervention. This means absolute silence and communication with a writing pad or electronic device. The patient must be instructed not to whisper, as this may be an even more traumatic vocal activity than speaking softly. However, exceptions can be made for patients who do not make vocal fold contact when they whisper, as determined during flexible laryngoscopy. Whistling through the lips also involves vocal fold contact in many people and should not be permitted unless laryngoscopy has confirmed that the instrumentalist does not make vocal fold contact while playing. The playing of many musical wind instruments also should not be permitted. Absolute voice rest is necessary only for serious vocal fold injury such as hemorrhage or mucosal disruption (Fig. 4.3). Even then, it is virtually never indicated for more than 7–10 days. Three days are often sufficient. Some excellent laryngologists do not believe voice rest should be used at all. However, absolute voice rest for a few days may be helpful in patients with laryngitis, especially those gregarious, verbal singers who find it difficult to moderate their voice use to comply with relative voice rest instructions. In many instances, considerations of finances and reputation mitigate against a recommendation of voice rest. In advising performers to minimize vocal use, Punt counseled, "Don't say a single word for which you are not being paid" [4].

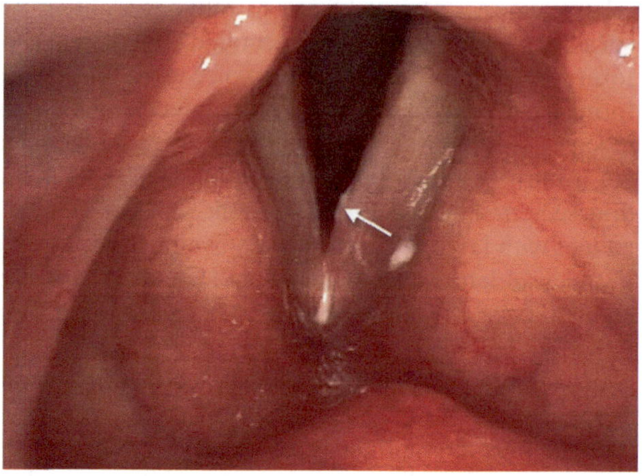

Fig. 4.3 Mucosal tear (arrow) of the vibratory margin of the left vocal fold in a 27-year-old tenor with sudden voice change. This lesion resolved completely with voice rest. (Figure 58–1 from Sataloff et al. [118]. Republished from Sataloff et al. [118]; with permission)

This admonition frequently guides the ailing singer or speaker away from pre-performance conversations and backstage greetings and allows a successful series of performances. Patients also should be instructed to speak softly and as infrequently as possible, often at a slightly higher pitch than usual; to avoid excessive telephone use; and to speak with abdominal support as they would in singing. This is relative voice rest, and it is helpful in most cases. An urgent session with a speech-language pathologist is extremely helpful for discussing vocal hygiene and providing guidelines to prevent voice abuse. Nevertheless, the patient must be aware that some risk is associated with performing with laryngitis even when performance is possible. Inflammation of the vocal folds is associated with increased capillary fragility and increased risk of vocal fold injury or hemorrhage. Many factors must be considered in determining whether a given speech or concert is important enough to justify the potential consequences.

Steam inhalations deliver moisture and heat to the vocal folds and tracheobronchial tree and may be useful. Some people use nasal irrigations, although these have little proven value for voice disorders. Gargling has no proven efficacy, but it is probably harmful only if it involves loud, abusive vocalization as part of the gargling process. Some physicians and patients believe it to be helpful in "moistening the throat," and it may have some relaxing or placebo effect. Ultrasonic treatments, local massage, psychotherapy, and biofeedback directed at relieving anxiety and decreasing muscle tension may be helpful adjuncts to a broader therapeutic program. However, psychotherapy and biofeedback, in particular, must be expertly supervised if used at all.

Voice lessons given by an expert teacher are invaluable. When technical dysfunction is suggested, the singer or actor should be referred to his or her teacher or to a singing voice specialist in a medical setting. Even when an obvious organic abnormality is present, referral to a voice teacher is appropriate, especially for younger actors and singers. Numerous "tricks of the trade" permit a voice professional to overcome some of the impairments of mild illness safely. If a singer plans to proceed with a performance during an illness, he or she should not cancel voice lessons as part of the relative voice rest regimen; rather, a short lesson to ensure optimal technique is extremely useful.

4.2.4 *Sinusitis*

Chronic inflammation of the mucosa lining the sinus cavities commonly produces thick secretions known as postnasal drip. Postnasal drip can be particularly problematic because it causes excessive phlegm, which interferes with phonation, and because it leads to frequent throat clearing, which may inflame the vocal folds. Sometimes chronic sinusitis is caused by allergies and can be treated with medications. However, many medications used for this condition cause side effects that are unacceptable in professional voice users, particularly mucosal drying. When medication management is not satisfactory, functional endoscopic sinus surgery may be appropriate [5]. Acute purulent sinusitis is a different matter. It requires aggressive treatment with antibiotics, sometimes surgical drainage, treatment of underlying conditions (such as dental abscess), and occasionally surgery [5].

4.2.5 *Lower Respiratory Tract Infection*

Lower respiratory tract infection may be almost as disruptive to a voice as upper respiratory tract infection. Bronchitis, pneumonitis, pneumonia, and especially reactive airway disease impair the power source of the voice and lead to vocal strain and sometimes injury. Lower respiratory tract infections should be treated aggressively, pulmonary function tests should be considered, and bronchodilators (preferably oral rather than inhaled) should be used as necessary. Coughing is also a very traumatic vocal activity, and careful attention should be paid to cough suppression. If extensive voice use is anticipated, nonnarcotic antitussive agents are preferable because narcotics may dull the sensorium and lead to potentially damaging voice or instrument performance technique.

4.2.6 *COVID-19*

COVID-19, or SARS-CoV-2 infection, also known as the novel corona virus, may be asymptomatic, may cause mild URI symptoms, or may cause devastating symptoms including death. Cough, fever and chills, shortness of breath, sore throat, fatigue, nausea and vomiting, diarrhea, and other symptoms are common. Loss of taste and smell were recognized early as symptoms of COVID-19. However, COVID-19 also may cause many other neurological effects including vocal fold paresis and paralysis. When the disease affects the lower respiratory tract severely, it can impair respiratory function permanently. This undermines the support needed to provide power for phonation (speaking, as well as singing) and wind instrument performance. Such problems lead commonly to compensatory hyperfunction. If the respiratory compromise is severe enough, it may disable a performer permanently; and since excellent respiratory function is required for singing, projected speech and wind performance (as well as for high-level athletic activity), relatively "mild" pulmonary compromise can be severe enough to impair or end a performance career.

4.2.7 *Tonsillitis*

Tonsillitis also impairs the voice through alterations of the resonator system and through technical changes secondary to pain. Although there is a tendency to avoid tonsillectomy, especially in professional voice users, the operation should not be withheld when clear indications for tonsillectomy are present. These include, for example, documented severe bacterial tonsillitis six times per year. However, patients must be warned that tonsillectomy may alter the sound of the voice, even though there is no change at the vocal fold (oscillator) level.

4.2.8 *Lyme Disease*

Lyme disease, as it is known today, has been reported for over a hundred years, but the bacteria responsible for the disease was not identified until 1982. It was discovered in Lyme, Connecticut, when a group of children contracted arthritis inexplicably; and research was initiated to identify the cause [6]. Due to its ability to appear similar to many other diseases and its wide range of nonspecific symptoms, Lyme disease often goes undiagnosed. If not recognized and treated, this condition can have profound consequences including damage to the inner ear, the eighth cranial nerve, and the facial nerve as reviewed by Sataloff and Sataloff (from which a portion of this section has been modified, with permission) [7]. It also can affect laryngeal nerves. Lyme disease is one of many common illnesses that can cause special problems for singers and other voice professionals. Lyme disease is an increasingly prevalent infection in many parts of the United States and elsewhere. It can affect the larynx directly by causing unilateral or bilateral vocal fold paresis/paralysis or interfere with other parts of the vocal tract by causing joint pains that impair posture and support, temporomandibular joint pain that leads to technical changes, and in other ways [8]. It is important for health care providers and music professionals to be familiar with this common problem in order to improve the chances of prompt diagnosis and treatment.

4.2.8.1 Epidemiology

In the United States, Lyme disease is known to be endemic particularly in northeastern, mid-Atlantic, and north-central states, with expansion into some parts of the southwest [9]. Approximately 60% of initial infections occur during the summer when it is warm and people are outside [10]. Lyme disease has no sex or age predilection.

4.2.8.2 Etiology

Lyme disease is an illness caused by a spirochete infection. Like syphilis, another spirochete infection, the clinical presentations may vary. Sir William Osler once termed syphilis "the great imitator," and likewise, Lyme disease has a broad clinical spectrum.

Lyme disease had many different names given to it until Steere, in 1977, recognized it as a multistage systemic disease [11]. In 1982, Burgdorfer et al. isolated the infectious organism from the belly of a tick, while studying a group of children with unexplained arthritis in Lyme, Connecticut [12]. He named this spirochete *Borrelia burgdorferi*. *Borrelia burgdorferi* is the primary cause of Lyme disease. However, *Borrelia garinii* and *Borrelia afzelii* also have been implicated and reported as common causes of Lyme neuroborreliosis in Europe [13]. Many different vectors have been listed as contributors to this disease. However, the tick seems to be the main culprit transmitting the spirochete. In the Northeast, the tick *Ixodes dammini* is the most common, and in the West, *Ixodes pacificus* has been implicated [9]. The ticks carry the disease in their stomachs and transmit it while feeding on the blood of their victims which can take up to 2 days. In many cases, the ticks are noticed and removed or washed away before the disease can be spread; but sometimes a tick is small enough to avoid notice. Even when definitive symptoms occur, the tick often is not found, and the classic target rash may have been absent or gone unnoticed. Therefore, the opportunity for early diagnosis often is missed, and many people carry Lyme disease into later stages of the disorder, during which nerve and vascular problems can occur, before the condition is diagnosed [7].

The tick life cycle has three stages: larva, nymph, and adult [11]. In each stage the tick acquires a blood meal and may obtain the spirochete from an infected host such as the white-tailed deer or white-footed mouse.

The exact nature of injury to humans is not known, but evidence exists for three possible mechanisms. These theories include direct invasion, immunological attack, and vasculitis [14].

4.2.8.3 Otolaryngologic Findings

The clinical spectrum of Lyme disease is broken down into three stages. In stage 1, a rash named erythema chronicum migrans follows the tick bite in 6–80% of cases [15]. The rash has an outer red circular or oval border with a clear central area. These lesions are called "target rash." The outer red zone is felt to represent the best area for biopsy when trying to isolate the organism for culture. This rash may follow or precede cold or flu-like symptoms. The rash usually occurs within a few days of the tick bite but may show up as long as a month later [16].

Other symptoms during this stage include fatigue, fever, chills, sore throat, headache, cough, chest pain, abdominal pain, muscle aches, loss of appetite, dizziness, lymphadenopathy, backache, conjunctivitis, enlarged liver and spleen, arthritis, and low-grade fever.

The patient usually calls on an otolaryngologist during stage 2 of Lyme disease. Although facial paralysis is the most common complaint in these patients, other symptoms may occur [10, 17]. They include hoarseness from involvement of the recurrent laryngeal nerve or inability to sustain a high note or project the voice due to injury to the superior laryngeal nerve among other symptoms. In 1988, Schroeter reported a case of a 45-year-old singer who developed left vocal fold paralysis and had positive antibodies to *Borrelia burgdorferi* [18]. The patient was treated with antibiotics for 6 weeks, during which time there was resolution of the vocal fold paralysis and dramatic reduction of the Lyme titers.

Stage 2 also may include a skin lesion called lymphadenosis benigna cutis. This lesion has another name, *Borrelia lymphocytoma*, and is characterized by lymphocytic infiltration of the dermis or subcutaneous tissue [19]. The lesion has a blue-red color with gross swelling.

Patients may have involvement of the temporomandibular joint and complain of ear pain or pain when chewing. Other joints may be involved such as the neck, knees, hips, shoulders, ankles, and elbows. Finger, wrist, elbow, shoulder, and neck involvement can be troubling particularly for wind and other instrumentalists.

Patients also may have involvement of the cardiovascular system and may develop arrhythmias and/or lightheadedness. Failure to recognize these lesions may lead to increased morbidity and possible death.

Another skin lesion is seen in stage 3 of Lyme disease. It is termed acrodermatitis chronic atrophicans [19]. This lesion usually is seen in elderly patients and is often misdiagnosed as scleroderma or vascular insufficiency.

4.2.8.4 Diagnosis and Treatment

The ELISA test is the most sensitive and is used widely for Lyme disease [14]. Western blot technique is used to confirm the diagnosis. Other assays such as immunofluorescence antibody and cultures have been utilized with varying success. Results of all of these studies vary from lab to lab, and blood samples should be sent to labs that do large volumes of testing and have experience. The IgM antibody is seen early and is less specific. However, it is useful when reinfection or reactivation is suspected. The IgG antibody may take 6 weeks to appear and is good for assessing stages 2 and 3. False-positive tests occur in patients with mononucleosis, syphilis, or rheumatic fever [9, 14]. False negatives may be seen in patients on antibiotics or patients who are immunocompromised by diseases such as cancer or AIDS.

Antibiotics are the recommended treatment. For adults, doxycycline or tetracycline is effective. When intolerance to these medications is encountered, amoxicillin is used. Amoxicillin is preferred in children. Chloramphenicol may be used when there is allergy to cephalosporin or penicillin. When resistance to these medications is found, intravenous medication such as ceftriaxone is used. Lyme disease is complex; with proper recognition, it is treatable and has an excellent prognosis.

4.2.9 Autoimmune Deficiency Syndrome (AIDS)

AIDS is a potentially lethal disease that has become common. Its incidence in the artistic community is probably somewhat higher than in the general public. Physicians should consider this diagnosis along with other causes of chronic debilitation and recurrent infections in the proper clinical setting in professional voice users. Dry mouth and hoarseness are common complaints in patients with HIV infection. Candida infection of the oral cavity or tracheobronchial tree should make the clinician particularly suspicious. When fungal infections are encountered, particularly fungal laryngitis, it is important not only to treat the infection, but also to rule out serious predisposing causes such as HIV infection and other conditions that suppress the immune system. Recurrent respiratory tract infection and infection with unusual organisms also raise one's suspicions, but it should be remembered that infections with Haemophilus influenza, Streptococcus pneumonia, and common viruses are the most frequent pathogens in HIV-infected patients, just as they are in patients without HIV. Acute infectious laryngitis and epiglottis may occur in AIDS patients, but they are less common than mild chronic laryngitis, dry mouth, and frequent or persistent symptoms of a "cold."

4.3 Systemic Conditions

4.3.1 Aging

This subject is so important that it has been covered extensively in other literature [20]. Many characteristics associated with vocal aging are actually deficits in conditioning, rather than irreversible aging changes. For example, in singers, such problems as a "wobble," pitch inaccuracies (singing flat), and inability to sing softly are rarely caused by irreversible aging changes, and these problems usually can be managed easily through voice therapy and training.

4.3.2 Hearing Loss

Hearing loss is often overlooked as a source of vocal problems. Auditory feedback is fundamental to speaking and singing. Interference with this control mechanism may result in altered vocal production, particularly if the person is unaware of the hearing loss. Distortion, particularly pitch distortion (diplacusis), also may pose serious problems for the singer. This appears to cause not only aesthetic difficulties in matching pitch but also vocal strain, which accompanies pitch shifts [21]. Hearing impairment can cause vocal strain, particularly if a person has sensorineural hearing loss (involving the nerve or inner ear) and is unaware of it. This condition may lead people to speak or sing more loudly than they realize.

4.3.3 Respiratory Dysfunction

The importance of "the breath" has been well recognized in the field of voice pedagogy. Respiratory disorders are discussed at length in other literature [22].

Even a mild degree of obstructive pulmonary disease can result in substantial voice problems. Unrecognized exercise-induced asthma is especially problematic in singers and actors, because bronchospasm may be precipitated by the exercise and airway drying that occurs during voice performance. In such cases, the bronchospastic obstruction on exhalation impairs support. This commonly results in compensatory hyperfunction.

Treatment requires skilled management and collaboration with a pulmonologist and a voice team [23]. Whenever possible, patients should be managed primarily with oral medications; the use of inhalers should be minimized. Steroid inhalers should be avoided altogether whenever possible for professional voice users. It is particularly important to recognize that asthma can be induced by the exercise of phonation itself [24], and in many cases a high index of suspicion and methacholine challenge test are needed to avoid missing this important diagnosis.

4.3.4 Allergy

Even mild allergies are more incapacitating to professional voice users than to others. This subject can be reviewed elsewhere [25]. Briefly, patients with mild intermittent allergies can usually be managed with antihistamines, although they should never be tried for the first time immediately prior to a voice performance. Because antihistamines commonly produce unacceptable side effects, trial and error may be needed in order to find a medication with an acceptable balance between effect and side effect for any individual patient, especially a voice professional. Patients with allergy-related voice disturbances may find hyposensitization a more effective approach than antihistamine use if they are candidates for such treatment. For voice patients with unexpected allergic symptoms immediately prior to an important voice commitment, corticosteroids should be used rather than antihistamines, in order to minimize the risks of side effects (such as drying and thickening of secretions) that might make voice performance difficult or impossible. Allergies commonly cause voice problems by altering the mucosa and secretions and causing nasal obstruction.

4.3.5 Laryngopharyngeal Reflux

Laryngopharyngeal reflux (LPR) is extremely common among voice patients, especially singers [26]. This is a condition in which the sphincter between the stomach and esophagus is inefficient, and acidic stomach secretions reflux (reach the laryngeal tissues), causing inflammation. The most typical symptoms are hoarseness in the morning, prolonged vocal warm-up time, postnasal drip, halitosis, and a bitter taste in the morning, a feeling of a "lump in the throat," frequent throat clearing, chronic irritative cough, and frequent tracheitis or tracheobronchitis. Any or all of these symptoms may be present. Heartburn is not common in these patients, so the diagnosis is often missed. Prolonged reflux also is associated with the development of Barrett's esophagus, esophageal carcinoma, and laryngeal carcinoma [26].

Physical examination usually reveals erythema (redness) of the arytenoids mucosa. A barium swallow radiographic study with water siphonage may provide additional information but is not needed routinely. However, if a patient complies strictly with treatment recommendations and does not show marked improvement within a month, or if there is a reason to suspect more serious pathology, a more comprehensive evaluation should be carried out. Twenty-four-hour pH impedance monitoring of the esophagus or pharyngeal pH monitoring is often effective in establishing a diagnosis. The results are correlated with a diary of the patient's activities and symptoms. Endoscopic examination of the esophagus should be considered for many patients. Bulimia should also be considered in the differential diagnosis when symptoms are refractory to treatment and other physical and psychologic signs are suggestive.

The mainstays of treatment for reflux laryngitis are elevation of the head of the bed (not just sleeping on pillows), antacids, proton pump inhibitors and H2 blockers, low acid diet, alkaline water, alginate, and avoidance of eating for 3–4 h before going to sleep. This is often difficult for singers and actors because of their performance schedules, but if they are counseled about minor changes in eating habits (such as eating larger meals at breakfast and lunch), usually they can comply. Avoidance of alcohol, caffeine, and specific foods is beneficial. Medications that decrease or block acid production may be necessary. It must be recognized that control of acidity is not the same as control of reflux. In many cases, reflux is provoked during singing because of the increased abdominal pressure associated with support. In these instances, it often causes excessive phlegm and throat clearing during the first 10 or 15 min of a performance or lesson, as well as other common laryngopharyngeal symptoms, even when acidity has been neutralized effectively. Laparoscopic Nissen fundoplication has proven extremely effective and should be considered a reasonable alternative to lifelong medication in this relatively young patient population [26].

4.3.6 Endocrine Dysfunction

Endocrine (hormonal) problems warrant special attention. The human voice is extremely sensitive to endocrinologic changes. Many of these are reflected in alterations of fluid content of the lamina propria just beneath the laryngeal mucosa. This causes alterations in the bulk and shape of the vocal folds and results in voice change. Hypothyroidism is a well-recognized cause of such voice disorders, although the mechanism is not understood fully [27–30]. Hoarseness, voice fatigue, muffling of the voice, loss of range, and a sensation of a lump in the throat may be present even with mild hypothyroidism. Even when thyroid function tests results are within the low normal range, this diagnosis should be considered, especially if thyroid-stimulating hormone levels are in the high-normal range or are elevated. Thyrotoxicosis may result in similar voice disturbances [30, 31].

Voice changes associated with sex hormones are encountered commonly in clinical practice and have been investigated more thoroughly than have other hormonal changes. Although a correlation appears to exist between sex hormone levels and depth of male voices (higher testosterone and lower estradiol levels in basses than in tenors) [32], the most important hormonal considerations in males occur during the maturation process.

When castrato singers were in vogue, castration at about age 7 or 8 years resulted in failure of laryngeal growth during puberty, and voices that stayed in the soprano or alto range and boasted a unique quality of sound [33]. Failure of a male voice to change at puberty is uncommon today and is often psychogenic in etiology [1]. However, hormonal deficiencies such as those seen in cryptorchidism, delayed sexual development, Klinefelter syndrome, or Fröhlich syndrome may be responsible. In these cases, the persistently high voice may be the complaint that causes the patient to seek medical attention.

Voice problems related to sex hormones are most common in female singers [34]. Although voice changes associated with the normal menstrual cycle may be difficult to quantify with current experimental techniques, unquestionably they occur [2, 34–38]. Most of the ill effects seen in the immediate premenstrual period are known as laryngopathia premenstrualis. This common condition is caused by physiologic, anatomic, and psychologic alterations secondary to endocrine changes. The vocal dysfunction is characterized by decreased vocal efficiency, loss of the highest notes in the voice, voice fatigue, slight hoarseness, and some muffling of the voice. It is often more apparent to the singer than to the listener. It was recognized long ago that submucosal hemorrhages in the larynx are more common in the premenstrual period

[36], and premenstrual vascular changes have been confirmed over the ensuing decades. In many European opera houses, singers used to be excused from singing during the premenstrual and early menstrual days ("grace days"). This practice was not followed in the United States and is no longer in vogue anywhere. Premenstrual changes cause significant vocal symptoms in approximately one-third of singers. Although ovulation inhibitors were shown long ago to mitigate some of these symptoms [37], in some women (about 5%) first-generation birth control pills used to deleteriously alter voice range and character even after only a few months of therapy [39–43]. However, modern oral contraceptives usually do not produce such problems and may even improve voice [42]. Under crucial performance circumstances, oral contraceptives may be used to alter the time of menstruation, but this practice is justified only in unusual situations. Symptoms similar to laryngopathia premenstrualis also occur in some women at the time of ovulation.

Pregnancy results frequently in voice alterations known as laryngopathia gravidarum. The changes may be similar to premenstrual symptoms or may be perceived as desirable changes. In some cases, alterations produced by pregnancy are permanent [44, 45]. Although hormonally induced changes in the larynx and respiratory mucosa secondary to menstruation and pregnancy are discussed widely in the literature, references to the important alterations in abdominal support are scarce. Abdominal distention during pregnancy also interferes with abdominal muscle function. Any singer whose abdominal support is compromised substantially should be discouraged from strenuous practice or performance until the abdominal impairment has resolved.

Estrogens are helpful in postmenopausal singers and should be administered supervision of a gynecologist or endocrinologist as potential systemic side effects have been described. Under no circumstances should androgens be given to female singers even in small amounts if any reasonable therapeutic alternative exists. Clinically, these drugs are used most commonly to treat endometriosis or postmenopausal loss of libido. Androgens cause unsteadiness of the voice, rapid changes of timbre, and lowering of the fundamental frequency (masculinization) [46–50]. These changes have been known for decades but still occur not only from illicit drug use for body building, but also iatrogenically. These changes are usually permanent.

Recently, we have seen increasing abuse of anabolic steroids among bodybuilders and other athletes. In addition to their many other hazards, these medications may alter the voice. They are (or are closely related to) male hormones; consequently, they are capable of producing masculinization of the voice. Lowering of the fundamental frequency and coarsening of the voice produced in this fashion are similar to a boy's voice change at puberty and generally are irreversible.

Other hormonal disturbances may also produce voice dysfunction. In addition to the thyroid gland and the gonads, the parathyroid, adrenal, pineal, and pituitary glands are included in this system. Other endocrine disturbances may alter voice, as well. For example, pancreatic dysfunction may cause xerophonia (dry voice), as in diabetes mellitus. Thymic abnormalities can lead to feminization of the voice [51], and thymomas may cause laryngeal myasthenia gravis that produces voice instability and fatigue.

4.3.7 Neurologic Disorders

Numerous neurologic conditions may adversely affect the voice. They are discussed in other literature [2]. Some of them, such as myasthenia gravis, are amenable to medical therapy with drugs such as pyridostigmine (Mestinon). Such therapy frequently restores the voice to normal. An exhaustive neurolaryngologic discussion is beyond the scope of this chapter. Nevertheless, when evaluating voice dysfunction, health care providers must consider numerous neurologic problems, including Parkinson's disease, essential tremor, various other disorders that produce tremor, drug-induced tremor, multiple sclerosis, dystonias, and many other conditions. Spasmodic dysphonia (SD), a laryngeal dystonia, presents particularly challenging problems. This subject is covered in detail elsewhere [2]. Focal dystonias that effect the mouth and lips can be troublesome for singers and other voice professionals, but they can be devastating for wind instrumentalists. The same is true for velopharyngeal insufficiency, a condition that is common among instrumentalists who play clarinet, oboe, saxophone, bassoon, French horn, trumpet, coronet, and other wind instruments. People who play these instruments often develop velopharyngeal insufficiency (VPI) which also is more likely to disable a wind player than a singer. In addition, wind instrumentalists (some of whom are also singers) develop a variety of other problems such as pneumoparotitis. Stuttering also provides unique challenges. Although still poorly understood, this condition is noted for its tendency to affect speech while sparing singing.

4.3.8 Vocal Fold Hypomobility

Vocal fold hypomobility may be caused by paralysis (no movement), paresis (partial movement), arytenoid dislocation, cricoarytenoid joint dysfunction, tumor, laryngeal fracture, and other causes. Differentiating among these conditions is often more complicated than it appears to be at first glance. A comprehensive discussion is beyond the scope of this chapter, and the reader is referred to other literature [2]. In addition to a comprehensive history and physical examination, evaluation commonly includes strobovideolaryngoscopy, objective voice assessment, laryngeal electromyography, and high-resolution computed tomography (CT) or magnetic resonance imaging (MRI) of the larynx and related neurological structures. Most vocal fold motion disorders are amenable to treatment. Voice therapy should be used first in virtually all cases. Even in many patients with recurrent laryngeal nerve paralysis, voice therapy alone is often sufficient. When therapy fails to produce adequate voice improvement in the patient's opinion, surgical intervention is appropriate and usually is effective.

4.4 General Health

As with any other athletic activity, optimal voice use requires reasonably good general health and physical conditioning. Abdominal and respiratory strength and endurance are particularly important. If a person becomes short of breath from climbing two flights of stairs, he or she certainly does not have the physical stamina necessary for proper respiratory support for a speech, let alone a strenuous musical production. This deficiency usually results in abusive vocal habits used in vain attempts to compensate for the deficiencies.

Systemic illnesses, such as anemia, Lyme disease, mononucleosis, AIDS, chronic fatigue syndrome, or other diseases associated with malaise and weakness, may impair the ability of vocal musculature to recover rapidly from heavy use and may also be associated with alterations of mucosal secretions. Other systemic illnesses may be responsible for voice complaints, particularly if they impair the abdominal muscles necessary for breath support. For example, diarrhea and constipation that prohibit sustained abdominal contraction may be reasons for the physician to prohibit a strenuous singing or acting engagement. Health care providers should be familiar with laryngeal manifestations of system disease [52].

Any extremity injury, such as a sprained ankle, may alter posture and therefore interfere with customary abdominothoracic support. Voice patients are often unaware of this problem and develop abusive, hyperfunctional compensatory maneuvers in the neck and tongue musculature as a result. These technical flaws may produce voice complaints such as voice fatigue and neck pain that bring the performer to the physician's office for assessment and care. They even can produce structural lesions such as hemorrhage and nodules.

4.4.1 Obesity

Singers, actors, and many other professional voice users are verbal, oral people. Most enjoy singing, talking, and a good bowl of pasta after the show. However, before indulging our passions for culinary excess, it is important to understand the impact of obesity not only on singing performance, but also on general health and longevity [53].

For medical reasons, when obesity becomes extreme, serious measures may be necessary to accomplish weight loss. The most severely overweight patients have an entity called "morbid obesity." This condition is diagnosed when a person is more than 100 pounds or 100% over ideal body weight. Morbid obesity is extremely common in our society. It is estimated that 34 million adult Americans (1 of every 5 people over the age of 19) have significant obesity. As little as 20% excess over desirable body weight may be enough to constitute a health hazard. Doctors have long been aware of the difficulty in controlling weight problems with medical treatment alone. Of all patients who lose weight, 90% regain it at some point in their lives, and many even exceed their original weight. This led doctors to consider surgery as an option in treating this problem in selected cases.

In February 1985, a panel of experts from the National Institutes of Health looked at health problems associated with obesity [54]. Opinions have not changed substantially since that time. They concluded that obesity has adverse effects on health and longevity.

1. Obesity creates enormous psychological stress, which is a problem not well understood by the general population. Large people are unpopular, discriminated against in the workplace, and considered lazy.
2. Obesity is associated with high blood pressure. Obese people have high blood pressure three times more often than nonobese people.
3. Obesity is associated with higher levels of cholesterol.
4. Obesity is associated with diabetes. As with high blood pressure, this is seen three times more commonly in obese individuals.
5. Obesity is a factor in the development of heart disease.
6. Obesity increases the risk of developing certain cancers, specifically those of the uterus, breast, cervix, and gall bladder in women, and the colon, rectum, and prostate in men.
7. Obese individuals have a shorter life span.
8. Obesity is related to respiratory problems and arthritis.

With weight loss, all of these problems can be improved substantially, and prolongation of life is possible.

The best treatment for obesity is avoidance of the problem. Early in training, singers and other voice professionals, as well as all other performers, should learn the importance of good physical and aerobic conditioning. This is important to the voice professional's general health, vocal health, and art. Even a moderate degree of obesity may affect the respiratory system adversely, undermining support. Weight reduction is recommended for people who are 20% or more above ideal weight. In the singer, weight should be lost slowly through modification of eating and lifestyle habits. Loss of 2 or 3 pounds per week is plenty. More rapid loss of weight causes fluid shifts and hormonal alterations that may result in changes in vocal quality and endurance. Although these changes appear to be temporary, the effects of weight loss on vocal function have not been studied adequately; therefore, we do not have answers to all the pertinent questions. It is certainly possible for a singer to lose weight too quickly, but we are not yet sure how much weight loss is too much. Studies should be encouraged to learn more about this problem. However, it appears that maintenance of ideal body weight is probably as healthy for the voice as it is for the rest of the body. For people 20–100% above ideal body weight, weight loss can be accomplished with a medically supervised diet and exercise. However, people who are morbidly obese frequently are unable to lose weight by dietary or medical means alone. Morbidly obese patients may be candidates for surgery to help control their weight problems.

Although several kinds of obesity operations exist, the older procedures have troublesome side effects. At present, the best methods are a form of gastric restrictive surgery, known as the gastric bypass and gastric banding. Postoperatively, weight loss occurs over 12–18 months and stops as ideal body weight is approached. In most cases, singing may be resumed at about 6 weeks following abdominal surgery. Although the effects on the voice are not yet documented fully, there does not appear to be any significant problem associated with slow weight loss in patients with morbid obesity. Although further study is necessary to confirm these impressions, in singers or actors with this degree of weight problem, considerations of longevity, heart condition, blood pressure, and other critical health matters may outweigh immediate voice concerns.

For most singers, an extra 10, 20, or 30 pounds is not perceived as much of a problem. However, as 20 becomes 30, and 30 becomes 40, substantial adverse effects occur in the body in general and the vocal tract specifically. In training, singers and actors should be encouraged to treat their entire bodies with the same reverence with which they regard their vocal folds. Self-respect as a professional athlete is a sound basis for a long vocal career—and a long life.

4.4.2 Anxiety

Voice professionals, especially singers and actors, are frequently sensitive and communicative people. When the principal cause of vocal dysfunction is anxiety, the physician often can accomplish much by assuring the patient that no organic problem is present and by stating that the diagnosis of anxiety reaction. The patient should be counseled that anxiety is normal and that recognition of it as the principal problem frequently allows the performer to overcome it. Tranquilizers and sedatives are rarely necessary and often are undesirable because they may interfere with fine motor control. For example, beta-adrenergic blocking agents such as propranolol hydrochloride have become popular among performers for the treatment of preperformance anxiety. Beta-blockers are not recommended for regular use; they have significant effects on the cardiovascular system and many potential complications, including hypotension, thrombocytopenic purpura, mental depression, agranulocytosis, laryngospasm with respiratory distress, and bronchospasm. In addition, their efficacy is controversial. Although they may have a favorable effect in relieving performance anxiety, beta-blockers may produce a noticeable adverse effect on singing performance [55].

Although these drugs have a place under occasional, extraordinary circumstances, their routine use for this purpose not only is potentially hazardous but also violates an important therapeutic principle. Performers have chosen a career that exposes them to the public. If such persons are so incapacitated by anxiety that they are unable to perform the routine functions of their chosen profession without chemical help, this should be considered symptomatic of an important underlying psychologic problem. For a performer to depend on drugs to perform is neither routine nor healthy, whether the drug is a benzodiazepine, a barbiturate, a beta-blocker, or alcohol. If such dependence exists, psychologic evaluation by an experienced arts-medicine psychologist or psychiatrist should be considered [56]. Obscuring the symptoms by fostering the dependence is insufficient. However, if the patient is on tour and will only be under a particular otolaryngologist's care for a week or so, the physician should not try to make major changes in his or her customary regimen. Rather, the physician should communicate with the performer's primary otolaryngologist or family physician to coordinate appropriate long-term care.

As professional voice users constitute a subset of society as a whole, all the psychiatric disorders encountered among the general public are seen from time to time in voice professionals. In some cases, professional voice users require modification of the usual psychologic treatment, particularly with regard to psychotropic medications. Detailed discussion of this and related subjects can be found elsewhere [57].

When voice professionals, especially singers and actors, have a significant vocal impairment that results in voice loss (or the prospect of voice loss), they often go through a psychologic process similar to grieving [56]. In some cases, fear of discovering that the voice is lost forever may unconsciously prevent patients from trying to use their voices optimally following injury or treatment. This can dramatically impede or prevent recovery of function following a perfect surgical result, for example. It is essential that otolaryngologists, performers, and their teachers be familiar with this fairly common scenario, and it is ideal to include an arts-medicine psychologist and/or psychiatrist as part of the voice team.

Psychogenic voice disorders, incapacitating psychologic reactions to organic voice disorders, and other psychologic problems are encountered commonly in young voice patients. They are discussed in other literature [56].

4.4.3 Substance Abuse

The list of substances ingested, smoked, or "snorted" by many people is disturbingly long. Whenever possible, patients who care about vocal quality and longevity should be educated about the deleterious effects of such habits upon their voice and upon the longevity of their careers by their physicians and teachers. A few specific substances have already been discussed.

4.4.4 Other Diseases That May Affect the Voice

The larynx is subject to numerous acute and chronic infections. Some of them may be mistaken for malignancy and may be biopsied unnecessarily, exposing the patient (and sometimes the physician) to unnecessary risk. Tuberculosis, for example, is still seen in modern practice. Although laryngeal lesions used to be associated with extensive pulmonary infection, they are now usually associated with much less virulent disease, often only a mild cough. Laryngeal tuberculosis lesions usually are localized [58, 59]. Sarcoidosis, another granulomatous disease, causes laryngeal symptoms in roughly 3–5% of cases [60]. Noncaseating granulomas are found in the larynx, and the false vocal folds are frequently involved, producing airway obstruction rather than dysphonia. Less common diseases including leprosy [61, 62], syphilis [63], scleroderma [64], typhoid [65], typhus, anthrax, and other conditions can produce laryngeal lesions that might lead the laryngologist to obtain a possibly unnecessary biopsy. Confusing lesions also may be caused by a variety of mycotic infections including histoplasmosis [66–68], coccidioidomycosis [69], cryptococcosis [70], blastomycosis [68–72], actinomycosis [73, 74], candidiasis [75], aspergillosis [76–78], mucormycosis [79], rhinosporidiosis [80], and sporotrichosis [81]. Parasitic diseases may also produce laryngeal masses. The most prominent example is leishmaniasis [82]. More detailed information about most of the conditions discussed above is available in a text by Michaels [83] and elsewhere in this book [2].

Collagen vascular diseases and other unusual problems may produce laryngeal masses. Rheumatoid arthritis may produce not only fixation of the cricoarytenoid and cricothyroid joints, but also consequent neuropathic muscle atrophy [84] and rheumatoid nodules of the larynx [85]. Rheumatoid arthritis with or without nodules may produce respiratory obstruction. Gout may cause laryngeal arthritis. In addition, gouty tophi may appear as white submucosal masses of the true vocal fold. They consist of sodium urate crystals in fibrous tissue and have been documented well [86–88]. Amyloidosis of the larynx is rare but well recognized [89–91]. Urbach-Wiethe disease (lipoid proteinosis) [92] often involves the mucous membrane of the larynx, usually the vocal folds, aryepiglottic fold, and epiglottis. Other conditions, such as granulomatosis with polyangiitis (Wegener granulomatosis) and relapsing polychondritis, also may involve the larynx. They are less likely to produce discrete nodules, but the diffuse edema associated with chondritis and necrotizing granulomas may produce substantial laryngeal and voice abnormalities. Amyloidosis of the larynx is rare and usually involves the false vocal folds, but it can extend onto the true vocal folds. Unusual laryngeal masses also may be caused by trauma. Trauma is discussed in detail elsewhere [2], but the physician must be careful to inquire about laryngeal trauma, the consequences of which may not be recognized until months or years after the injury.

A few rare skin lesions also may involve the larynx producing symptomatic lesions, and sometimes airway obstruction. These include pemphigus vulgaris, seen in adults between 40 and 60 years of age. Pemphigus lesions may involve the mucosa, including the epiglottis [93]. Epidermolysis bullosa describes a group of congenital vesicular disorders usually seen at birth or shortly thereafter. This condition may cause laryngeal stenosis, or large, bleb-like vocal fold masses with detachment of the epithelium. Some viral conditions may cause laryngeal structural pathology, most notably papillomata. However, herpes, variola, and other organisms also have been implicated in laryngeal infection.

There are numerous other conditions, many of which are not covered comprehensively in this chapter, that may affect voices adversely. Most of them are not common problems among professional voice users. However, the laryngologist should remember that laryngeal manifestations of many systemic diseases may cause voice changes that bring the patient to medical attention for the first time [52, 53]. We must remain alert for their presence and think of them particularly when more common, obvious etiologies are not identified, or when patients do not respond to treatment as expected. The voice may be affected by the following problems not discussed above (among others): acromegaly, Arnold-Chiari malformations, blood dyscrasias, neurologic disease (vocal fold paralysis), collagen vascular disease (including rheumatoid arthritis, systemic lupus erythematosus, scleroderma, Sjögren's syndrome, and others), deafness, gout, Hodgkin's disease, leprosy, lymphoma, Madelung's disease, malignancies, myopathies, a myriad of infectious diseases (bacterial, viral, granulomatous, and fungal), mononucleosis, numerous syndromes (Basedow's, adrenogenital syndrome, Down's syndrome, hereditary angioedema, Kleinfelter's syndrome, Melkersson-Rosenthal syndrome, pachyonychia congenita, short stature syndromes, Shy-Drager syndrome, and many others), syphilis, sarcoidosis, tuberculosis, Crohn's disease, Wilson's disease, and other chronic diseases.

Dentofacial anomalies also may impact voice substantially, as reviewed elsewhere (REFERENCE).

4.5 Structural Abnormalities of the Larynx

4.5.1 Nodules

Nodules are callous-like masses of the vocal folds that are caused by vocally abusive behaviors and are a dreaded malady of singers and actors. Occasionally, laryngoscopy reveals asymptomatic vocal nodules that do not appear to interfere with voice production; in such cases, the nodules need not be treated. Some famous and successful singers have had untreated vocal nodules throughout their careers. However, in most cases, nodules result in hoarseness, breathiness, loss of range, and voice fatigue. They may be caused by abusive speaking rather than improper singing technique. Voice therapy always should be tried as the initial therapeutic modality and will cure the vast majority of patients even if the nodules look firm and have been present for many months or years. Even apparently large, fibrotic nodules often shrink, disappear, or become asymptomatic with 6–12 weeks of expert voice therapy with good patient compliance. Even in those who eventually need surgical excision of the nodules, preoperative voice therapy is essential to prevent recurrence. Care must be taken in diagnosing nodules.

It is almost impossible to make the diagnosis accurately and consistently without strobovideolaryngoscopy and good optical magnification. Vocal fold cysts are commonly misdiagnosed as nodules, and treatment strategies are different for the two lesions. Vocal nodules are confined to the superficial layer of the lamina propria and are composed primarily of edematous tissue or collagenous fibers. Basement membrane reduplication is common. They are usually bilateral and fairly symmetric.

Caution must be exercised in diagnosing small nodules in patients who have been singing or speaking actively. In many singers, for example, bilateral, symmetric soft swellings at the junction of the anterior and middle thirds of the vocal folds develop after heavy voice use. No evidence suggests that patients with such "physiologic swelling" are predisposed to develop vocal nodules. At present, the condition is generally considered to be within normal limits. The physiologic swelling usually disappears with 24–48 h of rest from heavy voice use. The physician must be careful not to frighten the patient by misdiagnosing physiologic swellings as vocal nodules. Nodules carry a great stigma among voice professionals, and the psychologic impact of the diagnosis should not be underestimated. When nodules are present, these patients should be informed with the same gentle caution used in telling a patient that he or she has a life-threatening mass.

4.5.2 Submucosal Cysts

Submucosal cysts of the vocal folds are probably also traumatic lesions that are the result of a blocked mucous gland duct in many cases. However, they also may be congenital or occur from other causes. They often cause contact swelling on the contralateral side and can be misdiagnosed as nodules. They usually can be differentiated from nodules by strobovideolaryngoscopy when the mass is observed to be fluid filled. They also may be suspected when the nodule (contact swelling) on one vocal fold resolves with voice therapy while the mass on the other vocal fold does not resolve. Cysts may be discovered on one side (occasionally both sides) when surgery is performed for apparent nodules that have not resolved with voice therapy. The surgery should be performed superficially and with minimal trauma, as discussed in a separate chapter. Ordinarily, cysts are lined with thin squamous epithelium. Retention cysts contain mucus. Epidermoid cysts contain caseous material. Generally, cysts are located in the superficial layer of the lamina propria. In some cases, they may be attached to the vocal ligament.

4.5.3 Polyps

Vocal fold polyps, another type of vocal fold mass, usually occur on only one vocal fold. They often have a feeding blood vessel coursing along the superior surface of the vocal fold and joining (or originating from) the base of the polyp. The pathogenesis of polyps cannot be proven in many cases, but the lesion is thought to be traumatic and sometimes starts as a hemorrhage. Polyps may be sessile or pedunculated.

Typically, they are located in the superficial layer of the lamina propria and do not involve the vocal ligament. In those arising from an area of hemorrhage, the vocal ligament may be involved with posthemorrhagic fibrosis that is contiguous with the polyp. Histologic evaluation most commonly reveals collagenous fibers, hyaline degeneration, edema, thrombosis, and often bleeding within the polypoid tissue. Cellular infiltration also may be present. In some cases, even sizable polyps resolve with relative voice rest and a few weeks of low-dose steroid therapy (e.g., methylprednisone 4 mg twice a day). However, most require surgical removal. If polyps are not treated, they may produce contact injury on the contralateral vocal fold. Voice therapy should be used to ensure good relative voice rest and prevent abusive voice behavior before and after surgery. When surgery is performed, care must be taken not to damage the leading edge of the vocal fold, especially if a laser is used. In all laryngeal surgery, delicate microscopic dissection is the standard of care. Vocal fold "stripping" is an out-of-date surgical approach formerly used for benign lesions; and it often resulted in scar and/or poor unserviceable voice function. It is no longer an acceptable surgical technique in most situations.

4.5.4 Granulomas

Granulomas usually occur in the cartilaginous portion of the vocal fold near the vocal process or on the medial surface of the arytenoid. They are composed of collagenous fibers, fibroblasts, proliferated capillaries, and leukocytes. They are usually covered with epithelium. Granulomas are associated with gastroesophageal reflux laryngitis and trauma (including trauma from voice abuse and from intubation). The term is a misnomer, since these lesions are inflammatory, not true granulomas as would be seen in tuberculosis or sarcoidosis. Therapy should include reflux control, voice therapy, and surgery if the granuloma continues to enlarge or does not resolve after adequate time and treatment. Granular cell tumors also can occur in the larynx [94].

4.5.5 Reinke's Edema

Severe Reinke's edema is characterized by an "elephant ear," floppy vocal fold appearance. It is often observed during examination in many nonprofessional and professional voice users and is accompanied by a low, coarse, gruff voice. Reinke's edema is a condition in which the superficial layer of lamina propria (Reinke's space) becomes edematous. The lesion does not usually include hypertrophy, inflammation, or degeneration, although other terms for the condition include polypoid degeneration, chronic polypoid corditis, and chronic edematous hypertrophy. Reinke's edema is often associated with smoking, voice abuse, reflux, and hypothyroidism. Underlying conditions should be treated. However, the condition may require surgery if voice improvement is desired. The surgery should be performed only if there is a justified high suspicion of serious pathology such as cancer, if there is airway obstruction, or if the patient is unhappy with his or her vocal quality. For some voice professionals, abnormal Reinke's edema is an important component of the vocal signature. Although the condition is usually bilateral, surgery should generally be performed on one side at a time. Many patients have mild Reinke's edema on one or both vocal folds that does not require treatment.

4.5.6 Sulcus Vocalis

Sulcus vocalis is a groove along the edge of the membranous vocal fold. The majority are congenital, bilateral, and symmetric, although posttraumatic acquired lesions occur. When symptomatic (they often are not), sulcus vocalis can be treated surgically if sufficient voice improvement is not obtained through voice therapy.

4.5.7 Scar

Vocal fold scar is a sequela of trauma and results in fibrosis and obliteration of the layered structure of the vocal fold. It may impede vibration and consequently cause dysphonia. Recent surgical advances have made this condition much more treatable than it used to be [95, 96], but it is still rarely possible to restore voices to normal in the presence of scar.

4.5.8 Hemorrhage

Vocal fold hemorrhage is a potential disaster in singers. Hemorrhages resolve spontaneously in most cases, with restoration of normal voice. However, in some instances, the hematoma organizes and fibroses, resulting in scar [97]. This alters the vibratory pattern of the vocal fold and can result in permanent hoarseness. In selected cases, it may be best to avoid this problem through surgical incision and drainage of the hematoma. In all cases, vocal fold hemorrhage usually is managed with absolute voice rest until the hemorrhage has largely resolved (usually about 1 week) and relative voice rest until normal vascular and mucosal integrity have been restored. This often takes 6 weeks and sometimes longer. Recurrent vocal fold hemorrhages usually are caused by weakness in a specific blood vessel, which may require surgical cauterization of the blood vessel using a laser or microscopic resection of the vessel [98].

4.5.9 Papilloma

Laryngeal papillomas are epithelial lesions caused by human papilloma virus. Histology reveals neoplastic epithelial cell proliferation in a papillary pattern and viral particles. At the present time, symptomatic papillomas are treated surgically, although alternatives have been recommended to the usual laser vaporization approach [99, 100]. Cidofovir injected into the lesion has shown considerable promise [99, 101].

4.5.10 Cancer

A detailed discussion of cancer of the larynx is beyond the scope of this chapter. The prognosis for small vocal fold cancers is good, whether they are treated by radiation or surgery. Although it may seem intuitively obvious that radiation therapy provides a better chance of voice conservation than even limited vocal fold surgery, late radiation changes in the vocal fold may produce substantial hoarseness, xerophonia (dry voice), and voice dysfunction. Consequently, from the standpoint of voice preservation, optimal treatments remain uncertain. Prospective studies using objective voice measures and strobovideolaryngoscopy should answer the relevant questions in the future. Strobovideolaryngoscopy is also valuable for follow-up of patients who have had laryngeal cancers. It permits detection of vibratory changes associated with infiltration by the cancer long before they can be seen with continuous light. Stroboscopy has been used in Europe and Japan for this purpose for many years. In the United States, the popularity of strobovideolaryngoscopy for follow-up of patients with cancer has increased greatly since the mid-to-late 1980s.

The psychologic consequences of vocal fold cancer can be devastating, especially in a professional voice user. They may be overwhelming for nonvoice professionals, as well. These reactions are understandable and expected. In many patients, however, psychologic reactions may be as severe following medically "less significant" vocal fold problems such as hemorrhages, nodules, and other conditions that do not command the public respect and sympathy afforded to a cancer. In many ways, the management of related psychologic problems can be even more difficult in patients with these "lesser" vocal disturbances.

4.5.11 Laryngoceles and Pharyngoceles

The ventricle of Morgagni is located between the true and false vocal folds. The appendix of the ventricle of Morgagni is a blind pouch called the saccule in the anterior superior portion. Laryngoceles are abnormal dilations or herniations of the laryngeal saccule [102]. They communicate with the laryngeal lumen and generally are filled with air. They become apparent clinically when they are distended after air is forced into them or when they are filled with fluid. They are connected to the ventricle by a narrow stalk and form a sac lined with pseudostratified, ciliated columnar epithelium. The appendix of the ventricle is considered abnormal if it extends above the upper border of the thyroid cartilage.

Laryngoceles limited to the interior of the larynx are called internal; those that protrude outside the thyroid cartilage into the neck are called external. They also may be mixed (internal and external). Laryngoceles should be distinguished from pharyngoceles, which are not true pouches and which generally diminish in size in the absence of pharyngeal pressure (e.g., when not whistling or playing a wind instrument) [102]. Pharyngoceles are air-filled expansions of the pharynx that can be large enough to require musicians to wear shirts with extra large collar sizes or to play with the collar unbuttoned. Laryngoceles and pharyngoceles are most common in brass instrumentalists. In laryngoceles, outpouchings of the laryngeal ventricle can extend through the openings in the thyrohyoid membrane for the superior laryngeal vessels and nerve, and balloon outward and upward toward the submandibular triangle [103]. External and mixed laryngoceles are really variants of the internal laryngocele. Because laryngoceles arise from the region of the saccule within the larynx, if the lesion is a laryngocele, there must be an intralaryngeal component manifested at least as a tract connecting the lateral component with the ventricle, with or without internal dilation. Hence, pure external laryngoceles do not exist. Lesions without an intralaryngeal component should be classified differently (e.g., as pharyngoceles).

There are several proposed mechanisms for laryngocele formation. In neonates, they are presumed to be remnants of the lateral air sacs seen in other primates. In adults, they can represent a congenital enlargement of the saccule or an acquired lesion associated with increased intraluminal pressure. The association of laryngoceles with occupations that involve long periods of forced expiration supports this notion, and they also are associated with laryngeal carcinomas [104].

Brass and woodwind players are at risk for a variety of head and neck abnormalities as a result of increased intraluminal pressure during musical performances [105]. Transient ischemic attacks, temporomandibular joint dysfunction, and dental malocclusion have been reported. Injury to the orbicularis oris in brass players can require surgical repair [106]. Stress velopharyngeal incompetence has been documented in trumpeters, bassoonists, and others as noted above. Young trumpet players are at greatest risk for injury to oral and cervical tissues when they generate peak respiratory pressure averaging 151 torr [107].

Although laryngoceles usually are associated with brass instruments, several authors have examined laryngocele formation in woodwind players. Stephani and Tarab obtained plain x-rays on 25 wind instrument players and found laryngoceles in all of them [108]. Macfie found laryngoceles in 53 of 94 (56%) woodwind bandsmen [109]. Subclinical laryngoceles are common among horn players, and they rarely require surgical intervention.

Surgery for laryngoceles in young musicians poses several problems. The literature offers no definitive guidance regarding the timing of surgery, the healing period before playing can be resumed, and the risk of recurrence with continued performance. Furthermore, the cervical approach used commonly for the treatment of external laryngoceles can disrupt the normal function of the strap muscles, which is important for tone generation for instrumentalists and for singers [110]. The risks of infection and progression of the defect must be balanced against a young performer's desire for musical growth.

Since Ward's early reports on this subject [103], our understanding of laryngoceles and pharyngoceles has changed slightly. Both laryngoceles and pharyngoceles can change size and appearance with variations in internal pressure. Although the classical definitions of laryngocele remain valid, combinations of both can occur. Air-filled masses that arise in the pharynx (commonly in the region of the piriform sinuses) and lack a laryngeal component or origin should be called pharyngoceles. Those that arise in the laryngeal ventricle should be called laryngoceles. Considering the origins of pharyngeal pouches as reviewed in Ward's 1963 paper [102] as well as the forces involved, it appears likely that most lesions with a laryngeal component originated in the larynx and extended in the neck rather than vice versa, but it is not always possible to prove origin. It is also important to recognize that the therapeutic implications of the distinctions are not as clear-cut as they once were and that lesions that combine the features of laryngoceles and pharyngoceles occur [111]. The distinctions between laryngoceles and pharyngoceles were quite important when we still believed laryngoceles usually required surgery and pharyngoceles required surgery only rarely. However, as arts-medicine has evolved, experience has shown that, in most cases, neither lesion requires surgery. Contrary to our earlier understandings, the vast majority of laryngoceles are asymptomatic.

4.5.12 *Other Conditions*

Numerous other conditions could be included in this chapter. For a more comprehensive discussion of the subjects covered above, the reader is referred [2].

4.6 Medical Management for Voice Dysfunction

Medical management of many problems affecting the voice involves not only care prescribed by an otolaryngologist but also voice therapy, which is provided by an interdisciplinary team. The roles and training of the principal members of the team are covered in detail elsewhere [2]. This chapter provides a brief introduction to their roles in the medical milieu.

4.6.1 Speech-Language Pathologist

An excellent speech-language pathologist is an invaluable asset in caring for professional voice users and other voice patients. However, otolaryngologists and singing teachers should recognize that, like physicians, speech-language pathologists have varied backgrounds and experience in the treatment of voice disorders. In fact, most speech-language pathology programs teach relatively little about caring for professional speakers and nothing about professional singers. Moreover, few speech-language pathologists have vast experience in this specialized area, and no fellowships in this specialty exist. Speech-language pathologists often subspecialize. A speech-language pathologist who expertly treats patients who have had strokes, stutter, have undergone laryngectomy, or have swallowing disorders will not necessarily know how to manage professional voice users optimally or even other less demanding voice patients. The otolaryngologist must learn the strengths and weaknesses of the speech-language pathologist with whom he or she works. After identifying a speech-language pathologist who is interested in treating professional voice users, the otolaryngologist should work closely with the speech-language pathologist to develop the necessary expertise. Assistance may be found through otolaryngologists who treat large numbers of singers or through educational programs such as the Voice Foundation's Symposium on Care of the Professional Voice. In general, therapy should be directed toward vocal hygiene, relaxation techniques, voice function exercised breath management, and abdominal support.

Speech (voice) therapy may be helpful even when a singer has no obvious problem in the speaking voice but significant technical problems singing. Once a person has been singing for several years, a singing teacher may have difficulty convincing him or her to correct certain technical errors. However, singers are much less protective of their speaking voices. A speech-language pathologist may be able to teach proper support, relaxation, and voice placement in speaking. Once mastered, these techniques can be carried over fairly easily into singing through cooperation between the speech-language pathologist and singing teacher or singing voice specialist. This "back door" approach has been extremely useful. For the actor, coordinating speech-language pathology sessions with acting voice lessons, and especially with training of the speaking voice provided by the actor's voice teacher or coach, is often helpful. We have found this combination so helpful that we have added an acting voice trainer to our medical staff. Information from the speech-language pathologist, acting voice trainer, and singing teacher or singing voice specialist should be symbiotic and should not conflict. If major discrepancies exist, bad training from one of the team members should be suspected, and changes should be made.

4.6.2 Singing Voice Specialist

Singing voice specialists are singing teachers who have acquired extra training to prepare them for work with injured voices, in collaboration with a medical voice team. They are indispensable for singers and very valuable for nonsingers with voice disorders.

In selected cases, singing lessons may be extremely helpful to nonsingers with voice problems. The techniques used to develop abdominal and thoracic muscle strength, breath control, laryngeal and neck muscle strength, and relaxation are similar to those used in voice therapy. Singing lessons often expedite therapy and appear to improve the outcome in some patients.

Otolaryngologists who care for singers frequently are often asked to recommend a voice teacher. This may put them in an uncomfortable position, particularly if the singer is already studying with someone in the community. Most physicians do not have sufficient expertise to criticize a voice teacher, and we must be extremely cautious about recommending that a singer change teachers. However, no certifying agency standardizes or ensures the quality of a singing teacher. Although one may be slightly more confident of a teacher associated with a major conservatory or music school or one who is a member of the National Association of Teachers of Singing (NATS), neither of these credentials ensures excellence, and many expert teachers have neither affiliation. However, with experience, an otolaryngologist can develop valid impressions. The physician should record the name of the voice teacher of every patient and observe whether the same kinds of voice abuse occur with disproportionate frequency in the pupils of any given teacher. Technical problems can cause organic abnormalities such as nodules; therefore, any teacher who has a high incidence of nodules among his or her students should be viewed with cautious concern, but the physician also needs to determine whether the teacher attracts a student cohort that has a high incidence of nodules before the students have started lessons, as may be seen among some populations of rock and popular music singers who have performed extensively without voice training. The physician should be particularly wary of teachers who are reluctant to allow their students to consult a doctor. The best voice teachers usually are quick to refer their students to an otolaryngologist if they hear anything disturbing in a student's voice. Similarly, voice teachers and voice professionals should compare information on the nature and quality of medical care received and its success. No physician cures every voice problem in every patient, just as no singing teacher produces premiere stars from every student who walks into the studio. Nevertheless, voice professionals must be critical, informed consumers and accept nothing less than the best medical care and voice training.

After seeing a voice patient, the otolaryngologist should speak with and/or write a letter to the voice teacher (with the patient's permission) describing the findings and recommendations as he or she would to a physician, speech-language pathologist, or any other referring professional. An otolaryngologist seriously interested in caring for singers should take the trouble to talk with and meet local singing teachers. Taking a lesson or two with each teacher provides enormous insight, as well. Taking voice lessons regularly is even more helpful. In practice, the otolaryngologist will usually identify a few teachers in whom he or she has particular confidence, especially for patients with voice disorders, and should not hesitate to refer singers to these colleagues, especially singers who are not already in training.

Pop singers may be particularly resistant to the suggestion of voice lessons, yet they are in great need of training. The physician should assure patients that a good voice teacher can teach a pop singer how to protect and expand the voice without changing its quality or making it sound "trained" or "operatic." It is helpful to point out that singing, like other athletic activities, requires exercise, warm-up, and coaching for anyone planning to enter the "big league" and stay there. Just as no major league baseball pitcher would play without a pitching coach and warm-up time in the bullpen, no singer should try to build a career without a singing teacher and appropriate strength and agility exercises. This approach has proved palatable and effective. Physicians also should be aware of the difference between a voice teacher and a voice coach.

A voice teacher trains a singer in singing technique and is essential. A voice coach is responsible for teaching songs, interpretation, language, diction, style, operatic roles, and so on, but is not responsible for exercise and basic technical development of the voice.

4.6.3 Acting-Voice Trainer

The use of acting-voice trainers (drama voice coaches) as members of the medical team is relatively new [2]. This addition to the team has been extremely valuable to patients and other team members. Like singing voice specialists, professionals with education in theatre arts use numerous vocal and body movement techniques that not only enhance physical function but also release tension and break down emotional barriers that may impede voice function. Tearful revelations to the acting-voice trainer are not uncommon; and, like the singing teacher, this individual may identify psychological and emotional problems that interfere with professional success and have been skillfully hidden from other professionals on the voice team and in the patient's life.

4.6.4 Others

A psychologist, psychiatrist, neurologist, pulmonologist, endocrinologist, gastroenterologist, and others with special interest and expertise in arts-medicine are also invaluable to the voice team. Every comprehensive center should seek out such people and collaborate with them, even if they are not full-time members of the voice team.

4.7 Surgery

A detailed discussion of laryngeal surgery is beyond the scope of this chapter and may be found elsewhere [2, 112]. However, a few points are worthy of special emphasis. Surgery for vocal nodules should be avoided whenever possible and should almost never be performed without an adequate trial of expert voice therapy, including patient compliance with therapeutic suggestions. A minimum of 6–12 weeks of observation should be allowed while the patient is using therapeutically modified voice techniques under the supervision of a speech-language pathologist and ideally a singing voice specialist. Proper voice use rather than voice rest (silence) is correct therapy. The surgeon should not perform surgery prematurely for vocal nodules under pressure from the patient for a "quick cure" and early return to performance. Permanent destruction of voice quality is a very real potential complication.

Even after expert surgery, voice quality may be diminished by submucosal scarring, resulting in an adynamic segment along the vibratory margin of the vocal fold. This situation produces a hoarse voice with vocal folds that appear normal on indirect examination under routine light, although under stroboscopic light, the adynamic segment is obvious. No reliable cure exists for this complication. Even large, apparently fibrotic nodules of long standing should be given a chance to resolve without surgery. In some cases, the nodules remain but become asymptomatic, and voice quality is normal. Stroboscopy in such patients usually reveals that the nodules are on the superior surface rather than the leading edge of the vocal folds during proper, relaxed phonation (although they may be on the contact surface and symptomatic when hyperfunctional voice technique is used and the larynx is forced down).

When surgery is indicated for vocal fold lesions, it should be limited as strictly as possible to the area of abnormality. Virtually no place exists for "vocal fold stripping" in patients with benign disease. Submucosal resection through a laryngeal microflap used to be advocated. The technique was introduced and first published by the author (RTS). Microflap technique involved an incision on the superior surface of the vocal fold, submucosal resection, and preservation of the mucosa along the leading edge of the vocal fold. The concept that led to this innovation was based on the idea that the intermediate layer of the lamina propria should be protected to prevent fibroblast proliferation. Consequently, it seemed reasonable to preserve the mucosa as a biologic dressing. This technique certainly produced better results than vocal fold stripping. However, close scrutiny of outcomes revealed a small number of cases with poor results and stiffness beyond the limits of the original pathology. Consequently, the technique was abandoned in favor of a new technique called minimicroflap, or a method of local resection strictly limited to the region of pathology [113]. Lesions such as vocal nodules should be removed to a level even with the vibratory margin rather than deeply into the submucosa. This minimizes scarring and optimizes chances for return to good vocal function. Naturally, if concern about a serious neoplasm exists, proper treatment takes precedence over voice preservation. Surgery should be performed under microscopic control. Preoperative and postoperative objective voice measures are essential to allow outcome assessment and self-critique. Only through such study can we improve surgical technique. Outcome studies are especially important in voice surgery as all our technical pronouncements are anecdotal because there is no experimental model for vocal fold surgery. The human adult is the only species with our complex, layered lamina propria.

Lasers are an invaluable adjunct in the laryngologists' armamentarium, but they must be used knowledgeably and with care. Considerable early evidence suggested that healing time was prolonged and the incidence of adynamic segment formation was higher with the laser on the vibratory margin than with traditional instruments. Two early studies raised serious concerns about dysphonia after laser surgery [114, 115]. Such complications may result from using too low a wattage causing dissipation of heat deeply into the vocal fold; thus, high power density for short duration has been recommended. Small spot size is also helpful. More recent experience has shown that expert laser surgery on the vibratory margin can produce excellent results. Nevertheless, many laryngologists caring for voice professionals avoid laser surgery to eliminate the risk of thermal injury to the vocal ligament. If a laser is used when biopsy specimens are needed, they should be taken before vaporizing the lesion with a laser. If a lesion is to be removed from the leading edge, the laser beam should be centered in the lesion, rather than on the vibratory margin, so that the beam does not create a divot in the vocal fold. The CO_2 laser used to be used for cauterizing isolated blood vessels responsible for recurrent hemorrhage or other problems, and it still is used occasionally. At the suggestion of Jean Abitbol, MD, the author (RTS) has placed a small piece of ice on the vocal fold immediately before CO_2 laser use to help dissipate the heat and help prevent edema (personal communication, 1983). No studies on the efficacy of this maneuver exist, but the technique appears helpful.

Such vessels are often found at the base of a hemorrhagic polyp. Vascular lasers are better than CO_2 lasers for management of these lesions and other vascular abnormalities. They include the 532 nm KTP (Nd-YAG) laser and the 445 nm Blue Laser.

Voice rest after vocal fold surgery is controversial. Although some laryngologists do not recognize its necessity at all, many physicians recommend voice rest for approximately 1 week or until the mucosal surface has healed. Even after surgery, silence for more than 7–10 days is nearly never necessary and represents a real hardship for many patients.

Too often, the laryngologist is confronted with a desperate patient whose voice has been "ruined" by vocal fold surgery, recurrent or superior laryngeal nerve paralysis, trauma, or some other tragedy. Occasionally, the cause is as straightforward as a dislocated arytenoid that can be reduced [116, 117]. However, if the problem is an avulsed vocal process, an adynamic segment, decreased bulk of one vocal fold after "stripping," bowing caused by superior laryngeal nerve paralysis, or some other complication in a mobile vocal fold, great conservatism should be exercised. None of the available surgical procedures for these conditions is effective consistently. If surgery is considered, the procedure and prognosis should be explained to the patient realistically and pessimistically. The patient must understand that the chances of returning the voice to professional quality are very slim and that it might be made worse. Nevertheless, procedures for vocal fold scar have improved, and surgery is often possible (including vocal fold injection and other procedures) to at least decrease the severity of dysphonia and to lessen vocal effort.

Occasionally, voice professionals inquire about surgery for pitch alteration. Such procedures have been successful in specially selected patients (such as those undergoing gender modification surgery), but they do not consistently provide good enough voice quality and range to be performed on a professional voice user in most situations.

4.8 Discretion

The excitement and glamour associated with caring for voice patients, particularly famous performers, naturally tempt the physician to talk about a distinguished patient. However, this tendency must be tempered. Having it known that he or she has consulted a laryngologist, particularly for treatment of a significant vocal problem, is not always in a voice professional's best interest. Famous singers, actors, politicians, and other professional voice users are entitled ethically and legally to the same confidentiality we ensure for our other patients.

4.9 Voice Maintenance

Prevention of voice dysfunction should be the goal of all professionals involved in the care of professional voice users. Good vocal health habits should be encouraged in childhood. Screaming, particularly outdoors at athletic events, should be discouraged. Promising young singers who join choirs should be educated to compensate for the Lombard effect. The youngster interested in singing, acting, debating, or other vocal activities should receive enough training to prevent voice abuse and should receive enthusiastic support for performing works and activities suitable for his or her age and voice. Training should be continued during or after puberty, and the voice should be allowed to develop naturally without pressure to perform operative roles prematurely. Young instrumentalists should be managed with similar care, as discussed in this chapter.

Excellent regular training and practice are essential, and avoidance of irritants, particularly smoke, should be stressed early. Educating voice professionals and wind instrumentalists about hormonal and anatomic alterations that may influence the voice allows them to recognize and analyze voice dysfunction, compensating for it intelligently when it occurs. The body is dynamic, changing over a lifetime, and the voice is no exception. Continued voice education, training, and monitoring are necessary throughout a lifetime, even in the most successful and well-established voice professionals and instrumental musicians. Voice problems even in premiere singers commonly are caused by cessation of lessons, excessive schedule demands, and other correctable problems, rather than by irreversible alterations of aging. Anatomic, physiologic, and serious medical problems may affect the voices of patients of any age. Cooperation among the laryngologist, speech-language pathologist, acting teacher, voice specialist and music teacher and singing teacher provides an optimal environment for cultivation and protection of the vocal artist and for voice presentation in wind instrumentalists.

Acknowledgment Modified in part from Sataloff RT. Professional voice: the science and art of clinical care. 4th ed. San Diego: Plural Publishing, Inc; 2017; with permission.

References

1. Brodnitz F. Hormones and the human voice. Bull N Y Acad Med. 1971;47:183–91.
2. Sataloff RT. Professional voice: the science and art of clinical care. 4th ed. San Diego: Plural Publishing; 2017. p. 1–2099.
3. von Leden H. Presentation at: Seventh symposium on care of the professional voice. New York: The Juilliard School; June 16, 1978.
4. Punt NA. Applied laryngology—singers and actors. Proc R Soc Med. 1968;61:1152–6.
5. Anderson TD, Sataloff RT. Rhinosinusitis. In: Sataloff RT, editor. Professional voice: the science and art of clinical care. 4th ed. San Diego: Plural Publishing; 2017. p. 747–50.
6. Nachman SA, Pontrelli L. Central nervous system Lyme disease. Semin Pediatr Infect Dis. 2003;14(2):123–30.
7. Sataloff JB, Sataloff RT. Otologic manifestations of Lyme disease. In: Kountakis SE, editor. Encyclopedia of otolaryngology, head and neck surgery. New Delhi: Springer; 2013. p. 2015–20.
8. Goldfarb D, Sataloff RT. Lyme disease: a review for the otolaryngologist. Ear Nose Throat J. 1994;73(11):824–9.
9. Kugeler KJ, Farley GM, Forrester JD, Mead P. Geographic distribution and expansion of human Lyme disease, United States. Emerg Infect Dis. 2015;21(8):1455–7.
10. Clark JR, Carlson RD, Sasaki CT, Pachner AR, Steere AC. Facial paralysis in Lyme disease. NATS J. 1995;95:1341–5.
11. Steere AC, Grodzick MS, Kornblatt AN, et al. The spirochetal etiology of Lyme disease. N Engl J Med. 1983;308:733–40.
12. Burgdorfer WA, Barbour AG, Hayes SF, Benach JL, Grunwaldt E, David JP. Lyme disease-tick-borne spirochetosis. Science. 1982;216:1317–9.
13. Strle F, Ruzic-Sablijic E, Cimperman J, Lotric-Furlan S, Maraspin V. Comparison of findings for patients with Borrelia garinii and Borrelia afzelii isolated from cerebrospinal fluid. Clin Infect Dis. 2006;43(6):704–10.
14. Magnarelli LA. Serologic diagnostics of Lyme disease. Ann N Y Acad Sci. 1988;539:154–61.
15. Sehgal VN, Khurana A. Lyme disease/borreliosis as a systemic disease. Clin Dermatol. 2015;33:542–50.
16. Barbour AG. Diagnosis of Lyme disease: rewards and perils. Ann Intern Med. 1989;11(7):501–2.
17. Glassock ME, Pensak ML, Gulia AJ, Baker DC. Lyme disease: a cause of bilateral facial paralysis. Arch Otolaryngol. 1985;111:47–9.
18. Schroeter V. Paralysis of recurrent laryngeal nerve in Lyme disease. Lancet. 1988;2(8622):1245.

19. Steere AC, Malaawista SE, Hardin JA, Ruddy S, Askenase PW, Andiman WA. Erythema chronicum migrans and Lyme arthritis: the enlarging clinical spectrum. Ann Intern Med. 1988;86:685–98.
20. Sataloff RT, Johns MM, Kost KM. Geriatric otolaryngology. New York: Thieme; 2015.
21. Sundberg J, Prame E, Iwarsson J. Replicability and accuracy of pitch patterns in professional singers. In: David PJ, Fletcher NH, editors. Vocal fold physiology: controlling chaos and complexity. Sydney: Singular Publishing; 1996. p. 291–306.
22. Sataloff RT, Cohn JR, Hawkshaw M. Respiratory dysfunction. In: Sataloff RT, editor. Professional voice: the science and art of clinical care. 4th ed. San Diego: Plural Publishing; 2017. p. 751–64.
23. Spiegel JR, Sataloff RT, Cohn JR, et al. Respiratory function in singers. Medical assessment, diagnoses and treatments. J Voice. 1988;2(1):40–50.
24. Cohn JR, Sataloff RT, Spiegel JR, et al. Airway reactivity-induced asthma in singers (ARIAS). J Voice. 1991;5(4):332–7.
25. Cohn JR, Padams PA, Hawkshaw MJ, Sataloff RT. Allergy. In: Sataloff RT, editor. Professional voice: the science and art of clinical care. 4th ed. San Diego: Plural Publishing; 2017. p. 737–42.
26. Sataloff RT, Katz PO, Sataloff DM, Hawkshaw MJ. Reflux laryngitis and related disorders. 4th ed. San Diego: Plural Publishing; 2013. p. 1–210.
27. Ritter FN. The effect of hypothyroidism on the larynx of the rat. Ann Otol Rhinol Laryngol. 1964;67:404–16.
28. Ritter RN. Endocrinology. In: Paparella M, Shumrick D, editors. Otolaryngology, vol. 1. Philadelphia: Saunders; 1973. p. 727–34.
29. Michelsson K, Sirvio P. Cry analysis in congenital hypothyroidism. Folia Phoniatr. 1976;28:40–7.
30. Gupta OP, Bhatia PL, Agarwal MK, Mehrotra ML, Mishr SK. Nasal pharyngeal and laryngeal manifestations of hypothyroidism. Ear Nose Throat J. 1977;56(9):10–21.
31. Malinsky M, Chevrrie-Muller C, Cerceau N. Etude Clinique et electrophysiologique des alterations de la voix au cours des thyrotoxioses. Ann Endocrinol. 1977;38:171–2.
32. Meuser W, Nieschlag E. Sexual hormone und Stimmlage des Mannes. Dtsch Med Wochenschr. 1977;102:261–4.
33. Brodnitz F. The age of the castrato voice. J Speech Hear Disord. 1975;40:291–5.
34. Anderson TD, Anderson DD, Sataloff RT. Endocrine function. In: Sataloff RT, editor. Professional voice: the science and art of clinical care. 4th ed. San Diego: Plural Publishing; 2017. p. 655–70.
35. Schiff M. The influence of estrogens on connective tissue. In: Asboe-Hansen G, editor. Hormones and connective tissue. Copenhagen: Munksgaard Press; 1967. p. 282–341.
36. Lacina V. Der Einfluss der Menstruation auf die Stimme der Sangerinnen. Folia Phoniatr. 1968;20:13–24.
37. Wendler J. Cyclically dependent variations in efficiency of the voice and its influencing by ovulation inhibitors. Zyklusabhangige Leistungsschwankungen der Stimme und ihre Beeinflussung durch Ovulationshemmer. Folia Phoniatr. 1972;24(4):259–77.
38. Abitbol J, Abitbol P. The larynx: a hormonal target. In: Rubin J, Sataloff RT, Korovin G, editors. Diagnosis and treatment of voice disorders. 4th ed. San Diego: Plural Publishing, Inc; 2014. p. 431–56.
39. Dordain M. Etude Statistique de l'influence des contraceptifs hormonaux sur la voix. Folia Phoniatr. 1972;24:86–96.
40. Pahn V, Goretzlehner G. Stimmstorungen durch hormonale Kontrazeptiva. Zentralb Gynakol. 1978;100:341–6.
41. Schiff M. "The pill" in otolaryngology. Trans Am Acad Opthalmol Otolaryngol. 1968;72:76–84.
42. Rodney JP, Sataloff RT. The effects of hormonal contraception on the voice: history of its evolution in the literature. J Voice. 2016;30(6):726–30.

43. Brodnitz F. Medical care preventative therapy (panel). In: Lawrence V, editor. Transcripts of the seventh annual symposium, care of the professional voice, vol. 3. New York: Voice Foundation; 1978. p. 86.
44. Flach M, Schwickardi H, Simen R. Welchen Einfluss haben Menstruation and Schwangershaft auf die augsgebildete Gesangsstimme? Folia Phoniatr. 1968;21:199–210.
45. Deuster CV. Irreversible Stimmstorung in der Schwangersheft. HNO. 1977;25:430–2.
46. Damste PH. Virilization of the voice due to anabolic steroids. Folia Phoniatr. 1964;16:10–8.
47. Damste PH. Voice changes in adult women caused by virilizing agents. J Speech Hear Disord. 1967;32:126–32.
48. Saez S, Francoise S. Recepteurs d'androgenes: mise en evidence dans la fraction cytosolique de muqueuse normale et d'epitheliomas pharyngolarynges humains. C R Acad Sci (Paris). 1975;280:935–8.
49. Vuorenkoski V, Lenko HL, Tjernlund P, Vuorenkoski L, Perheentupa J. Fundamental voice frequency during normal and abnormal growth, and after androgen treatment. Arch Dis Child. 1978;53:201–9.
50. Bourdial J. Les troubles de la voix provoques par la therapeutique hormonale androgene. Ann Otolaryngol. 1970;87:725–34.
51. Imre V. Hormonell bedingte Stimmstorungen. Folia Phoniatr. 1968;20:394–404.
52. Hamdan A, Sataloff RT, Hawkshaw MJ. Laryngeal manifestations of systemic diseases. San Diego: Plural Publishing; 2019.
53. Hamdan A, Sataloff RT, Hawkshaw MJ. Obesity and voice. San Diego: Plural Publishing; 2020.
54. National Institutes of Health. Health implications of obesity. Consensus development conference statement. Bethesda: National Institutes of Health; 1986.
55. Gates GA, Saegert J, Wilson N, Johnson L, Sheperd A, Hearnd EM. Effects of beta-blockade on singing performance. Ann Otol Rhinol Laryngol. 1985;94:570–4.
56. Rosen DC, Sataloff RT. Psychology of voice disorders. San Diego: Singular Publishing; 1997.
57. Sataloff RT, Brandfonbrener A, Lederman R, editors. Performing arts medicine. 3rd ed. Narberth: Science and Medicine; 2010.
58. Bull TR. Tuberculosis of the larynx. Br Med J. 1966;2:991–2.
59. Hunter AM, Millar JW, Wrightman AJ, Horne NW. The changing pattern of laryngeal tuberculosis. J Laryngol Otol. 1981;95:393–8.
60. Divine KD. Sarcoidosis and sarcoidosis of the larynx. Laryngoscope. 1965;75:533–69.
61. Munor MacCormick CE. The larynx in leprosy. Arch Otolaryngol. 1957;66:138–49.
62. Binford CH, Meyers WM. Leprosy. In: Binford CH, Conor DH, editors. Pathology of tropical and extraordinary diseases, vol. 1. Washington, DC: Armed Forces Institute of Pathology; 1976. p. 205–25.
63. MacKenzie M. A manual of diseases of the throat and nose, Vol. 1. Diseases of the pharynx, larynx, and trachea. J. & A. Churchill: London; 1884.
64. Astacio JN, Goday GA, Espinosa FJ. Escleroma. Experiences en El Salvador. Seconda Mongrafia de Dermatologia iberolatino-americana. Suplemento AO No. 1, Lisboa, Portugal, 1971.
65. Hajek M. Pathologie unde Therapie der Erkrankungen des Kehlkopfes, der Luftrohre und der Bronchien. Leipzig: Verlag von Curt Kabitzsch; 1932.
66. Withers BT, Pappas JJ, Erickson EE. Histoplasmosis primary in the larynx. Report of a case. Arch Otolaryngol. 1977;77:25–8.
67. Calcaterra TC. Otolaryngeal histoplasmosis. Laryngoscope. 1970;80:111–20.
68. Sataloff RT, Wilborn A, Prestipino A, Hawkshaw M, Heuer RJ, Cohn JR. Histoplasmosis of the larynx. Am J Otolaryngol. 1993;14(3):199–205.
69. Friedmann I. Diseases of the larynx. Disorders of laryngeal function. In: Paparella MM, Shumrick DA, editors. Otolaryngology. 2nd ed. Philadelphia: WB Saunders; 1980. p. 2449–69.

70. Reese MC, Conclasure JB. Cryptococcosis of the larynx. Arch Otolaryngol. 1975;101:698–701.
71. Bennett M. Laryngeal blastomycosis. Laryngoscope. 1964;74:498–512.
72. Hoffarth GA, Joseph DL, Shumrick DA. Deep mycoses. Arch Otolaryngol. 1973;97:475–9.
73. Brandenburg JH, Finch WW, Kirkham WR. Actinomycosis of the larynx and pharynx. Otolaryngology. 1978;86:739–42.
74. Shaheen SO, Ellis FG. Actinomycosis of the larynx. J R Soc Med. 1983;76:226–8.
75. Tedeschi LG, Cheren RV. Laryngeal hyperkeratosis due to primary monilial infection. Arch Otolaryngol. 1968;82:82–4.
76. Rao PB. Aspergillosis of the larynx. J Laryngol Otol. 1969;83:377–9.
77. Ferlito A. Clinical records. Primary aspergillosis of the larynx. J Laryngol Otol. 1974;88:1257–63.
78. Keir SM, Flint A, Moss JA. Primary aspergillosis of the larynx simulating carcinoma. Hum Pathol. 1983;14:184–6.
79. Anand CS, Gupta MC, Kothari MG, Anand TS, Singh SK. Laryngeal mucormycosis. Indian J Otolaryngol. 1978;30:90–2.
80. Pillai OS. Rhinosporidiosis of the larynx. J Laryngol Otol. 1974;88:277–80.
81. Ferlito A. Clinical records. Primary aspergillosis of the larynx stimulating carcinoma. Hum Pathol. 1938;14:184–6.
82. Zinneman HH, Hall WH, Wallace FG. Leishmaniasis of the larynx. Report of a case and its confusion with histoplasmosis. Am J Med. 1961;31:654–8.
83. Michaels L. Pathology of the larynx. New York: Springer-Verlag; 1984.
84. Wolman L, Darke CS, Young A. The larynx in rheumatoid arthritis. J Laryngol. 1965;79:403–34.
85. Bridger MWN, Jahn AF, van Nostrand AWP. Laryngeal rheumatoid arthritis. Laryngoscope. 1980;90:296–303.
86. Virchow R. Seltene Gichtablagerungen. Virchows Arch Path Anat. 1868;44:137–8.
87. Marion RB, Alperin JE, Maloney WH. Gouty tophus of the true vocal cord. Arch Otolaryngol. 1972;96:161–2.
88. Epstein SS, Winston P, Friedmann I, Ormerod FC. The vocal cord polyp. J Laryngol Otol Lond. 1957;71:673–88.
89. Stark DB, New GB. Amyloid tumors of larynx, trachea or bronchi: report of 15 cases. Ann Otol Rhinol Laryngol. 1949;58:117–34.
90. Michaels L, Hyams VJ. Amyloid in localized deposits and plasmacytomas of the respiratory tract. J Pathol. 1979;128(1):29–38.
91. Pribtkin E, Friedman O, O'Hara B, et al. Amyloidosis of the upper aerodigestive tract. Laryngoscope. 2003;113:2095–101.
92. Urbach E, Wiethe C. Lipoidosis cutis et mucosae. Virchows Arch Path Anat. 1929;273:285–319.
93. Charow A, Pass F, Ruben R. Pemphigus of the upper respiratory tract. Arch Otolaryngol. 1971;93:209–10.
94. Sataloff RT, Hawkshaw M, Ressue J. Granular cell tumor of the larynx. Ear Nose Throat J. 1998;77(8):582–4.
95. Moore JE, Hawkshaw MJ, Sataloff RT. Vocal fold scar. Oxford: Compton Publishing, Ltd; 2016.
96. Moore JE, Sataloff RT. Vocal fold scar. In: Sataloff RT, editor. Professional voice: the science and art of clinical care. 4th ed. San Diego: Plural Publishing; 2017. p. 1605–10.
97. Sataloff RT, Hawkshaw M. Vocal fold hemorrhage. In: Sataloff RT, editor. Professional voice: the science and art of clinical care. 4th ed. San Diego: Plural Publishing; 2017. p. 1587–604.
98. Hochman I, Sataloff RT, Hillman R, Zeitels S. Ectasias and varices of the vocal fold: clearing the striking zone. Ann Otol Rhinol Laryngol. 1999;108(1):10–6.
99. Zeitels SM. Phonomicrosurgical techniques. In: Sataloff RT, editor. Professional voice: the science and art of clinical care. 4th ed. San Diego: Plural Publishing; 2017. p. 1479–500.

100. Zeitels SM, Sataloff RT. Phonomicrosurgical resection of glottal papillomatosis. J Voice. 1999;13(1):123–7.
101. Wellens W, Snoeck R, Desloovere C, et al. Treatment of severe laryngeal papillomatosis with intralesional injections of cidofovir [(S)-1-(3-Hydroxy-Phospho nylmethoxypropyl) Cytosine, HPMPC, Vistide]. In: McCafferty G, Coman W, Carroll R, editors. Proceedings of the XVI world congress of otorhinolaryngology head and neck surgery. Bologna: Monduzzi Editor; 1997. p. 455–549.
102. Holinger LD, Barnes DR, Smid LJ, Holinger PH. Laryngocele and saccular cysts. Ann Otol Rhinol Laryngol. 1978;87:675–85.
103. Ward PH, Frederickson J, Strandjord NM, Valvessori GE. Laryngeal and pharyngeal pouches. Surgical approach and the use of cinefluorographic and other radiologic techniques as diagnostic aids. Laryngoscope. 1963;73:564–82.
104. DeSanto LW. Laryngocele, laryngeal mucocele, large saccules, and laryngeal saccular cysts: a developmental spectrum. Laryngoscope. 1974;84:1291–6.
105. Norris CW. Pharyngoceles of the hypopharynx. Laryngoscope. 1979;89:1788–807.
106. Papsin BC, Maaske LA, McGrail JS. Orbicularis oris muscle injury in brass players. Laryngoscope. 1996;106:757–60.
107. Fiz JA, Aguilar J, Carreras A, et al. Maximum respiratory pressure in trumpet players. Chest. 1993;104:1203–4.
108. Stephanie A, Tarab S. Obscure and ventricular laryngocele. Schweiz Rundsch Med Prax. 1972;61:1520–3.
109. Macfie DD. Asymptomatic laryngoceles in wind instrument bandsmen. Arch Otolaryngol. 1966;83:270–5.
110. Backus J. The effect of the player's vocal tract on wood wind instrument tone. J Acoust Soc Am. 1985;78:17–20.
111. Isaacson G, Sataloff RT. Bilateral laryngoceles in a young trumpet player: case report. Ear Nose Throat J. 2000;4:272–4.
112. Sataloff RT, Chowdhury F, Portnoy J, Hawkshaw MJ, Joglekar S. Surgical techniques in otolaryngology – head and neck surgery: laryngeal surgery. New Delhi: Jaypee Brothers Medical Publishers; 2014.
113. Sataloff RT, Spiegel JR, Heuer RJ, et al. Laryngeal mini-microflap: a new technique and reassessment of the microflap saga. J Voice. 1995;9(2):198–204.
114. Abitbol J. Limitations of the laser in microsurgery of the larynx. In: Lawrence VL, editor. Transactions of the twelfth symposium: care of the professional voice. New York: The Voice Foundation; 1984. p. 297–302.
115. Strong MS, Jako GJ. Laser surgery in the larynx. Early clinical experience with continuous CO_2 laser. Ann Otol Rhinol Laryngol. 1972;81:791–8.
116. Sataloff RT, Feldman M, Darby KS, Carroll LM, Spiegel JR. Arytenoid dislocation. J Voice. 1988;1(4):368–77.
117. Sataloff RT, Bough ID, Spiegel JR. Arytenoid dislocation: diagnosis and treatment. Laryngoscope. 1994;104(10):1353–61.
118. Sataloff RT, Hawkshaw MJ, Sataloff JB, DeFatta RA, Eller RL. Atlas of laryngoscopy. 3rd ed. San Diego: Plural Publishing; 2012.

Part II
In-Office Surgery

Chapter 5
In-Office Voice Surgery: Basic Principles, Patient Selection, Safety, and Tolerance

5.1 Introduction

Endoscopic surgery may be performed in the operating room (OR) or in an office setting. External (transcervical) laryngeal surgery usually is performed in an OR. To provide optimal care, laryngologists must be familiar with the latest techniques in both approaches. Modern microsurgery of the voice is referred to widely as phonosurgery, although von Leden introduced that term originally in 1963 for procedures designed to alter vocal quality or pitch [1]. Voice surgery is a better term for delicate, precise laryngeal surgery, although phonomicrosurgery is used widely, as well. Usually, voice surgery is performed using a microscope, small, modern instruments, and with great respect for the induplicable anatomic complexity of the vibratory margin of the vocal fold. Similar precision can be achieved in an office setting for many procedures, using special instruments designed for in-office microsurgery such as those illustrated in Fig. 5.1.

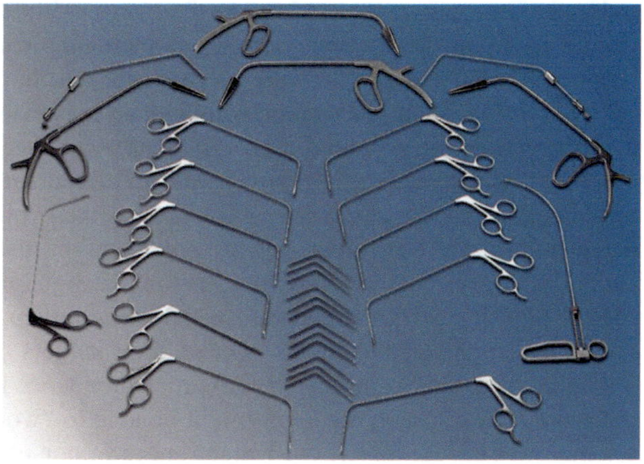

Fig. 5.1 Selected indirect laryngeal surgical instruments designed by the author (RTS). Manufactured by Integra LifeSciences (Princeton, NJ, USA)

A.-l. Hamdan et al., *Office-Based Laryngeal Surgery*,
https://doi.org/10.1007/978-3-030-91936-8_5

Most surgical procedures for voice disorders can be performed endoscopically, obviating the need for external incisions and minimizing the amount of tissue disruption. Although endoscopic microsurgery seems intuitively more "conservative," this supposition holds true only when the equipment provides good exposure of the surgical site and the abnormality can be treated meticulously and thoroughly with endoscopic instruments. When endoscopic visualization is not adequate because of patient anatomy, disease extent, or other factors, the surgeon should not compromise the results of treatment or risk patient injury by attempting to complete an endoscopic procedure in the office or in the OR. In such patients, it may be safer to leave selected benign lesions untreated or to treat the pathology through an external approach.

For a more comprehensive discussion of voice surgery, the reader is referred to other literature by Sataloff [2], a small portion of which has been modified in part for this chapter (with permission).

5.2 Patient Selection and Consent

Prior to performing voice surgery, it is essential to be certain that patient selection is appropriate, and that the patient understands the limits and potential complications of the surgery. Appropriate patients for voice surgery not only have voice abnormalities, but also really want to change their voice quality, effort, and/or endurance. Not all people with "pathological" voices are unhappy with them. Sports announcers, female trial attorneys with gruff, masculine voices, and others sometimes consult a physician only because of fear of cancer. If there is no suspicion of malignancy, restoring their voices to "normal" (e.g., by evacuating Reinke's edema) may be a disservice and might even jeopardize their careers. Similarly, it is essential to distinguish accurately between organic and functional or psychogenic voice disorders before embarking on laryngeal surgery. Although a breathy voice may be caused by numerous organic conditions including vocal fold paralysis, it is also found commonly in people with psychogenic dysphonia. The differentiation may require a very skilled voice team. Although all reasonable efforts should be made to avoid operative intervention in professional voice users, particularly singers, there are times when surgery is appropriate and necessary. Ultimately, the decision depends on a risk-benefit analysis. If a professional voice user is unable to continue adequately his or her career, and if surgery might restore vocal function, surgery should not be withheld. Sometimes, making such judgments can be challenging. A rock or pop singer with a mild paresis may have satisfactory voice quality with only minimal technical adjustments needed. Pop singers perform with amplification, obviating the need to sing loudly and project the voice in some cases (depending on the artist's style). Such a patient might be able to "work around" pathology safely for many years. However, even much more minor pathology can be disabling in some classical singers. For example, if a high soprano specializing in Baroque music develops a mild-to-moderate superior laryngeal nerve paresis, she may experience breathiness and instability. If she gives in to the temptation to compensate by slightly retracting her tongue and lowering her larynx, the breathiness will be controlled because of increased adductory forces, but she will lose the ability to perform rapid, agile runs and trills. Similar problems may occur from compensatory maladjustments in response to other benign lesions such as vocal fold cysts. In such instances, the artist may be served better by surgical correction of the underlying problem than by long-term use of hyperfunctional compensation (bad technique) that can itself cause other performance problems, as well as additional vocal fold pathology. The patient must understand all of these considerations clearly, including the risks of surgery. He or she needs to acknowledge the risk that any voice surgery may make the voice worse permanently even in the best of hands, and the patient must consider that risk acceptable in light of ongoing voice problems.

Other complications also must be discussed including (among others) complications of anesthesia, dental fracture, recurrence of laryngeal lesions, airway compromise, vocal fold web formation, and other untoward occurrences. In addition to the standard surgical consent, the author (RTS) provides patients with additional written information prior to surgery. The patient keeps one copy of the "Risks and Complications of Surgery" document, and the original signed copy remains in the chart. Specialized informed consent documents are used by the author (RTS) for other selected treatments such as injection of Cidofovir (Gilead Sciences, Inc. Foster City, California), and injection of botulinum toxin, even though such documents are not really required. If medications are used for treatment purposes (as opposed to research purposes) and are off-label uses of medicines approved by the United States Food and Drug Administration (FDA) for other purposes, their use does not require institutional review board (IRB) approval. However, it may be helpful and prudent to provide patients with as much information as possible and to document that they have been so informed. Our standard patient forms mention off-label medication use.

It is helpful for the laryngologist, speech-language pathologist, singing voice specialist, and patient to involve the patient's singing teacher in the surgery decision-making process. Everyone must understand not only the risks of surgery, but also the risks involved in deciding against surgery and relying upon technical maladjustments. In many cases, there is no "good" or "right" choice, and the voice care team must combine great expertise with insight into the career and concerns of each individual patient to help voice patients and especially voice professionals make the best decision.

5.3 Documentation

Preoperative objective voice assessment and documentation are invaluable in addition to routine documentation of informed consent discussions. As a bare minimum, a high-quality recording of the patient's voice should be made before surgery. Auditory memories of physicians and patients often are not good, and both the doctor and postoperative voice user are surprised frequently when they compare postoperative and preoperative recordings. Frequently, the preoperative voice is worse than either person remembers. In addition, such documentation is invaluable for medical-legal purposes. Photographs or videos of the larynx obtained during strobovideolaryngoscopy are extremely helpful. Ideally, complete objective laboratory voice assessment and evaluation by a voice team should be performed. Proper documentation is critical for assessing outcomes, even for the physician who is not interested in research or publication.

5.4 Timing of Voice Surgery

The timing of voice surgery is important and can be particularly challenging in professionals with demanding voice commitments. Many factors need to be considered including the menstrual cycle, pre- and postoperative voice therapy, concurrent medical conditions, psychological state, professional voice commitments, and others.

Hormonal considerations may be important, especially in female patients with symptomatic laryngopathia premenstrualis. In patients who have obvious premenstrual vocal fold vascular engorgement, or those who have a history of premenstrual vocal fold hemorrhages, it might be better to avoid elective surgery during the premenstrual period unless the surgery is intended to treat vessels that have hemorrhaged and that are prominent only prior to menses. In patients with conditions other than vascular lesions who have premenstrual symptoms and signs, it may be best to perform surgery between approximately days 4 and 21 of the menstrual cycle. Although it appears unnecessary to time surgery in this way for all patients, the issue has not been studied fully.

Timing of surgery with regard to voice therapy and performance commitments can be especially difficult in busy voice professionals. The surgeon must be careful to avoid letting the patient's professional commitments and pressures dictate inappropriate surgery or surgical timing that is not in the patient's long-term best interest. For example, some professional voice users will push for early surgery for vocal nodules and promise to appear for voice therapy later, after a busy concert season ends. This is not appropriate because therapy may cure the nodules and avoid surgical risks altogether. However, professional commitments often require that appropriate surgery be delayed until a series of concerts, the run of a play, a school year, political election, or other professional voice obligation is completed. In treating vocal fold cysts, polyps, paresis, and other conditions, such delays are often reasonable. They are made safer through ongoing voice therapy and close laryngologic supervision. Sometimes individualized treatments may help temporize. For example, injection of a temporary medialization material in the office or OR can provide temporary relief from symptoms, although the glottic incompetence is likely to return and require definitive surgery eventually. Injection of steroids into a cyst also may prove effective and might avoid the need for prolonged voice rest that may be required after excision.

At least a brief period of preoperative voice therapy is helpful, and the author (RTS) virtually never operates on benign vocal fold pathology or paresis without expert preoperative voice therapy. Even when therapy cannot cure a lesion, it ameliorates the abuses caused by compensatory hyperfunction, and good preoperative therapy is the best postoperative voice therapy. It is also invaluable in educating the patient about vocal function and dysfunction and in making sure that he or she is informed fully about surgery and other options. Following surgery, voice therapy is medically necessary for many conditions. It is extremely important for optimal, long-term surgical outcome to time surgery so that the patient will be able to comply with postoperative voice rest and postoperative rehabilitation with the voice team.

Many other conditions must be considered when deciding the timing of voice surgery. Concurrent medical conditions such as allergies that produce extensive coughing or sneezing (which may injure vocal folds following surgery), a coagulopathy (even temporary coagulopathy from aspirin use), and other physical factors may be important contributors to voice results. Psychological factors should be considered, as well. The patient must not only understand the risks and complications of surgery, but also be as psychologically prepared as possible to accept them and to commit to the therapeutic and rehabilitation process. Sometimes, psychological preparation requires a delay in surgical scheduling to allow increased time for the patient to work with the voice team and, in some cases, a psychological professional [3]. There are very few indications for benign voice surgery that contraindicate a delay of several weeks. It is generally worth taking the time to optimize the patient's comfort and preparedness. Indeed, in the author's (RTS) opinion, the patient is the most important part of the voice rehabilitation team. Realistic, committed collaboration by the patient is invaluable in achieving consistent, excellent surgical results.

5.5 Indirect Laryngoscopy

Laryngoscopic surgery generally is performed through direct laryngoscopy, as discussed elsewhere [2]. However, indirect laryngoscopic surgery has been performed for many years and still has value especially since technology has improved. It permits biopsy of lesions under local anesthesia, removal of selected foreign bodies, fairly meticulous resection of selected lesions using indirect laryngoscopic instruments, injection of fat, collagen and other substances, and other procedures. In patients whose necks will not flex or extend enough to permit rigid direct laryngoscopy (cervical arthritis, fracture, fusion), indirect laryngoscopic surgery may provide a safe alternative to external surgery.

For indirect laryngoscopic surgery, usually the patient is seated. Topical anesthesia is applied and may be augmented by regional blocks. The larynx is visualized either with a laryngeal mirror, laryngeal telescope, or flexible laryngoscope. The author (RTS) uses a flexible laryngoscope in nearly all cases, with an assistant managing the laryngoscope. When surgery is performed solely for injection (e.g., fat, collagen, or steroid), either an external or transoral technique may be used. External injection may be performed by passing the needle through the cricothyroid membrane and into the desired position in the vocal fold, through the thyroid lamina usually near the midpoint of the musculomembranous vocal fold about 7–9 mm above the inferior border of the thyroid cartilage, or through the thyrohyoid membrane. Transoral injection has been used most commonly, and the transoral technique is suitable also for biopsy and other procedures. Assistance usually is required for flexible laryngoscopic guidance. If a flexible laryngoscope is not used, the procedure can be monitored with indirect laryngoscopy. The patient's tongue is held with gauze, as for routine indirect laryngoscopy. Cooperative patients may be asked to hold the tongue themselves. This allows the surgeon to operate using both hands, but surgery can be performed safely even with a laryngeal mirror (Fig. 5.2) or telescope if no assistant available. If videolaryngoscopy is used during the procedure, and if the examination room has a second monitor behind the surgeon for the patient, the power is turned off during indirect surgical procedures. Angled instruments designed specifically for indirect laryngoscopic surgery are passed through the mouth and guided visually. Only a surgeon who is skilled in the necessary maneuvers should perform in-office procedures. The advantages of this technique include relatively easy access in anyone whose larynx can be visualized with a mirror or telescope, avoidance of the need for an OR procedure, and ready availability when delays in getting to a hospital and waiting for an OR might cause serious problems (e.g., a chicken bone or other foreign body perched above the laryngeal inlet). However, the procedure also has distinct disadvantages. Precise control is not as good as that accomplished with microlaryngoscopy under sedation or general anesthesia with paralysis, intraoperative loss of patient cooperation may result in injury, and the ability to handle complications such as bleeding and edema is limited. Nevertheless, an in-office, awake approach can be invaluable, and it should be in the armamentarium of the laryngological surgeon. In selected cases, we have found in-office surgery useful for suture removal, biopsy, resection of lesions (especially if the lesion is on the superior surface, or if the vocal fold edge is already scarred and perfect precision is less critical than it would be in the vibrating vocal fold of a voice professional), steroid injection into evolving vocal fold scar, augmentation, lysis of webs reforming early following surgery, CO_2 and vascular laser treatment, injection augmentation, arytenoid palpation, vocal process palpation, laryngeal dilatation, and other procedures.

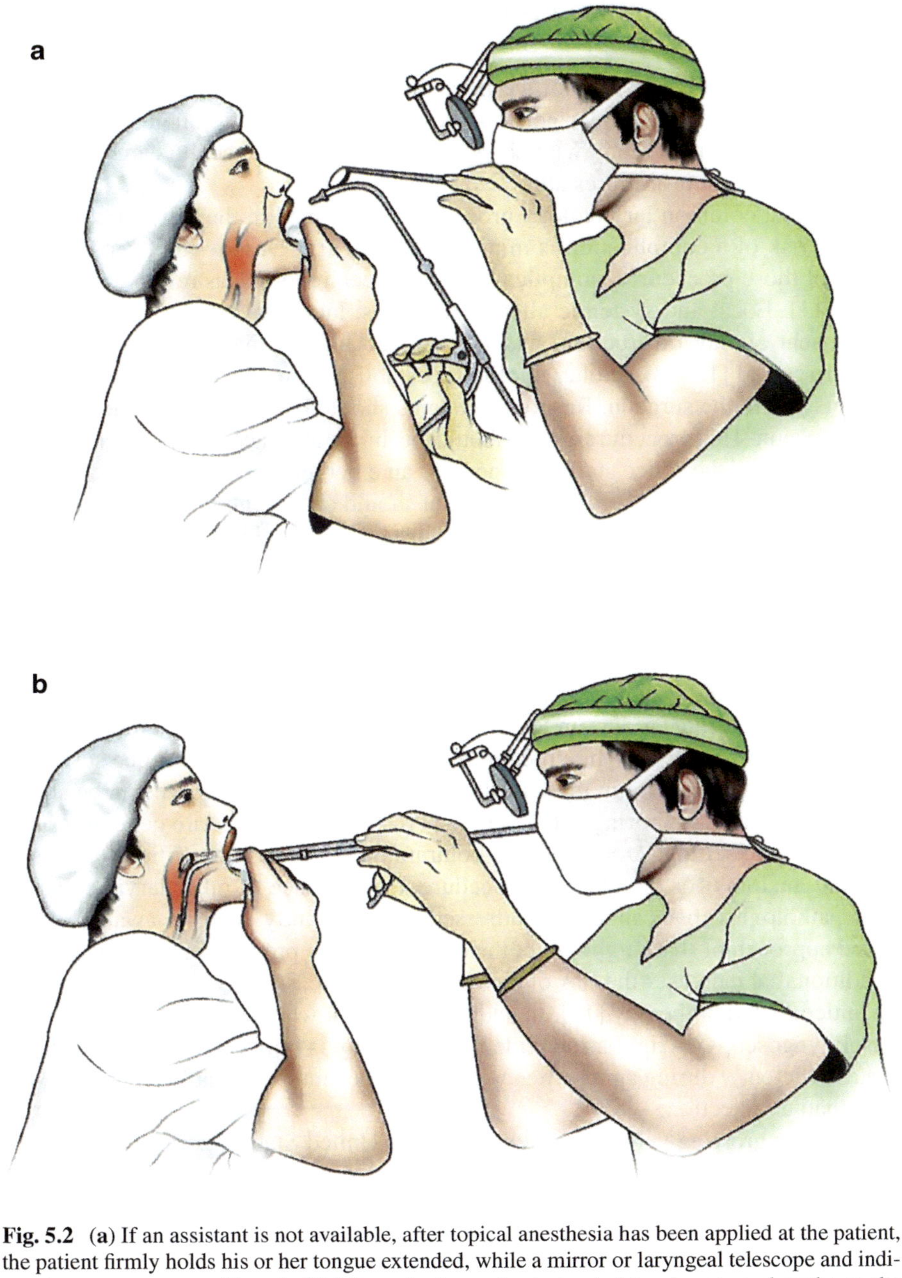

Fig. 5.2 (**a**) If an assistant is not available, after topical anesthesia has been applied at the patient, the patient firmly holds his or her tongue extended, while a mirror or laryngeal telescope and indirect instrument are positioned. (**b**) The patient may be instructed to phonate or breathe as the indirect surgery is performed. (Republished with permission. Sataloff et al. [80])

5.6 Safety of In-Office Procedures

The safety and efficacy of in-office procedures have been studied in comparison with similar procedures under general anesthesia [4, 5]. New policies for hospital inpatient management along with economic forces to reduce health care costs have made office-based procedures attractive alternatives [6].

The most common laryngology procedures performed in the office are safe and that the risk of a complication is minimal [4, 5, 7–10]. Despite the overwhelming safety of those procedures, complications have been reported, as reviewed by Ziade et al. [11]. Local and systemic allergic reactions, laryngeal edema, bleeding with subsequent airway obstruction, and mechanical and thermal tissue injuries have been described [12–18]. Otolaryngologists establish protocols to minimize harm to patients and to the surgeon. Response systems should be in place for when adverse events occur. The procedure room should be in an area accessible to emergency equipment, and the office staff to respond to an emergency [19].

As stated above, preoperative assessment should occur when evaluating and preparing a patient for an in-office procedure just as one would do for surgery scheduled in the OR. Appropriate patient selection remains critical in order to minimize risk and to improve outcomes with office-based procedures.

Allergy to the product being considered for vocal fold injection usually is an absolute contraindication to its use. Relative contraindications may be anatomic or physiologic in nature. For example, multiple severe, medical, comorbidities, especially those affecting cardiac and pulmonary function, are relative contraindications for in-office procedures. While they might seem to suggest that in-office surgery is preferable to a procedure in the OR, the in-office surgery experience can be stressful; and in-office monitoring and emergency response resources are generally superior in an OR setting. Other relative contraindications include difficult access to relevant anatomy for the planned procedure, the presence of other laryngopharyngeal pathologies that cannot be addressed concomitantly with an awake, office-based approach or that might affect the outcome of the procedure, and any medical condition that increases the risk of airway compromise, such as bleeding in patients on anticoagulation therapy [19]. In addition, a patient who does not tolerate flexible nasolaryngoscopy or rigid strobovideolaryngoscopy is unlikely to be able to cooperate sufficiently during an in-office vocal fold procedure, especially one more complex than an injection.

With the growing geriatric population in the United States, increasing consideration is being given to whether these patients are appropriate candidates for in-office procedures versus having the same procedure completed in an outpatient surgery center or in a hospital OR. As noted above, one cannot assume that any procedure with topical and/or local anesthesia in the office is "safer" than an equivalent procedure completed in the OR under sedation or general anesthesia. While this may be true for many patients, various factors must be considered.

5.6.1 Anesthesia Considerations

In the OR, the anesthesiologist can titrate the anesthetic or sedative agent(s) based on patient comfort, vital sign parameters, and the needs of the surgeon.

In some cases, topical/local anesthesia can pose more risk for airway compromise than general anesthesia with an endotracheal tube. Examples might include patients having difficulty managing their secretions, patients with increased risk of bleeding, and some patients with an airway foreign body.

The characteristics of the setting in which the procedure is to be performed can help the surgeon to decide on the appropriate facility. The availability of resources and personnel can vary greatly depending on the setting in which the procedure is being performed, and hospital ORs often are able to respond to emergencies faster and more comprehensively than physician offices.

There are patients who do better with in-office procedures because of the severity of their comorbid medical conditions such as ASA category 3 or 4, which can preclude a safe elective laryngeal procedure under general anesthesia in some patients [20]. A debilitating medical condition is not an absolute contraindication for office-based laryngeal procedures; however, any patient considered high risk for an OR procedure should be treated as high risk during office-based procedures. In general, patients considering in-office surgery should be considered for the same preoperative evaluations and medical clearances that they would need for surgery in the OR.

Assessment often includes vital signs; and a period of postprocedure monitoring often is appropriate [21, 22]. Rubin et al. have recommended that pulse oximetry, cardiac monitoring, and an intravenous access set should be ready for use at any time [19]. A "time-out" checklist should be completed prior to the procedure including confirmation of patient identifiers, patient allergies, procedure name, site and side of the procedure if applicable, confirmation that the consent form was completed and signed, and confirmation that all equipment, instruments, and medications are available.

5.6.2 Performance of Procedure

The successful completion of an in-office laryngologic procedure depends on preprocedure education of the patient, team support during the procedure, and expeditious surgery. Particularly when working during the limited effective time of topical and local anesthetics, efficiency is necessary. As the anesthetic begins to wear off, so may the cooperation of the patient. If the maximum dose of anesthetic already has been given, then the procedure may have to be terminated. If a procedure is expected to take longer than the usual duration of the topical anesthetic, performing it in the office may not be the best option.

5.6.3 *Recovery*

The amount of time that the patient spends in the office immediately following a procedure varies depending on the surgeon's practice, the patient's clinical status, and the procedure. With the risk of severe, early allergic reactions being exceedingly low for vocal fold injection using materials available currently, extended post-procedure observation usually is not necessary. In some cases, the patient should be advised to stay with a responsible adult for the first 24 h. Concerning signs and symptoms should be communicated to the patient and family/caregiver when possible, and the patient should be instructed to call the office or 9-1-1 (or the equivalent outside the United States) if an emergency occurs.

5.6.4 *Equipment*

The safety of equipment requires attention. Although some guidelines state that the risk of infection transmission from reprocessed medical devices such as endoscopes is very low (around one infection per 1.8 million endoscopic procedures), there is a higher transmission rate during outbreaks of infections such as influenza, and it is often overlooked [23, 24].

CDC Guidelines for equipment cleaning and sterilization may be followed and can be found online for various instruments and equipment (www.cdc.gov). According to the Spaulding classification of medical devices, flexible laryngoscopes are considered "semi-critical" medical devices, and high-level disinfection is recommended since they contact the nasopharyngeal mucosa without penetration [25]. They require manual cleaning, leak testing, cleaning with an enzymatic agent, high-level disinfection, and drying with vertical storage. Available methods for achieving high-level disinfection are (1) manual disinfection with a liquid disinfectant/sterilant used according to the set of instructions specified by the endoscope manufacturer, (2) an automated endoscope reprocessor, and (3) a disposable sheath [26–28]. Scopes should be cleaned thoroughly after they have been disinfected because some patients may be allergic to residual traces of disinfectant left inadvertently on an endoscope.

High-level disinfection destroys all microorganisms except for high numbers of bacterial spores. Heat-automated pasteurization (65–77 °C) over a period of 30 min can be used for heat-tolerant operative endoscopes and accessories. Liquid immersion in chemical sterilants [29–33] should be used for heat-sensitive endoscopes and accessories. Reprocessing procedures for each type of endoscope should be based on the medical device manufacturer's instructions for use. Annual infection control audits may help ensure adherence to the reprocessing standards and policies [31].

To avoid the transmission of infection between patients, considerations should include the parts of the device that were contaminated indirectly either during or after the examination [32]. Portions of the laryngoscope including the handle, eyepiece, and light cord can harbor organisms; therefore, these surfaces should be cleaned after use [32, 33].

5.7 In-Office Injection

A literature review on the safety of in-office injection laryngoplasty was completed using PubMed/Medline databases with the search terms "injection," "laryngoplasty," "vocal fold/vocal cord," "medialization," "safe," "safety," "in-office/office-based," and "complications." In total, 47 articles in English were identified from 1990 until January 2015 [11].

Injection laryngoplasty is one of the most commonly performed office-based laryngeal surgeries, and its indications have expanded to include treatment for vocal fold paralysis, paresis, atrophy, scar, and sulcus [7], as well as other procedures. It is discussed in greater detail elsewhere in this book.

Vocal fold injections have proven to be safe and effective [34, 35], but many case series and retrospective reviews have shown that the materials used and the procedure itself can lead to minor, or even serious, complications. Sulica et al. reviewed 460 in-office vocal fold injections using different techniques and injectable materials. Despite the overwhelming safety profile of vocal fold injections, they reported a case of vasovagal reaction and cases complicated by airway problems [21]. Zielke et al. concluded that adverse reactions can occur for all commercially available injectable materials. They found that the time interval between injection and the reaction, as well as the type of reaction, vary between different products [36]. For instance, hyaluronic acid can have local severe skin hypersensitivity and granulomatous reactions at the injection site when used for cosmetic reasons [37, 38]. Similar reactions can occur in the larynx. Also, cases of atrial fibrillation in a patient with underlying cardiac disease, airway inflammation, edema, hematoma, ulceration, and necrosis with subsequent airway obstruction were reported with the use of hyaluronic acid in laryngeal injections [12, 21, 39]. Anderson and Sataloff reported two cases of localized superficial lamina propria deposits of collagen after an injection laryngoplasty, and both patients were taken to the OR in order to remove the material [13]. A case of laryngeal abscess following injection laryngoplasty was reported by Zapanta et al. [40]. DeFatta et al. reported on 22 vocal fold injections using calcium hydroxylapatite in 16 patients resulting in 10 major complications including adynamic mucosa, severely decreased mucosal wave, and granulomas affecting the vibratory margin [41]. Furthermore, one case of severe laryngeal bleeding followed by pulmonary complications and death has been reported in the literature [14].

Rarely, unpredictable and unexpected complications may occur that may be challenging to manage in an office setting, such as breaking a laryngeal needle during indirect injection (Fig. 5.3) [42]. The laryngologist and office staff should be prepared to manage any eventuality.

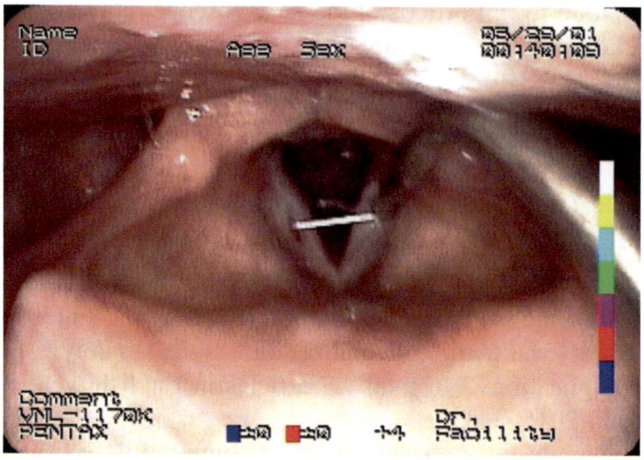

Fig. 5.3 This 20-year-old female underwent superficial dexamethasone injection for vocal fold stiffness approximately 2 weeks following resection of a vocal fold cyst. The injection went well, and good hydrodissection was accomplished. No unusual mechanical resistance was encountered. However, as the instrument was being removed, the tip of the injection needle broke off and lodged across the vocal folds, as illustrated. Although indirect alligator forceps were in the room, she had coughed and swallowed the foreign body before it could be retrieved. It passed without incident. (Republished with permission. Sataloff [81])

When considering a permanent augmentation, a trial vocal fold injection using a temporary material can be performed safely in the office [43]. In the author's (RTS) experience, when there is concern about potential airway compromise resulting from an in-office injection, it should either be done in the OR, or a trial saline in-office injection should be considered. The saline can be titrated to achieve optimal effect, but much of it will resorb within several hours, although effects occasionally last as long as 2 weeks. So, even saline injection should be performed and with caution. This trial injection allows the patient and surgeon to determine whether a longer-lasting injection or permanent medialization would result in a comfortable airway for the patient.

Botulinum toxin injection into the laryngeal muscles is carried out in the office setting most often for the treatment of laryngeal dystonias such as spasmodic dysphonia and tremor, as discussed in Chap. 9 [44, 45]. Botulinum toxin injections can result in complications related to technique or to effects on the muscles injected. Bilateral abductor paralysis resulting in airway obstruction may occur following bilateral injections for abductor spasmodic dysphonia. A rare case of abductor paralysis was reported following bilateral injection for adductor spasmodic dysphonia [46]. Botulinum toxin injection for abductor spasmodic dysphonia typically is done by many surgeons on one side at a time to avoid this complication. Rarely, botulinum toxin injected unilaterally can affect the contralateral posterior cricoarytenoid muscle inadvertently, resulting in temporary, bilateral abductor paralysis. Exposure of the cricopharyngeus muscle to botulinum toxin can result in dysphagia.

5.8 Injection of Substances Other Than Botulinum Toxin

Care should be taken not to inject superficially in the subepithelial plane, unless attempting hydrodissection for scar or to elevate a mass, too deep (inferiorly) causing infraglottic protrusion and increasing phonation threshold pressures in some cases, or to overinject an already compromised airway [34]. For medializations, the needle should be inserted at a slight angle to improve retention of the injected material. Some authors believe that 3 days of strict voice rest (including refraining from heavy lifting, straining, cough, and throat clearing) after the procedure will reduce the risk of extrusion, although others including the author (RTS) usually recommend voice rest for only 1–2 days. There is no convincing evidence to support either recommendation. Vocal fold injection is discussed in greater detail in Chap. 8.

5.9 In-Office Biopsy

A literature review on the safety of in-office laryngeal biopsy was completed using PubMed/Medline databases with the search terms: "laryngeal," "larynx," "vocal fold/vocal cord," "in-office/office-based," "safe," "safety," "biopsy," and "complications." In total, six articles in English were identified from 1990 until January 2015 [11]. This topic is revisited in greater detail in Chap. 12.

Advances in technology have allowed otolaryngologists to perform biopsies of the upper aerodigestive tract in the office safely, usually without the need for cardiopulmonary monitoring [8, 47, 48]. An important advantage is the ability to obtain a tissue diagnosis without going to the OR in many cases, which can reduce the time to diagnosis and treatment, avoid general anesthesia risks, and reduce health care costs [11].

Cohen et al. performed 102 in-office vocal fold biopsies, and the tissue was determined to be adequate for pathological studies in 96 patients (94.1%) [48]. The sensitivity of in-office biopsy ranges between 69.2% and 81.1%, while the specificity ranges between 96.1% and 100% [48, 49]. Lippert et al. reported a diagnosis rate of 83% for laryngopharyngeal biopsies obtained transnasally or transorally in the office [8]. Two of 116 patients did not tolerate the in-office procedure, and there were no complications reported. Time to treatment was reduced from an average of 48.8 days without successful in-office biopsy to 24.2 days with successful biopsy. Risk of bleeding following in-office laryngeal biopsy was investigated by Naidu et al. They performed 11 in-office vocal fold biopsies and concluded that mild bleeding after each procedure was common and self-limited, and no serious complications were encountered in any of the reported cases [50].

5.10 In-Office Laser Surgery

A literature review on the safety of in-office lasers for laryngeal pathology was completed using PubMed/Medline databases with the search terms: "in-office"/"office-based," "laser," "vocal cord/vocal fold," "larynx/laryngeal," "safe/safety," and "complications." In total, 40 articles in English were identified from 1995 until January 2015 [11]. This subject is addressed in Chap. 10.

Laser treatment is an integral component of the laryngologist's in-office armamentarium. In-office laser procedures can be carried out transnasally with the advantage of having an unobstructed view of the operative field with minimal tissue manipulation [51]. Lasers have been used safely to treat leukoplakia, localized laryngeal cancers, papillomas, small polyps, webs, ectasias, varices, and Reinke's edema successfully [52, 53]. Compared to cold knife surgery, lasers have been associated with improved hemostasis during the procedure and a decreased risk of post-operative bleeding [51, 54–56]. This can be particularly valuable for in-office surgery. If precautions regarding the use of laser technology are not followed, or if laser procedures are performed in less-than-expert hands, laser procedures can be associated with serious complications such as injury to adjacent tissues with subsequent edema and scar, as well as burns to the skin and mucosa, development of glottic webs, airway stenosis, and glottal incompetence [54, 56]. Even with the most expert surgical technique, such complications occur occasionally.

Many publications have provided laryngologists with advice about using lasers in the office safely. For example, it has been demonstrated that red rubber tubes are safer to use compared to plastic tubes, if a tube (such as a feeding tube) will be in place during the procedure [9, 57]. Using saline-soaked gauze or towels can add an additional barrier of protection from injury to the patient [56] but care should be taken to avoid drying and desiccation of the gauze since that may lead to a fire [57]. Proper eye protection, usually provided by the laser manufacturer, must be worn at all times by anyone in the room including the patient when the laser is in use.

5.11 In-Office Laryngeal Electromyography

Laryngeal electromyography (LEMG) is an office-based procedure that has become invaluable in the evaluation of vocal fold mobility and confirming placement of the needle during botulinum toxin injections [58]. It takes approximately 5 min to perform comprehensive diagnostic LEMG, and the most invasive part is the insertion of a 26-gage needle 37 mm in length for botulinum toxin injection or for diagnostic EMG, usually transcutaneously into selected intrinsic muscles of the larynx [21, 58]. In order to avoid transmission of blood-borne pathogens between patients and health care workers through needle stick, adequate safety and infection control protocols should be in place. Universal precautions and protective barriers are standard, as well as specific recommendations in the event that a health care worker should be exposed [59, 60].

This procedure has been associated with rare complications including infection, hematoma, vocal fold hemorrhage, and edema causing upper airway obstruction [21]. Therefore, bleeding disorders and use of blood thinners represent relative contraindications. Pre- and postprocedure cardiology evaluation for patients with pacemakers may be considered and repetitive stimulation studies usually are omitted in these patients. Caution should be exercised in a patient with glottic or subglottic stenosis in whom the airway is not protected with a tracheotomy. In this situation, LEMG of the thyroarytenoid muscles should be performed on one side at a time, as is usually the case, assuring that there is no symptomatic edema or hemorrhage before testing the other side [21].

Another potential risk is current leak and electrical injury. In order to avoid this complication, the patient should be grounded when appropriate, the equipment should have an isolation system that should be checked periodically for possible current leakage [61]. Moreover, extension cords should not be used, and the patient should remain isolated from other electrical devices during the evaluation [61].

5.12 In-Office Tracheoesophageal Puncture (TEP)

A literature review on the safety of tracheoesophageal puncture was completed using PubMed/Medline databases with the search terms: "in-office"/"office-based," "tracheoesophageal fistula/puncture," "TEP," "safe/safety," and "complications." In total, 20 articles in English were identified from 1995 through January 2015 [11].

Following total laryngectomy, tracheoesophageal prosthesis insertion is popular for alaryngeal speech. Traditionally, it was performed in the OR under general anesthesia, but with more widespread use of office-based, unsedated, transnasal esophagoscopy (TNE), several techniques for tracheoesophageal prosthesis placement in the office without sedation have been described [4, 10, 62–68]. It is considered to be a safe in-office procedure even for patients who underwent regional or free flap reconstruction [64]. It eliminates the need to extend the neck fully during the procedure, which can be difficult for patients who have undergone a complex reconstruction or who received radiation therapy [68]. However, creating a tracheoesophageal fistula can have complications associated with any of the steps during the procedure. These include the creation of a false tract, infection, bleeding, and pain [66].

The literature provides strategies to facilitate the procedure and minimize complications. A guide wire simplifies the procedure and helps ensure proper placement [67], especially in cases in which bulky reconstructions created a thick wall between the trachea and neopharynx [18]. Blind techniques for tracheoesophageal puncture should be avoided in most situations. It is preferable to see the tip of the needle in the esophageal lumen using an endoscope and to insufflate the esophageal lumen in order to minimize manipulation of the mucosa at the tracheoesophageal puncture site and avoid damage to the posterior esophageal wall [66, 68]. In addition, using a small needle (21 gage) may minimize damage to the mucosa, especially if many attempts are needed [68].

5.13 Patient Tolerance in Unsedated Office-Based Laryngeal Surgery

Patient cooperation is essential for successful office-based laryngeal surgery. Proper counseling and assuring that patient's expectations are reasonable can help improve patient tolerance and surgical outcome. The current literature indicates that despite advances in technology that facilitate treatment of upper aerodigestive system lesions using endoscopes with working channels, patient tolerance remains a concern. In 2004, in a review of 82 cases (30 laryngeal papilloma and 52 vocal fold dysplasia) treated in an office using pulse dye laser, Zeitels et al. reported the termination of 5 cases because of patient discomfort and/or poor visibility [69]. Postma et al. reviewed 611cases of transnasal esophagoscopy and reported termination of the procedure in 17 cases due to tight nasal passages. Moreover, two patients had vasovagal reactions that were self-limiting [70]. Trask et al. reported successful use of the transnasal approach for vocal fold augmentation in patients with vocal fold paralysis. The procedure was tolerated well by all the patients except one who developed a panic attack and dyspnea that necessitated a tracheotomy to secure the airway. The authors advocated the use of this approach as a safe and effective alternative to the transoral and percutaneous approaches for injection laryngoplasty [71]. Their results were supported by Hamdan et al. who reported the successful use of this approach in 16 patients. The procedure was tolerated well by all subjects with significant improvement in phonatory symptoms in two-thirds of their study group [72]. In 2006, Rees et al. investigated patient tolerance of in-office pulsed dye laser treatment and reported an overall average comfort score of 7.4 out of 10 (1 being the maximal discomfort). Only 13% of their study group (total 89 subjects) preferred to have the procedure done under general anesthesia if repeat surgery was needed in the future. Six out of fifty-four who had undergone similar treatment under general anesthesia reported more discomfort in the office setting. In the study group overall, discomfort was mostly in the throat and less in the nose. Almost one in two patients had problems with gagging [73]. In 2006, Amin reviewed patient tolerance in 10 patients who underwent vocal fold augmentation using the thyrohyoid approach and reported a mean tolerance score of 2.1 out of 10 with 1 being no problem. All procedures were completed successfully with marked improvement in voice handicap index score (21.3 preoperatively to 7.5 postoperatively), and in stroboscopic findings [74]. In 2013, Birkent et al. investigated patient tolerance of 35 patients who underwent in-office percutaneous injection laryngoplasty using the trans-cricothyroid approach. The patients were asked to rate their expected and experienced discomfort using a visual analog scale (1–10, with 1 being no pain) before the procedure and after. The patients' expectations were similar to what they reported immediately after surgery (4.57 vs. 4.41, respectively). The authors stressed the need to explain to the patient the different steps of the procedure in order to meet their expectations and improve patient tolerance [75]. A year later, Clary et al. described the use of a laryngeal introducer in injection laryngoplasty and reported a mean overall discomfort score of 4.53 + 1.82 out of 10 (10 being the worst). Similar to the study by Rees et al., the discomfort was more in the throat than in the nose [76]. Gadkaree et al. compared patient tolerance, anxiety, and discomfort in patients undergoing injection laryngoplasty using the peroral vs. thyrohyoid approach and reported higher (worse) scores in the thyrohyoid group. However, anesthesia-related discomfort was worse in those who underwent the peroral approach in comparison to the thyrohyoid approach [77]. In 2018, Bensoussan and Anderson reported patient intolerance and anxiety as exclusion criteria in office-based laryngeal surgery in their review on current practice of unsedated, in-office laryngeal procedures [78]. The review included 16 of 22 Canadian laryngologists. In 2021, Hamdan et al. reported patient tolerance in 178 office-based procedures using three different surgical approaches, including transnasal, peroral, and percutaneous [79]. The average tolerance score on a scale of 1–5 with 1 being very comfortable, was 1.68 ± 1.05 for the transnasal, 1.6 ± 0.91 for the transoral fiberoptic, and 1.84 ± 0.95 for the percutaneous approach, with no significant difference between the three (p value 0.77). There was also no significant difference between the three approaches in anesthesia discomfort and anxiety. The procedure was tolerated well by all patients except one who developed a vasovagal attack necessitating termination of the procedure.

In all the above reports, patient tolerance was key, for completion and success of office-based surgery. The importance of proper patient selection taking into account the patient's mental readiness and psychological state, and thorough preoperative counseling explaining the different steps of the surgical procedure and what to expect, cannot be overemphasized. Other important key success factors for better patient tolerance include adequate topical anesthesia of the upper airway, choice of the surgical approach accounting for anatomic variations such as tight nasal vault and obscure cervical landmarks, and the surgeon's training and experience. Excellent surgical dexterity and short duration of the procedure can improve patient tolerance and probably voice outcome, although research is needed to confirm that speculation.

5.14 Conclusion

The most commonly performed laryngologic in-office procedures have a low risk for complications. Nevertheless, a high level of office preparedness to handle rare but potentially serious complications is important. Balancing the systematic approach to preoperative assessment with the individual needs of the patient will allow the surgeon to select appropriate candidates for in-office procedures, protocols to minimize risks and treat complications; and safe, effective in-office laryngeal surgery.

Acknowledgments Portions of this chapter have been modified in part from Sataloff RT. Voice surgery. In: Sataloff RT, editor. Professional voice: the science and art of clinical care. 4th ed. San Diego; Plural Publishing; 2017. p. 1371–478.

References

1. von Leden H. A cultural history of the larynx and voice. In: Sataloff RT, editor. Professional voice: the science and art of clinical care. 4th ed. San Diego: Plural Publishing; 2017. p. 9–88.
2. Sataloff RT. Voice surgery. In: Sataloff RT, editor. Professional voice: the science and art of clinical care. 4th ed. San Diego: Plural Publishing; 2017. p. 1371–478.
3. Rosen DC, Sataloff JB, Sataloff RT. Psychology of voice disorders. 2nd ed. San Diego: Plural Publishing; 2021.
4. Koufman JA. Introduction to office-based surgery in laryngology. Curr Opin Otolaryngol Head Neck Surg. 2007;15(6):383–6.
5. Shah MD, Johns MM 3rd. Office-based laryngeal procedures. Otolaryngol Clin N Am. 2013;46(1):75–84.
6. Bové MJ, Jabbour N, Krishna P, et al. Operating room versus office-based injection laryngoplasty: a comparative analysis of reimbursement. Laryngoscope. 2007;117(2):226–30.
7. Rosen CA, Amin MR, Sulica L, et al. Advances in office-based diagnosis and treatment in laryngology. Laryngoscope. 2009;119(suppl 2):S185–212.
8. Lippert D, Hoffman MR, Dang P, McCulloch TM, Hartig GK, Dailey SH. In-office biopsy of upper airway lesions: safety, tolerance, and effect on time to treatment. Laryngoscope. 2015;125(4):919–23.
9. Franco RA Jr. In-office laryngeal surgery with the 585nm pulsed dye laser. Curr Opin Otolaryngol Head Neck Surg. 2007;15(6):387–93.
10. Bach KK, Postma GN, Koufman JA. In-office tracheoesophageal puncture using transnasal esophagoscopy. Laryngoscope. 2003;113(1):173–6.
11. Ziade G, Jaworek A, Sataloff RT. Safety of laryngology procedures commonly performed in the office. In: Sataloff RT, editor. Professional voice: the science and art of clinical care. 4th ed. San Diego: Plural Publishing; 2017. p. 1521–31.
12. Shamanna SG, Bosch JD. Injection laryngoplasty: a serious reaction to hyaluronic acid. J Otolaryngol Head Neck Surg. 2011;40(5):E39–42.
13. Anderson TD, Sataloff RT. Complications of collagen injection of the vocal fold: report of several unusual cases and review of the literature. J Voice. 2004;18(3):392–7.
14. Powell J, Carding P, Birdi R, Wilson JA. Injection laryngoplasty in the outpatient clinic under local anaesthetic: a case series of sixty-eight patients. Clin Otolaryngol. 2014;39(4):224–7.
15. Sanderson JD, Simpson CB. Laryngeal complications after lipoinjection for vocal fold augmentation. Laryngoscope. 2009;119(8):1652–7.
16. Sataloff RT, Spiegel JR, Hawkshaw M, Jones A. Laser surgery of the larynx: the case for caution. Ear Nose Throat J. 1992;71(11):593–5.
17. Koufman JA, Rees CJ, Frazier WD, et al. Office-based laryngeal laser surgery: a review of 443 cases using three wavelengths. Otolaryngol Head Neck Surg. 2007;137(1):146–51.
18. Britt CJ, Lippert D, Kammer R, et al. Secondary tracheoesophageal puncture in-office using Seldinger technique. Otolaryngol Head Neck Surg. 2014;150(5):808–12.
19. Rubin JBM, Harries M, Harris T, et al. Laryngeal intervention clinic: guidelines for development of a laryngeal intervention clinic (LInC). ENT-UK Newsl ENT Prof. 2010;20(6):3.
20. Mayhew D, Mendonca V, Murthy BVS. A review of ASA physical statistics – historical perspectives and modern developments. Anaesthesia. 2019;74:373–9.
21. Sulica L, Rosen CA, Postma GN, et al. Current practice in injection augmentation of the vocal folds: indications, treatment principles, techniques, and complications. Laryngoscope. 2010;120(2):319–25.
22. Volk GF, Hagen R, Pototschnig C, et al. Laryngeal electromyography: a proposal for guidelines of the European Laryngological Society. Eur Arch Otorhinolaryngol. 2012;269(10):2227–45.
23. Alfa MJ. Monitoring and improving the effectiveness of cleaning medical and surgical devices. Am J Infect Control. 2013;41(5 suppl):S56–9.
24. Simmons SA. Laryngoscope handles: a potential for infection. AANA J. 2000;68(3):233–6.

25. Spaulding E. Chemical disinfection of medical and surgical materials. In: Lawrence CA, editor. Disinfection, sterilization, and preservation. Philadelphia: Lea and Febiger; 1968.
26. Rutala WA, Weber DJ. Disinfection and sterilization: an overview. Am J Infect Control. 2013;41(5 suppl):S2–5.
27. Collins WO. A review of reprocessing techniques of flexible nasopharyngoscopes. Otolaryngol Head Neck Surg. 2009;141(3):307–10.
28. Liming B, Funnell I, Jones A, Demons S, Marshall K, Harsha W. An evaluation of varying protocols for highlevel disinfection of flexible fiberoptic laryngoscopes. Laryngoscope. 2014;124(11):2498–501.
29. Ayliffe G, Minimal Access Therapy Decontamination Working Group. Decontamination of minimally invasive surgical endoscopes and accessories. J Hosp Infect. 2000;45(4):263–77.
30. Bhattacharyya N, Kepnes LJ. The effectiveness of immersion disinfection for flexible fiberoptic laryngoscopes. Otolaryngol Head Neck Surg. 2004;130(6):681–5.
31. Rutala WA, Weber DJ. New developments in reprocessing semicritical items. Am J Infect Control. 2013;41(5 suppl):S60–6.
32. Bhatt JM, Peterson EM, Verma SP. Microbiological sampling of the forgotten components of a flexible fiberoptic laryngoscope: what lessons can we learn? Otolaryngol Head Neck Surg. 2014;150(2):235–6.
33. Muscarella LF. Prevention of disease transmission during flexible laryngoscopy. Am J Infect Control. 2007;35(8):536–44.
34. Chhetri DK, Jamal N. Percutaneous injection laryngoplasty. Laryngoscope. 2014;124(3):742–5.
35. Lisi C, Hawkshaw MJ, Sataloff RT. Viscosity of materials for laryngeal injection: a review of current knowledge and clinical implications. J Voice. 2013;27(1):119–23.
36. Zielke H, Wölber L, Wiest L, Rzany B. Risk profiles of different injectable fillers: results from the Injectable Filler Safety Study (IFS Study). Dermatol Surg. 2008;34(3):326–35; discussion 335.
37. Lupton JR, Alster TS. Cutaneous hypersensitivity reaction to injectable hyaluronic acid gel. Dermatol Surg. 2000;26(2):135–7.
38. Fernandez-Acenero MJ, Zamora E, Borbujo J. Granulomatous foreign body reaction against hyaluronic acid: report of a case after lip augmentation. Dermatol Surg. 2003;29(12):1225–6.
39. Chang J, Courey MS, Al-Jurf SA, Schneider SL, Yung KC. Injection laryngoplasty outcomes in irradiated and nonirradiated unilateral vocal fold paralysis. Laryngoscope. 2014;124(8):1895–9.
40. Zapanta PE, Bielamowicz SA. Laryngeal abscess after injection laryngoplasty with micronized AlloDerm. Laryngoscope. 2004;114(9):1522–4.
41. DeFatta RA, Chowdhury FR, Sataloff RT. Complications of injection laryngoplasty using calcium hydroxylapatite. J Voice. 2012;26(5):614–8.
42. Chia P, Jaworek A, Sataloff RT. Airway foreign body during in-office vocal fold injection. Ear Nose Throat J. 2017;96(3):97–8.
43. Carroll TL, Rosen CA. Trial vocal fold injection. J Voice. 2010;24(4):494–8.
44. Watts C, Nye C, Whurr R. Botulinum toxin for treating spasmodic dysphonia (laryngeal dystonia): a systematic Cochrane review. Clin Rehabil. 2006;20(2):112–22.
45. Stong BC, DelGaudio JM, Hapner ER, Johns MM 3rd. Safety of simultaneous bilateral botulinum toxin injections for abductor spasmodic dysphonia. Arch Otolaryngol Head Neck Surg. 2005;131(9):793–5.
46. Venkatesan NN, Johns MM, Hapner ER, DelGaudio JM. Abductor paralysis after botox injection for adductor spasmodic dysphonia. Laryngoscope. 2010;120(6):1177–80.
47. Verma SP. Office-based laryngopharyngeal biopsy. Oper Tech Otolaryngol. 2012;23:203–5.
48. Cohen JT, Safadi A, Fliss DM, Gil Z, Horowitz G. Reliability of a transnasal flexible fiberoptic in-office laryngeal biopsy. JAMA Otolaryngol Head Neck Surg. 2013;139(4):341–5.
49. Castillo Farias F, Cobeta I, Souviron R, et al. In-office cup biopsy and laryngeal cytology versus operating room biopsy for the diagnosis of pharyngolaryngeal tumors: efficacy and cost-effectiveness. Head Neck. 2015;37(10):1483–7.

50. Naidu H, Noordzij JP, Samim A, Jalisi S, Grillone GA. Comparison of efficacy, safety, and cost-effectiveness of in-office cup forcep biopsies versus operating room biopsies for laryngopharyngeal tumors. J Voice. 2012;26(5):604–6.
51. Hermens JM, Bennett MJ, Hirshman CA. Anesthesia for laser surgery. Anesth Analg. 1983;62(2):218–29.
52. McMillan K, Shapshay SM, McGilligan JA, Wang Z, Rebeiz EE. A 585-nanometer pulsed dye laser treatment of laryngeal papillomas: preliminary report. Laryngoscope. 1998;108(7):968–72.
53. Franco RA Jr, Zeitels SM, Farinelli WA, Faquin W, Anderson RR. 585-nm pulsed dye laser treatment of glottal dysplasia. Ann Otol Rhinol Laryngol. 2003;112(9, pt 1):751–8.
54. Reinisch L, Ossoff RH. Laser applications in otolaryngology. Otolaryngol Clin N Am. 1996;29(6):891–2.
55. Centric A, Hu A, Heman-Ackah YD, Divi V, Sataloff RT. Office-based pulsed-dye laser surgery for laryngeal lesions: a retrospective review. J Voice. 2014;28(2):262.e9–262.e12.
56. Ossoff RH. Laser safety in otolaryngology—head and neck surgery: anesthetic and educational considerations for laryngeal surgery. Laryngoscope. 1989;99(8, pt 2, suppl 48):1–26.
57. Strong MS, Jako GJ, Vaughan CW, Healy GB, Polanyi T. The use of CO2 laser in otolaryngology: a progress report. Trans Sect Otolaryngol Am Acad Ophthalmol Otolaryngol. 1976;82(5):595–602.
58. Sataloff RT, Praneetvatakul P, Heuer RJ, et al. Laryngeal electromyography: clinical application. J Voice. 2010;24(2):228–34.
59. Occupational Safety and Health Administration. Occupational exposure to bloodborne pathogens; Final rule. Fed Regist. 1991;(29 CFR Part 1910.1030):64004–182.
60. Panlilio AL, Panlilio AL, Cardo DM, Grohskopf LA, Heneine W, Ross CS. Updated U.S. Public Health Service guidelines for the management of occupational exposures to HIV and recommendations for postexposure prophylaxis. MMWR Recomm Rep. 2005;54(RR-9):1–17.
61. Perlman A. Electromyography in oral and pharyngeal motor disorders. GI Motility. 2006. https://doi.org/10.1038/gimo32.
62. Doctor VS, Enepekides DJ, Farwell DG, Belafsky PC. Transnasal oesophagoscopy-guided in-office secondary tracheoesophageal puncture. J Laryngol Otol. 2008;122(3):303–6.
63. Sidell D, Ghadiali M, Chhetri DK. Unsedated officebased tracheoesophageal puncture using a novel guidewire technique. Otolaryngol Head Neck Surg. 2010;142(2):284–5.
64. Bergeron JL, Jamal N, Erman A, Chhetri DK. Office-based tracheoesophageal puncture: updates in techniques and outcomes. Am J Otolaryngol. 2014;35(5):549–53.
65. Ng RW, Lam P, Wong BY. Insertion of Provox2 voice prosthesis using the anterograde technique immediately after the secondary tracheoesophageal puncture. J Laryngol Otol. 2005;119(12):988–90.
66. Morrison MP, Chheda NN, Postma GN. The tough tracheoesophageal puncture. Am J Otolaryngol. 2012;33(1):113–5.
67. Allen J, Belafsky PC. Seldinger technique for in-office tracheoesophageal puncture. Ear Nose Throat J. 2010;89(8):355–6.
68. Fukuhara T, Fujiwara K, Nomura K, Miyake N, Kitano H. New method for in-office secondary voice prosthesis insertion under local anesthesia by reverse puncture from esophageal lumen. Ann Otol Rhinol Laryngol. 2013;122(3):163–8.
69. Zeitels SM, Franco RA Jr, Dailey SH, Burns JA, Hillman RE, Anderson RR. Office-based treatment of glottal dysplasia and papillomatosis with the 585-nm pulsed dye laser and local anesthesia. Ann Otol Rhinol Laryngol. 2004;113(4):265–76.
70. Postma GN, Cohen JT, Belfsky PC, et al. Transnasal esophagoscopy: revisited (over 700 consecutive cases). Laryngoscope. 2005;115(2):321–3.
71. Trask DK, Shellenberger DL, Hoffman HT. Transnasal, endoscopic vocal fold augmentation. Laryngoscope. 2005;115(12):2262–5.
72. Hamdan AL, Ziade G, Jaffal H, Skaff G. Transnasal injection laryngoplasty. Ann Otol Rhinol Laryngol. 2015;124(6):474–9.

73. Rees CJ, Halum SL, Wijewickrama RC, Koufman JA, Postma GN. Patient tolerance of in-office pulsed dye laser treatments to the upper aerodigestive tract. Otolaryngol Head Neck Surg. 2006;134(6):1023–7.
74. Amin MR. Thyrohyoid approach for vocal fold augmentation. Ann Otol Rhinol Laryngol. 2006;115(9):699–702.
75. Birkent H, Sardesai M, Hu A, Merati AL. Prospective study of voice outcomes and patient tolerance of in-office percutaneous injection laryngoplasty. Laryngoscope. 2013;123(7):1759–62.
76. Clary MS, Milam BM, Courey MS. Office-based vocal fold injection with the laryngeal introducer technique. Laryngoscope. 2014;124(9):2114–7.
77. Gadkaree SK, Best SR, Walker C, Akst LA, Hillel AT. Patient tolerance of transoral versus percutaneous thyrohyoid office-based injection laryngoplasty: a case-controlled study of forty-one patients. Clin Otolaryngol. 2015;40(6):717–21.
78. Bensoussan Y, Anderson J. In-office laryngeal procedures (IOLP) in Canada: current safety practices and procedural care. J Otolaryngol Head Neck Surg. 2018;47:23.
79. Hamdan AL, Jabbour C, Khalifee E, Ghanem A, El Hage A. Tolerance of patients using different approaches in laryngeal office-based procedures. J Voice. 2021:S0892-1997(20)30456-2. Advance online publication. https://doi.org/10.1016/j.jvoice.2020.12.009.
80. Sataloff RT, Chowdhury F, Portnoy JE, Hawkshaw MJ, Joglekar S. Laryngeal surgery. New Delhi: Jaypee Brothers; 2014. p. 18.
81. Sataloff RT. Professional voice: the science and art of clinical care. 4th ed. San Diego: Plural Publishing; 2017. p. 1525.

Chapter 6
Topical Anesthesia in Office-Based Laryngeal Surgery

6.1 Introduction

Office-based laryngeal surgery dates back to the nineteenth century and has been used continuously to some extent. It was replaced for most procedures by direct laryngoscopy in the second half of the twentieth century [1]. However, office-based laryngeal surgery has regained popularity over the last few decades. This resurgence is ascribed in part to the advent of the flexible nasopharyngoscope with a working channel, and in part to the successful application of topical anesthesia to the upper airway. Topical anesthetic in otolaryngology practice has been used for more than a century and was reviewed for airway use more than 50 years ago [2]. Numerous procedures currently done in the operating room under general anesthesia used to be performed in an office setting while the patient was awake [3]. The main advantage of topical anesthesia to the upper airway is that it allows the patient to remain conscious, and hence breathe spontaneously. Additionally, the surgeon can communicate with the patient asking him/her to swallow, breathe slowly, or perform different phonatory tasks that may improve the surgical outcome. Other benefits include hastened recovery and improved time efficiency for both the surgeon and the patient [4–6].

Adequate topical anesthesia to the upper airway is essential for the success of any office-based laryngeal procedure. Appropriate patient selection taking into account the tolerance level and willingness to collaborate is crucial. Patients with high anxiety traits and low threshold for pain and patients with hyperactive gag reflexes may not be ideally suited for unsedated office-based laryngeal surgery. The choice of topical anesthetic, as well as the mode of administration, are important. Several topical anesthetics have been developed over the last century and are readily

Supplementary Information The online version contains supplementary material available at [https://doi.org/10.1007/978-3-030-91936-8_6].

A.-l. Hamdan et al., *Office-Based Laryngeal Surgery*,
https://doi.org/10.1007/978-3-030-91936-8_6

available for use by otolaryngologists. These are classified as amides such as lidocaine, prilocaine, and etidocaine, and esters such as tetracaine, benzocaine, and procaine. Each of these topical anesthetics has a recommended dosage, time of onset of action, and duration. For instance, lidocaine, which is the most commonly used topical anesthetic, is administered in concentrations of 2% and 4%. The effect starts within 90 s and lasts 15–20 min before starting to abate. Pontocaine is also commonly used in a 2% concentration solution and carries a longer half-life than that of lidocaine. Cocaine is used less frequently despite its added value in terms of high potency and vasoconstriction. The decline in its usage is ascribed to associated adverse reactions and fear of toxicity [6]. The mode of application of topical anesthesia to the upper airway is also important. The method of choice must take into consideration the surgeon's expertise and the patients' anatomic features. A severe septal deviation may preclude the administration of local anesthetic via the working channel of a nasopharyngoscope, whereas a large base of tongue and/or restricted temporomandibular joint movement may hinder administration of the anesthetic orally. Similarly, a strong gag reflex may impair the efficacy of topical anesthesia to the hypopharynx and lower airway. Other patients' related factors that should be considered while applying topical anesthesia to the upper airway are age and the presence of co-morbidities. For example, an elderly with cardiovascular disease undergoing office-based laryngeal surgery requires diligent monitoring and readiness for emergency intervention.

This chapter reviews the methods used to apply topical anesthesia to the upper airway. The effect of topical anesthesia on the sensation and function of the laryngopharyngeal complex is reviewed and associated systemic toxicities are discussed.

6.2 Topical Anesthesia to the Upper Airway; Anatomic Sites and Methods of Application

6.2.1 Topical Anesthesia to the Nasal Cavity

The use of topical anesthesia to the nose while performing diagnostic and therapeutic office-based nasopharyngolaryngoscopy is common practice although questioned by some [7–9]. The local anesthetic is applied usually with a decongestant (0.05% oxymetazoline) or preceded by application of a decongestant that provides widening of the nasal passage and improved hemostasis in case of adverse injury to the mucosal lining. If cocaine is used, adding a vasoconstrictor is unnecessary given the high vasoconstrictor effect of this topical anesthetic. The effect of topical anesthesia on the nasal mucosa varies with the type of anesthetic used and its mode of application. In a study of 200 patients who underwent diagnostic transnasal fiberoptic laryngoscopy, Özkırış et al. reported less pain in the group who used lidocaine and prilocaine in comparison to those who received bupivacaine and ropivacaine [8]. In another study, Bourolias et al. compared the efficacy of lidocaine 10% vs.

tetracaine 2% applied to the nasal mucosa for 10 min, and showed less pain in those who had topical anesthesia using tetracaine. The study group consisted of 48 patients who underwent office-based transnasal laryngoscopy [9]. The effect of topical anesthesia also varies with the mode of administration. Anesthesia to the nasal cavity is commonly applied using anesthetic spray, gel, or cotton pledgets soaked with the local anesthetic and inserted into the nasal cavity for 10–15 min [5, 6, 10]. There is no consensus in the literature on the most effective mode of application. Zainudin et al. compared nasal gel anesthesia vs. nasal spray anesthesia (lignocaine) in 55 patients undergoing fiberoptic bronchoscopy. The authors reported more discomfort and/or pain in those who had lignocaine spray vs. those who had lignocaine gel [11]. In another prospective, randomized, controlled study of 240 patients undergoing ultrathin esophagogastro-duedonoscopy, Hu reported less nasal pain using cotton-tipped pledgers vs. endoscopic-guided aerosolized spray to the nasal cavity. Moreover, the overall patient tolerance was higher in the former group [12].

6.2.2 Topical Anesthesia to the Pharynx

Successful topical anesthesia to the pharynx is a prerequisite for successful office-based endoscopic procedures on the upper aero-digestive system inferior to the nose. The topical anesthetic is commonly administered by spraying the oral cavity, oropharynx, and hypopharynx with 2% or 4% lidocaine, although some physicians prefer other medications such as Cetacaine (Cetylite, Pennsauken, NJ), a combination of benzocaine 14%, butamben 2%, and tetracaine hydrochloride 2%. The first 2 s of spraying usually aim at the base of the tongue, hypopharynx, soft palate, and posterior pharyngeal wall. The patient may be asked to swallow and pant or inhale deeply while additional spray is applied. Deep inhalation during spraying allows some of the anesthetics to reach the larynx and trachea. Spraying may be repeated intermittently at 3–4 min intervals (8–14 sprays on average) [6, 11]. Topical anesthesia to the hypopharynx also may be applied directly using a cotton ball held by a curved forcep. This technique allows access to the base of the tongue, epiglottis, and even pyriform sinuses [6]. For safety, a cotton ball with a string attached should be considered in case the cotton ball is dislodged from the forceps (Fig. 6.1). Alternatively, patients may be asked to gargle the anesthetic solution for few minutes or to use an anesthetic gel. Sohmer et al. reported their experience with lidocaine 2.5% and prilocaine 2.5% cream application to the base of tongue in 57 patients undergoing bronchoscopy. The procedure was tolerated well by almost all patients without the need for other forms of anesthesia except for lidocaine liquid in the larynx [13]. Similarly, Amornyotin et al. compared the effect of viscous lidocaine solution vs. lidocaine spray on pharyngeal anesthesia in a large group of patients undergoing esophagogastroduodenoscopy. The authors reported better clinical efficacy and less pain in those who were anesthetized using spray in comparison to those who were anesthetized using viscous lidocaine [14]. Another less frequently

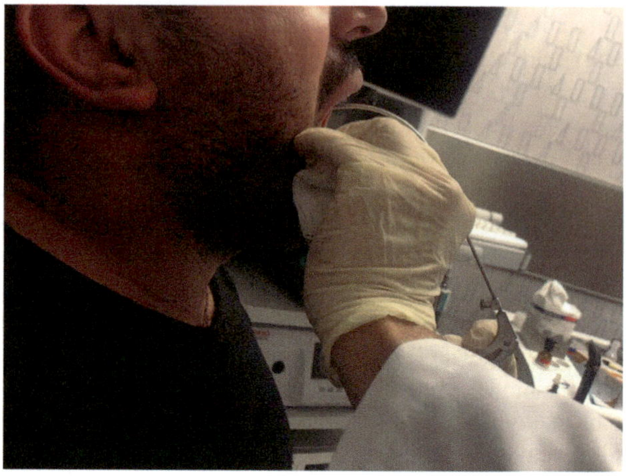

Fig. 6.1 Cotton swab at the base of the tongue introduced orally using a curved cup forceps

used option is asking the patient to suck anesthetic lozenges. Chan et al. compared the effectiveness of anesthetic lozenges vs. xylocaine spray in 191 patients undergoing unsedated esophagogastroduodenoscopy. Patients and physicians had comparable satisfaction rates using either form of local anesthetic. However, those who had their pharynx sprayed had less gag and better tolerance than those who sucked lozenges, but those who used lozenges had better taste experience [15].

6.2.3 *Local Anesthesia to the Larynx*

As noted above, topical anesthesia to the larynx for office procedures is not new; and topical anesthesia of the larynx also has been advocated for patients undergoing general anesthesia. In 1985, Colman and Reynolds reported the topical application of 10% cocaine solution to the larynges of adults and children undergoing endoscopy to the upper airway and digestive system under general anesthesia. The aim was to prevent laryngeal spasm following removal of the endotracheal tube [16]. With the advent of instrumentations and technology, topical anesthesia to the larynx has become the norm for all office-based laryngeal procedures. The objective is to secure a calm surgical bed for 15–20 min, during which there is a decrease in laryngeal sensation and attenuation of the brisk adductor reflexes that occur during unanesthetized stimulation such as surgical manipulation. Several modes of administration are described in the literature. These include dripping the local anesthetic via the working channel of the flexible nasopharyngoscope, dispersing the local anesthetic via a small catheter introduced through the working channel of the flexible nasopharyngoscope, or delivering the local anesthetic via a curved suction or cannula introduced perorally. Other commonly described techniques include the use of a pressurized nebulizer to inhale the anesthetic, or injection of the local anesthetic into the airway using a 25-gage needle that is inserted percutaneously via the cricothyroid membrane or trachea. Nerve block of the internal laryngeal branches of the superior laryngeal nerves is used less frequently but can be extremely effective.

1. *Administration of topical anesthetic to the larynx via the flexible nasopharyngoscope*. In this technique, the flexible nasopharyngoscope is introduced into the nasal cavity and is positioned behind the soft palate just above the base of tongue and tip of the epiglottis. Then, the topical anesthetic, most commonly lidocaine 2% or 4%, is dripped through the working channel of the flexible nasopharyngoscope while the patient is asked to sustain an /i/ or sniff (Fig. 6.2). Following that, the tip of the flexible nasopharyngoscope is introduced further down the laryngeal inlet to just above the vocal folds, and the patient is asked to phonate while the local anesthetic is dripped. This maneuver is referred sometimes to as "laryngeal gargle" (Fig. 6.3, Video 6.1) [17]. Alternatively, the topical anesthetic

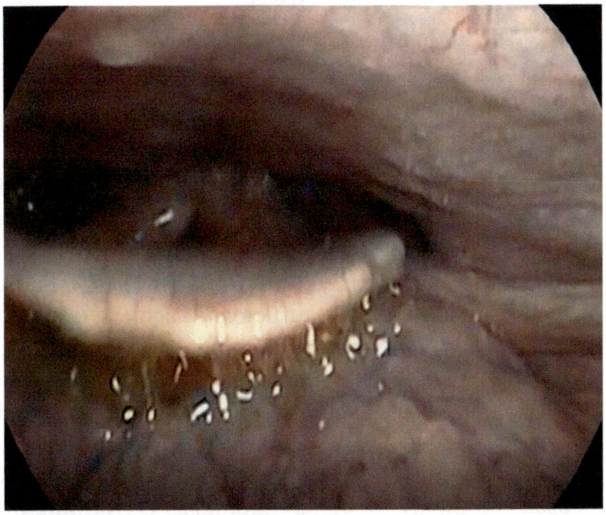

Fig. 6.2 Laryngeal endoscopic view showing local anesthesia (lidocaine 2%) dripped at the base of tongue and supraglottis during sniffing

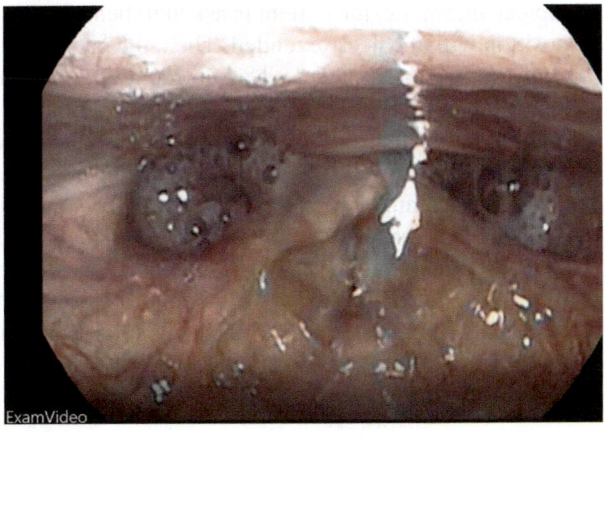

Fig. 6.3 "Laryngeal gargle" using lidocaine 2% seen on laryngeal endoscopy. Note how the liquid solution is dispersed throughout the laryngeal cavity and pyriform sinuses

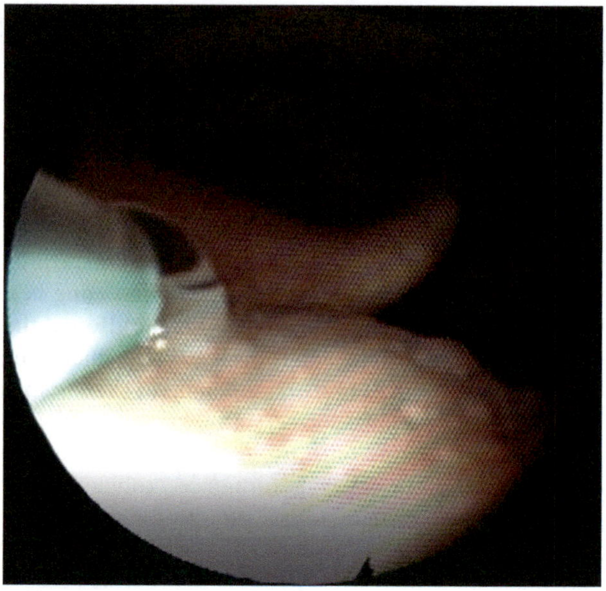

Fig. 6.4 Topical anesthesia solution (2% lidocaine) applied to the base of tongue and epiglottis using a Teflon catheter introduced through the working channel of flexible endoscope

can be delivered via a small catheter that is introduced through the working channel of the fiberoptic nasopharyngoscope (Fig. 6.4). Based on a review of regional anesthesia for office-based procedures in otolaryngology, Wang and Simpson reported that a total of 2–4 ml of 4% lidoacine installed as aliquots to the laryngeal surface is sufficient to achieve topical anesthesia to the larynx [5]. During the administration of anesthesia to the larynx, some of the local anesthetics may reach the subglottis and trachea. The elicited cough allows further dispersion of the anesthetic solution in the larynx and pharynx [6, 18].

2. *Administration of the local anesthetic to the larynx via the oral route.* Administration of topical anesthesia to the larynx using the peroral approach is used commonly by otolaryngologists performing office-based laryngeal procedures. After having sprayed the oral cavity with lidocaine 2% or 4%, or another topical anesthetic, the patient is asked to bend forward and assume the "sniffing" position with the neck extended. Then, the patient is asked to open his/her mouth while an Abraham cannula is advanced to the oropharyngeal cavity in one hand, and the tongue is grasped with the other hand. Visualization may be achieved with an assistant controlling a flexible laryngoscope. Alternatively, the patient may be asked to hold his/her tongue using a gauze while the physician introduces the cannula perorally. This frees the surgeons hand to visualize with a laryngeal mirror, as was done for many decades before flexible laryngoscopy became available in the 1970s. The topical anesthetic is then dripped at the base of the tongue and at the tip of the epiglottis [5, 6, 11, 18]. A few seconds later, while a direct visualization of the larynx is secured using a flexible nasopharyngoscope (or using a mirror) that is positioned behind the palate, the cannula is introduced further down the laryngeal inlet, and the local anesthetic is applied.

The patient is asked to phonate to allow better distribution of the anesthetic to the entire laryngeal mucosa. If the patient inhales during application of the anesthetic, excellent anesthesia of the vibratory margins and subglottic area is achieved. See Video 6.2.

3. *Administration of the local anesthetic to the larynx via a nebulizer device.* Nebulized anesthesia to the nose, pharynx, larynx, and tracheobronchial tree was described initially by Thawley in 1987 as a safe alternative to other methods of local anesthesia to the upper airway [19]. The authors advocated the safety of this technique and its added value in avoiding laryngeal manipulation and hence trauma and/or discomfort to the patient (Fig. 6.5). Since then the efficacy of nebulized anesthesia has been reported by numerous authors. In a review of 273 patients undergoing examination of the larynx and tracheobronchial tree, Christoforidis et al. reported good or excellent topical anesthesia using ultrasonic nebulizer in 94% of cases. The authors used 4–7 ml of lidocaine 4% [20]. Noitasaeng et al. compared lidocaine spray (5 puffs over 20 min) vs. nebulized lidocaine (250 mg over for 15 min) in patients undergoing esophagogastroduodenoscopy (EGD) and reported better patient acceptance of the procedure in those who used the nebulizer [21]. Another major advantage of using a nebulizer to deliver topical anesthesia to the upper airway is the even distribution of the aerosol to the entire mucosal lining of the larynx and lower airway. It is important to note that the effect of the nebulizer is partially determined by the size of the aerosol particles. Large particle atomizers are more likely to deposit in the larynx and pharynx, whereas small particle atomizers are more likely to deposit in the lungs. As beautifully described by Erickson, larger particles will "rain out" and coalesce in the hypopharynx and larynx whereas the smaller ones will reach

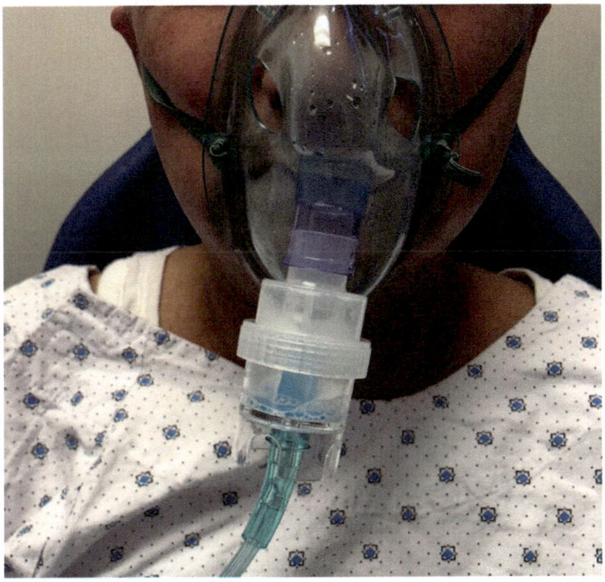

Fig. 6.5 Two cc of 2% lidocaine topical anesthesia administered using a nebulizer

the lungs [2]. Supporting this observation, Perkins et al. investigated the deposition patterns of different-sized particles of inhaled corticosteroids in the larynx using a computational fluid dynamic model. The authors noted that large particles had higher glottic deposition than small particles [22].

4. *Administration of topical anesthesia to the larynx via the transcervical approach.* The administration of local anesthetic directly into the trachea is used commonly by many otolaryngologists who advocate the cricothyroid approach. By grasping the larynx with the thumb and index finger of one hand, 1-inch to 1.5-inch needle, attached to a syringe that contains the local anesthetic, is used to puncture the cricothyroid membrane or trachea. Surgeon preference ranges from 18-gage to 25-gage needle size. The surgeon is advised to make sure that air is withdrawn from the syringe before the injection. The presence of air bubbles on aspiration confirms the position of the needle in the airway. Alternatively, an assistant can provide a view of the larynx using a flexible laryngoscope. Following the injection of the topical anesthetic, the patient usually coughs. This allows the spread of the anesthetic to the larynx and pharynx (Fig. 6.6a, b, Video

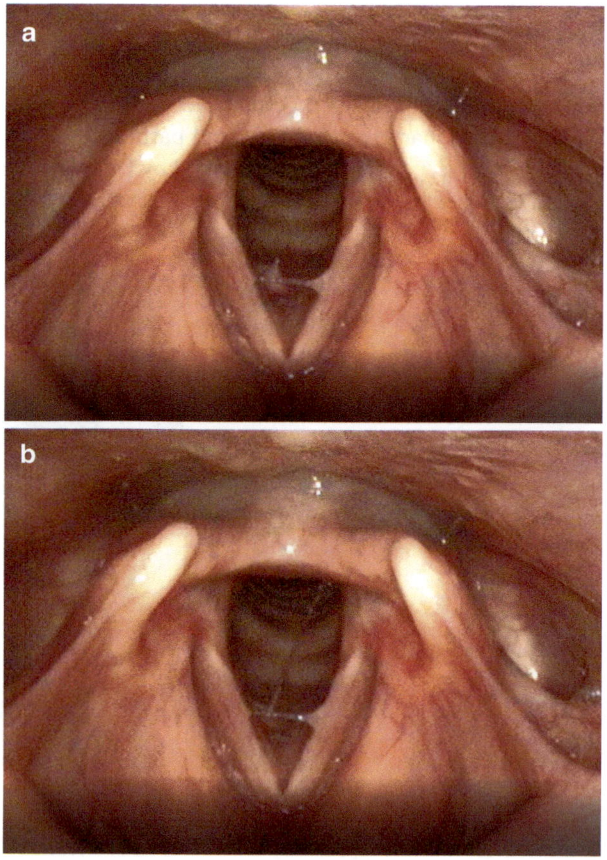

Fig. 6.6 Topical anesthesia administered via a 25-gauge needle inserted through the cricothyroid membrane (**a**) showing the tip of the needle penetrating the airway, (**b**) showing the injection of the lidocaine into the airway

6.3) [5, 6]. Very rarely, forceful cough with the needle in place can lead to pneumomediastinum. Topical anesthetic also can be applied using a spinal needle inserted through the thyrohyoid membrane with fiberoptic visualization.

5. *Administration of laryngeal anesthesia via superior laryngeal nerve block.* Superior laryngeal nerve block is an option reserved for outpatient surgery patients who are refractory to or fail the delivery of topical anesthesia via the discussed above approaches. The physician starts by identifying the superior cornu of the thyroid cartilage and the greater cornu of the hyoid bone. The hyoid bone is then displaced or tilted laterally toward the side where the injection is intended, about 1 cm anterior to the line between these two anatomic landmarks, and the local anesthetic is injected in the space between the thyroid cartilage and hyoid bone at the laryngeal entry of the internal branch of the superior laryngeal nerve [2, 5]. Unlike the percutaneous cricothyroid approach in which the needle pierces the cricothyroid membrane, while performing superior laryngeal anesthesia through topical medication, the needle does not penetrate the laryngeal lumen. It is important to note that superior laryngeal nerve block provides anesthesia to the supraglottic region and not the infraglottic region.

There is no clear consensus in the literature on the best anesthetic approach/technique for unsedated office-based laryngeal surgery. The choice of approach/technique is left to the discretion of the surgeon who needs to take into consideration patient related-factors such as anatomy and tolerance, as well as comorbidities. Patients with hyperactive gag reflex, abnormal oropharyngeal anatomy such as hypertrophic tonsils or prominent cervical osteophytes may not be eligible for peroral administration of topical anesthesia. Moreover, for some such patients, unsedated office-based surgery might not be the best approach. If there are compelling reasons to use office-based surgery, mild sedation may help overcome some of these problems, especially the hyperactive gag response. Often diazepam 5–10 mg the night before and 1 h before the procedure will be sufficient. Similarly, patients with obscure cervical landmarks may not be the ideal candidates for transcervical delivery of local anesthetic. Naunheim and Woo investigated the difference in patient satisfaction using three anesthetic techniques [23]. One hundred patients had topical anesthetic (lidocaine) delivered to the upper airway via either a nebulizer ($n = 32$), a cannula ($n = 35$), or a tracheal puncture ($n = 33$). Among the 90 patients who had surgery and had completed the survey, the highest satisfaction score was achieved in the tracheal puncture group, followed by the cannula group and the nebulizer group. Patients who received trans-tracheal topical anesthesia had the least amount of pain and nausea. Moreover, patient satisfaction correlated with the surgeons' satisfaction, which also was higher in the tracheal group in comparison to the other groups. In a recent study of 154 patients who underwent 176 different office-based laryngeal procedures, Hamdan et al. reported no significant difference in anesthesia discomfort between those who underwent the transnasal, peroral fiberoptic, and trans-tracheal approaches (2.16 ± 1.39 vs. 2.4 ± 1.29 vs $2.21 + 1.13$, respectively, p-value (0.825)). Similarly, there was no significant difference in the anesthesia time between the three groups [24].

In summary, the success in achieving topical anesthesia to the upper airway is determined in part by the patient's readiness for the office-based laryngeal procedure. The absence of a gag reflex, decreased sensation in the laryngeal mucosa, and attenuated adductor reflex, are invariably reassuring signs that the larynx and pharynx are well anesthetized. Economy of time is paramount during surgery as the time window for full anesthesia effect from lidocaine rarely exceeds 15–20 min. Administration of local anesthesia a second time may be needed in selected cases. Alternatively, a longer acting agent such as Cetacaine may be used.

6.3 Effect of Topical Anesthesia on the Pharynx and Larynx

Local anesthetics act by blocking the voltage-gated sodium channels at the surface membrane of the neural structure with a subsequent decrease in action potential propagation. In the pharynx, the decrease in chemosensory input results in impaired oral sensation and difficulty swallowing. The delay in the sensation of swallowing leads to prolongation of swallowing time and an increase in the interval between swallows [25]. Raphael et al. investigated the effect of lignocaine (sprayed or nebulized) and oral benzocaine lozenges on the upper airway reflexes and reported a significant elevation in sensitivity threshold [26]. The effect varied in intensity and duration with the method of delivery and type of local anesthetic used. Topical application of an anesthetic to the upper airway also has been shown to affect upper airway reflex regulation and airflow resistance. The change in airflow resistance is attributed to blockage of the airway receptors with subsequent impairment in reflexes. In a study of 16 healthy volunteers, Liistro et al. reported transient airway obstruction following extensive upper airway anesthesia using 10% lidocaine. The airway obstruction occurred during forced inspiratory and expiratory vital capacity maneuvers. There was also a decrease in maximal inspiratory flow rate 15 min after applying the anesthetic. The authors attributed their findings to dysregulation in upper airway reflexes responsible for maintenance of upper airway patency [27]. These findings are in agreement with a case report by Ho et al. published in 2004, who described complete upper airway obstruction in a 69-year old man following the application of local anesthesia to the upper airway [28]. Several studies have shown that local anesthesia to the upper airway also has an impact on the laryngeal behavior following tracheal extubation. Administration of topical anesthetic (lidocaine or lignocaine) to the larynx and trachea helps reduce postoperative laryngeal spasm, coughing, and sore throat [29, 30]. Mihara et al. conducted a meta-analysis looking at the efficacy of topical and/or systemic lidocaine administration in reducing the prevalence of laryngeal spasm and reported a significant preventive role with a risk ratio of 0.42. The analysis included 787 patients who had undergone general anesthesia [31].

Despite impairment in sensation following administration of a topical anesthetic to the upper airway, motor function of the larynx and pharynx are not affected. Rubin et al. investigated the impact of topical anesthesia on vocal fold motion in ten patients using transnasal flexible endoscopy and reported no significant effect. The briskness of vocal fold motion and the longitudinal tension of the vocal folds were assessed by five trained laryngologists using a visual analog scale [32]. Similarly, Mahajan et al. reported no change in peak cough flow and velocity following administration of topical anesthesia to the upper airway. The measurements were taken using tussometry which displays airflow rate against time [33]. In another prospective, cross-over, randomized, double-blind placebo-controlled study, Maxwell et al. showed no significant difference in electrographic parameters between subjects who gargled with placebo vs. those who gargled with lidocaine 2% and 4%. However, there was a difference in the logarithmic ratio of noise/signal energy for mid-range /i/ between the control group and the test group (lidocaine and placebo). Although there was no significant effect on the voice, mild dysarthria was noted in those who gargled with lidocaine [34]. Yang and Chen investigated the effect of topical anesthesia on the acoustic parameters of 30 subjects who were asked to sustain, the vowel /i/. The results indicated a nonsignificant decrease in the fundamental frequency in the anesthetized condition vs. control condition (125.7 + 19.7 Hz vs. 130.1 + 18.5 Hz) [35].

In summary, topical anesthesia to the larynx and pharynx leads to impaired sensation, and may lead to delayed swallowing and decreased airway reflexes. Alterations in airflow volume and resistance may ensue. Motor function of the pharyngeal and laryngeal muscles is not affected. Voice quality is unchanged perceptually and acoustic changes are not significant.

6.4 Systemic Toxicity of Topical Anesthesia to the Upper Airway

Systemic toxicity following administration of topical anesthesia to the upper airway has not been reported in office-based laryngeal surgery. In a review of 611 cases of transnasal esophagoscopy performed under topical anesthesia, Postma et al. reported safety of topical anesthesia in all patients without a single case of toxicity [36]. The lack of systemic toxicity following topical anesthesia to the upper airway also was reported by Sulica et al. in their review of 236 cases of office-based injection laryngoplasty. None of the cases had toxicity attributed to the use of topical anesthesia [37]. The lack of local anesthetic toxicity reports in office-based laryngeal surgery can be attributed to the paradigm shift away from the use of medicinal cocaine over the last 25 years. In a large survey on the use of cocaine by otolaryngologists, Long et al. reported a decline mostly due to the adverse reactions associated with its usage. These included hemodynamic alterations such as tachycardia and hypertension leading to cardiac arrest, in addition to neurologic sequel such as seizures [38].

Despite the replacement of cocaine by synthetic local anesthetics, and despite the behavioral modification in the application of topical anesthesia in terms of timing and dosage (intermittent vs. continuous, decrease in dosage) [39], the possibility of overdose and toxicity following the use of local anesthetic in any office-based procedure should not be disregarded. The severity of toxicity depends primarily on the plasma concentration of the local anesthetic administered, which varies with the agent used, the amount given, its extent of absorption at the site of application, and the efficacy of detoxification in the body, i.e., the excretory process. All these parameters should be taken into consideration when the topical anesthetic is administered in an office setting. For lidocaine, the maximal dose that can be given safely to a healthy adult is estimated to be 4.5 mg/kg, which amounts to an average of 200–300 mg. The dose may be increased to 500 mg if the anesthetic is mixed with a vasoconstrictor [37, 40, 41]. In a review by Wellenstein et al., the authors advocated the safe use of lidocaine in the range of 200–600 mg [10]. Another important determinant of plasma level is the absorption rate which varies with the site of installation of the local anesthetic. The rate of absorption has been reported to be higher in the pyriform sinuses and lower airway in comparison to the nasopharynx and hypopharynx. In addition, the mode of administration, in a single dose vs. stepwise application, also matters. Rosenberg et al. investigated the blood concentration of lidocaine after stepwise application of lidocaine spray to the upper airway and reported a peak level of lidocaine (1 pg/ml) in 20–30 min after spraying [41]. To avoid the summation of plasma peak level, the authors advocated the installation of the anesthetic at a 5-min interval.

When the plasma level of topical anesthetic reaches the toxic level (above 5 μg/ml in the case of lidocaine), symptoms and signs of toxicity appear. The toxic reactions are classified primarily as neurologic and/or cardiovascular. The neurologic symptoms include confusion, anxiety, auditory disturbances such as tinnitus, lightheadedness, muscle twitching, circumoral paresthesia, and, at times, tremors. In severe cases, the patient may develop signs of cortical stimulation and medullary depression leading to respiratory distress and convulsions [2, 6, 42]. The convulsion is ascribed to "*disinhibition of nerve conduction at the gamma aminobutyric acid (GABA) receptor complex*" as reported by McCaughey in 1992 [43, p. 178]. Hemodynamically, patients may experience hypotension, bradycardia, and peripheral vasodilation with possible collapse. Lidocaine toxicity also may exert an inotropic effect on cardiac muscle function resulting in decreased contractility and arrhythmias. Once recognized, neurologic and hemodynamic toxicities usually are treated with prompt administration of oxygen. Oxygen reduces the progression of hypoxia and acidosis and decreases the severity of the associated symptoms. Other possible complications of topical anesthetic include anaphylactic reaction and methemoglobinemia. This is a very rare condition characterized by oxidation of hemoglobin which makes it unable to bind or carry oxygen. The risk is higher when more potent topical anesthetics such as benzocaine are used. Benzocaine-induced methemoglobinemia is well-reported in the literature with significant morbidity if not addressed promptly [44–46]. A reasonable alternative commonly used by the author (RTS) is Cetacaine, which combines benzocaine, butamben, and tetracaine. Nevertheless, the availability of methylene blue for emergency treatment of methemoglobinemia should be available. Whited et al. reported a 71-year-old woman who developed methemoglobin of 10.5% following routine administration of tetracaine hydrochloride 1.0% for evaluation of hoarseness and dysphagia [47].

In summary, systemic toxicity following administration of topical anesthesia to the upper airway is extremely rare. Nevertheless, hemodynamic changes, as well as neurologic signs and symptoms, must alert the physician performing office-based laryngeal procedures to the possible adverse effects of the topical anesthetic. Stepwise administration of the topical anesthetic and not exceeding the recommended dose help avoid toxicity.

References

1. Zeitels SM. The history and development of phonomicrosurgery. In: Sataloff RT, editor. Professional voice: the science and art of clinical care. 4th ed. San Diego: Plural Publishing; 2017. p. 1347–69.
2. Erickson JC III. Surface anesthesia of the airway and larynx. Int Anesthesiol Clin. 1964;2(3):709–24.
3. Bredenkamp JK, Abemayor E, Wackym PA, Ward PH. Tonsillectomy under local anesthesia: a safe and effective alternative. Am J Otolaryngol. 1990;11(1):18–22.
4. Jourdy DN, Kacker A. Regional anesthesia for office-based procedures in otorhinolaryngology. Anesthesiol Clin. 2010;28(3):457–68.
5. Wang SX, Simpson CB. Anesthesia for office procedures. Otolaryngol Clin N Am. 2013;46(1):13–9.
6. Woo P. Office-based laryngeal procedures. Otolaryngol Clin N Am. 2006;39(1):111–33.
7. Frosh AC, Jayaraj S, Porter G, Almeyda J. Is local anaesthesia actually beneficial in flexible fibreoptic nasendoscopy? Clin Otolaryngol Allied Sci. 1998;23(3):259–62.
8. Özkırış M, Aydın R, Gencer ZK, Saydam L. Comparison of topical anesthetic effects of lidocaine, prilocaine, ropivacaine, and bupivacaine in transnasal fiberoptic nasopharyngolaryngoscopy. Am J Rhinol Allergy. 2014;28(3):e141–3.
9. Bourolias C, Gkotsis A, Kontaxakis A, Tsoukarelis P. Lidocaine spray vs tetracaine solution for transnasal fiber-optic laryngoscopy. Am J Otolaryngol. 2010;31(2):114–6.
10. Wellenstein DJ, van der Wal RA, Schutte HW, et al. Topical anesthesia for endoscopic office-based procedures of the upper aerodigestive tract. J Voice. 2019;33(5):732–46.
11. Zainudin BM, Rafia MH, Sufarlan AW. Topical nasal anaesthesia for fibreoptic bronchoscopy: lignocaine spray or gel? Singap Med J. 1993;34(2):148–9.
12. Hu CT. Gauze pledgetting versus endoscopic-guided aerosolized spray for nasal anesthesia before transnasal EGD: a prospective, randomized study. Gastrointest Endosc. 2010;71(1):11–20.
13. Sohmer B, Bryson GL, Bencze S, Scharf MM. EMLA cream is an effective topical anesthetic for bronchoscopy. Can Respir J. 2004;11(8):587–8.
14. Amornyotin S, Srikureja W, Chalayonnavin W, Kongphlay S, Chatchawankitkul S. Topical viscous lidocaine solution versus lidocaine spray for pharyngeal anesthesia in unsedated esophagogastroduodenoscopy. Endoscopy. 2009;41(07):581–6.
15. Chan CK, Fok KL, Poon CM. Flavored anesthetic lozenge versus Xylocaine spray used as topical pharyngeal anesthesia for unsedated esophagogastroduodenoscopy: a randomized placebo-controlled trial. Surg Endosc. 2010;24(4):897–901.
16. Colman MF, Reynolds R. The use of topical cocaine to prevent laryngospasm after general anesthesia on endoscopy procedures. Laryngoscope. 1985;95(4):474.
17. Hogikyan ND. Transnasal endoscopic examination of the subglottis and trachea using topical anesthesia in the otolaryngology clinic. Laryngoscope. 1999;109(7):1170–3.

18. Rosen CA, Amin MR, Sulica L, et al. Advances in office-based diagnosis and treatment in laryngology. Laryngoscope. 2009;119(2):S185–212.
19. Thawley SE. Nebulized anesthesia for the nose, pharynx, larynx, and trachea. Laryngoscope. 1987;97(4):499–500.
20. Christoforidis AJ, Tomashefski JF, Mitchell RI. Use of an ultrasonic nebulizer for the application of oropharyngeal, laryngeal and tracheobronchial anesthesia. Chest. 1971;59(6):629–33.
21. Noitasaeng P, Vichitvejpaisal P, Kaosombatwattana U, Tassanee J, Suwannee S. Comparison of spraying and nebulized lidocaine in patients undergoing esophago-gastro-duodenoscopy: a randomized trial. J Med Assoc Thail. 2016;99(5):462–8.
22. Perkins EL, Basu S, Garcia GJ, Buckmire RA, Shah RN, Kimbell JS. Ideal particle sizes for inhaled steroids targeting vocal granulomas: preliminary study using computational fluid dynamics. Otolaryngol Head Neck Surg. 2018;158(3):511–9.
23. Naunheim MR, Woo P. Topical anesthetic techniques in office-based laryngeal surgery: a comparison of patient preferences. Laryngoscope. 2020;130(1):166–70.
24. Hamdan A, Ghanem A, Khalifeh E. Tolerance of patients using different approaches in laryngoscopic office-based procedure. J Voice. 2021:S0892-1997(20)30456-2. https://doi.org/10.1016/j.voice.2020.12.009.
25. Chee C, Arshad S, Singh S, Mistry S, Hamdy S. The influence of chemical gustatory stimuli and oral anaesthesia on healthy human pharyngeal swallowing. Chem Senses. 2005;30(5):393–400.
26. Raphael JH, Stanley GD, Langton JA. Effects of topical benzocaine and lignocaine on upper airway reflex sensitivity. Anaesthesia. 1996;51(2):114–8.
27. Liistro G, STtãnescu DC, Veriter C, Rodenstein DO, D'Odemont JP. Upper airway anesthesia anduces airflow aimitation in awake humans. Am Rev Respir Dis. 1992;146(3):581–5.
28. Ho AM, Chung DC, To EW, Karmakar MK. Total airway obstruction during local anesthesia in a non-sedated patient with a compromised airway. Can J Anesth. 2004;51(8):838–41.
29. Davies DW, Moylan SL, O'Sullivan G. Topical anaesthesia of the larynx: cocaine or lignocaine? Eur J Anaesthesiol. 1992;9(5):393–7.
30. Altintaş F, Bozkurt P, Kaya G, Akkan G. Lidocaine 10% in the endotracheal tube cuff: blood concentrations, haemodynamic and clinical effects. Eur J Anaesthesiol. 2000;17(7):436–42.
31. Mihara T, Uchimoto K, Morita S, Goto T. The efficacy of lidocaine to prevent laryngospasm in children: a systematic review and meta-analysis. Anaesthesia. 2014;69(12):1388–96.
32. Rubin AD, Shah A, Moyer CA, Johns MM. The effect of topical anesthesia on vocal fold motion. J Voice. 2009;23(1):128–31.
33. Mahajan RP, Murty GE, Singh P, Aitkenhead AR. Effect of topical anaesthesia on the motor performance of vocal cords as assessed by tussometry. Anaesthesia. 1994;49(12):1028–30.
34. Maxwell MJ, English JD, Moppett IK, McGlashan JA, Norris AM. Vocalization assessed by electrolaryngography is unaffected by topical lidocaine anesthesia: a prospective, crossover, randomized, double-blind placebo-controlled study. Anesth Analg. 2012;114(4):785–90.
35. Yang CC, Chen SH. Impact of topical anesthesia on acoustic characteristics of voice during laryngeal telescopic examination. Otolaryngol Head Neck Surg. 2005;132(1):110–4.
36. Postma GN, Cohen JT, Belafsky PC, et al. Transnasal esophagoscopy: revisited (over 700 consecutive cases). Laryngoscope. 2005;115(2):321–3.
37. Sulica L, Rosen CA, Postma GN, et al. Current practice in injection augmentation of the vocal folds: indications, treatment principles, techniques, and complications. Laryngoscope. 2010;120(2):319–25.
38. Long H, Greller H, Mercurio-Zappala M, Nelson LS, Hoffman RS. Medicinal use of cocaine: a shifting paradigm over 25 years. Laryngoscope. 2004;114(9):1625–9.
39. Schenck NL. Local anesthesia in otolaryngology: a re-evaluation. Ann Otol Rhinol Laryngol. 1975;84(1):65–72.
40. Kouba DJ, LoPiccolo MC, Alam M, et al. Guidelines for the use of local anesthesia in office-based dermatologic surgery. J Am Acad Dermatol. 2016;74(6):1201–19.
41. Rosenberg PH, Heinonen J, Takasaki M. Lidocaine concentration in blood after topical anaesthesia of the upper respiratory tract. Acta Anaesthesiol Scand. 1980;24(2):125–8.

42. Schmalbach CE. Patient safety and anesthesia considerations for office-based otolaryngology procedures. Otolaryngol Clin N Am. 2019;52(3):379–90.
43. McCaughey W. Adverse effects of local anaesthetics. Drug Saf. 1992;7(3):178–89.
44. Vessely MB, Zitsch RP III. Topical anesthetic-induced methemoglobinemia: a case report and review of the literature. Otolaryngol Head Neck Surg. 1993;108(6):763–7.
45. Hieger MA, Afeld JL, Cumpston KL, Wills BK. Topical benzocaine and methemoglobinemia. Am J Ther. 2017;24(5):e596–8.
46. Taleb M, Ashraf Z, Valavoor S, Tinkel J. Evaluation and management of acquired methemoglobinemia associated with topical benzocaine use. Am J Cardiovasc Drugs. 2013;13(5):325–30.
47. Whited C, Cohen SM. Nasal tetracaine spray–induced methemoglobinemia. Otolaryngol Head Neck Surg. 2012;146(4):678–9.

Chapter 7
Surgical Techniques and Operative Approaches in Office-Based Laryngeal Surgery

7.1 Introduction

The last two decades have witnessed a major trend in laryngology practice toward office-based surgery. In part, this change is due to radical improvement in instrumentation [1, 2]. Technological innovations, particularly the advent of endoscopes with working channels and distal chip camera, have allowed the use of flexible needles and lasers for treatment of structural and functional voice disorders traditionally managed in the operating room. This shift toward office-based laryngeal surgery has spared many patients the need for general anesthesia and the morbidities associated with suspension microlaryngoscopy. It also has allowed surgeons to monitor the patient's voice during surgery. Awake patients may assist the surgeon by performing various phonatory tasks that can help gauge glottic closure and vocal fold movement. Patients are instructed on how to control their breathing to help minimize brisk abductor or adductor movements that might hinder surgery [3–6]. The increased use of office-based laryngeal surgery also has affected health care spending favorably. Based on a review that included 13 studies, Schimberg et al. reported a lower cost of office-based laryngeal surgery in comparison to laryngeal surgery performed under general anesthesia [7]. In another comparative study on patients with recurrent respiratory papillomatosis, Rees et al. reported an estimated saving of at least $5000 per procedure [8]. However, this decrease in cost per procedure might be counterbalanced by an increase in the number of surgical interventions per case and a low threshold for surgery. Surgeons whose clinics are well equipped for unsedated office-based laryngeal surgery might be more inclined to operate on small or early lesions in comparison to those who do not have this option.

Despite the many potential advantages listed above, the success of office-based laryngeal surgery hinges on several important factors. In addition to proper patient

---

Supplementary Information The online version contains supplementary material available at [https://doi.org/10.1007/978-3-030-91936-8_7].

A.-l. Hamdan et al., *Office-Based Laryngeal Surgery*,
https://doi.org/10.1007/978-3-030-91936-8_7

selection, adequate preoperative counseling, and successful topical anesthesia to the upper airway, the choice of the surgical approach is crucial for the completion of any procedure. This chapter reviews the approaches commonly used in office-based laryngeal surgery. The surgical details and limitations of each approach are discussed. A detailed review of the literature on the surgical outcome and complications of the different office-based laryngeal surgeries is available to the readers in Chaps. 8, 9, 10, 11, and 12 of this book.

7.2 Surgical Technique and Approaches

The spectrum of office-based laryngeal surgery has expanded markedly since 1990s to include a large number of procedures. These include injection laryngoplasty for the treatment of vocal fold paralysis/paresis and other causes of glottic insufficiency; vocal fold injection of steroid or other substances in patients with vocal fold scar or benign lesion; cidofovir injections in patients with recurrent respiratory papillomatosis; botulinum toxin injection for the treatment of laryngeal movement disorders; laser therapy for benign, premalignant, and early malignant lesions of the vocal folds; laryngeal biopsy; excision of vocal fold masses; removal of laryngeal sutures or stents; dilation of laryngeal stenosis; and other procedures [4–6, 9]. All these procedures are performed commonly using one of three approaches, namely, the peroral often referred to as transoral approach, the transcervical or percutaneous approach via the cricothyroid membrane, thyroid cartilage or thyrohyoid membrane, and the transnasal approach. The choice of approach depends on the type of procedure, the surgeon's experience and preference, the patient's anatomy and tolerance, and the availability of equipment and medical resources. Physicians performing in-office laryngeal surgery should be familiar with all these techniques.

7.2.1 The Peroral or Transoral Approach

The peroral approach is the oldest approach depicted in surgery of the upper airway under local anesthesia. It was described initially in 1852 by Green who used the technique to resect a laryngeal polyp from an 11-year-old [10]. It also was used by Kirstein in 1895 [11]. It became used more widely after it was reintroduced in 1911 by Bruening and later promoted by Arnold in the treatment and rehabilitation of vocal fold paralysis [12, 13]. Over the last century, application of the peroral approach has increased to include office-based treatment of patients with many voice disorders. Dedo et al. reviewed their experience with 135 patients who underwent injection laryngoplasty using the peroral approach and reported improvement in 96% and full recovery in 81% of the cases [14]. Halderman et al. reported the use of the peroral approach in their case series of 82 office-based injection medializations with good patient tolerance. Only six cases were aborted and had to be injected under direct laryngoscopy [15]. The peroral approach also has been described for office-based removal of vocal fold masses. Shahshahan et al. reported in-office removal of a vocal fold polyp in an 84-year-old woman with no recurrence after 6 months [9]. Similarly, Lan et al. reported office-based resection of vocal fold polyps using small cup forceps introduced orally under video-stroboscopic examination [16]. Omori et al. described their experience with 114 patients who underwent video-endoscope-assisted laryngeal surgery performed perorally [17]. The peroral approach has been adopted in vocal fold injection of pharmaceutical agents, as well. Tateya et al. reported complete or partial regression of vocal fold nodules following vocal fold steroid injection using the peroral approach under fiberoptic guidance [18]. Similarly, Mortensen and Woo showed 82% improvement following peroral vocal fold steroid injection in patients with vocal fold scar/nodules/polyps [19]. Ford et al. reported good patient tolerance and no major complications using the peroral approach while injecting botulinum toxin in 16 patients with spasmodic dysphonia [20], and Johanna and Woo used the peroral approach for cidofovir injection in five patients with recurrent respiratory papillomatosis. The authors reported successful treatment with improvement in voice function [21].

The wide use of the peroral approach in office-based laryngeal surgery is partially ascribed to the versatility of this approach in allowing access to the glottis and supraglottic structures. The shaft of the curved needle introduced orally also may be used to retract tissues to improve visualization of the site of injection. Additionally, the peroral approach offers direct visualization of the tip of the needle while performing laryngeal injections. A major limitation in some patients is poor tolerance. Patients with hyperactive gag reflex may not be able to tolerate the introduction of the curved needle through the oral cavity and are not good candidates for this technique.

Surgical technique: After having applied topical anesthesia to the pharynx and larynx (see Chap. 6) and while the patient is in the sitting position leaning forward, the tongue is held with the one hand, while the curved needle attached to a syringe or orotracheal injector device is introduced with the other hand. The curved needles usually are 22- to 25-cm-long. Depending on the material to be injected, needles may be from 18 to 27 gauge. The surgeon needs to navigate the tip of the needle with extreme caution across the tonsillar pillars down the laryngeal inlet [4–6]. The needle may be either disposable or nondisposable [22, 23]. The use of a malleable needle easy to curve according to the patient's anatomy is very helpful in averting potential injury to the mucosa. It is important to pass the needle beyond the base of tongue under vision. Use of a flexible nasopharyngoscope with a distal chip camera guided by an assistant is very helpful. The tip of the endoscope is usually positioned behind the palate above the epiglottis. This not only provides a good, wide field of view, but it also helps prevent the needle from injuring the laryngoscope. After the needle tip enters the laryngeal inlet, the tip of the laryngoscope may be advanced closer to the vocal folds. Once the tip of the needle is visualized, it is directed toward the site of injection. In patients with glottic insufficiency, the tip of the needle is placed just anterior and lateral to the vocal process (Fig. 7.1). In cases of vocal

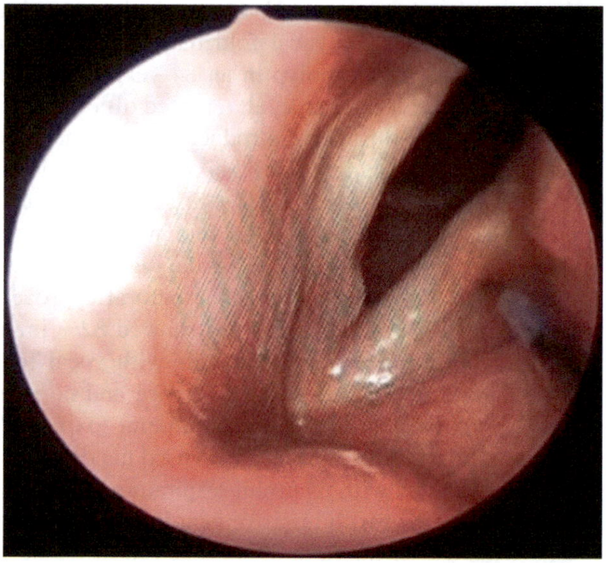

Fig. 7.1 Peroral approach in a patient with left vocal fold paralysis. A flexible endoscopic view showing the insertion site of the injecting needle within the thyroarytenoid muscle and lateral to the vocal process. Note that the shaft of the needle is used to retract the false vocal fold laterally. Note a polypoid lesion on the right vocal fold

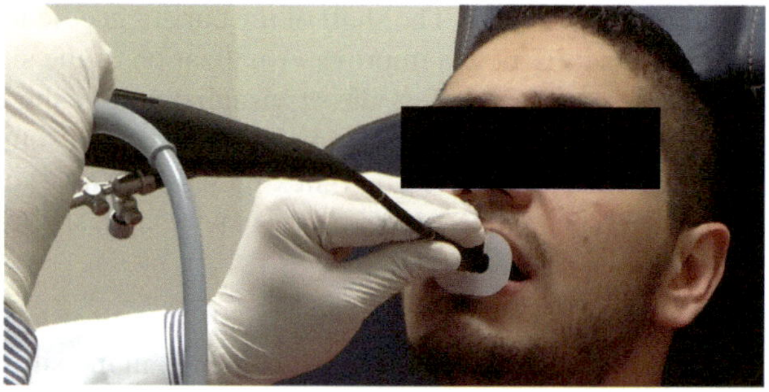

Fig. 7.2 View of the flexible endoscope introduced through the modified oral airway (Guedel)

fold injection with steroid, saline, 5-fluorouracil (5-FU) or other substances, the tip is placed in the superficial layer of the lamina propria, whereas in patients undergoing botulinum toxin injection, the needle is inserted within the body of the medial belly of the thyroarytenoid muscle. Alternatively, the injection can be made in the false vocal folds as in cases of laryngeal tremor or for other purposes. In patients undergoing office-based removal of vocal fold masses using the peroral approach, curved instruments (cup forceps, knife, heart-shaped forceps, scissors, etc.) are introduced orally instead of the needle [23]. Details about laryngeal biopsy and removal of vocal fold masses are available in Chap. 12.

The transoral flexible endoscopic technique described by Hamdan et al. is used less frequently [24]. While the patient is seated and the head in neutral position, topical anesthetic in the form of gel or spray is applied to the base of tongue and oropharynx. Few minutes later, the patient is instructed to insert the modified Guedel oral airway in his/her mouth and bite on it (Fig. 7.2). The flexible nasopharyngoscope with a working channel is then introduced through the modified Guedel oral airway, and more topical anesthetic is administered through the working channel of the endoscope. Once the pharyngeal and laryngeal surfaces are anesthetized, the flexible needle (size of which varies with the type of injection) is introduced through the working channel and directed toward the site of injection (Fig. 7.3). The main value of this approach is the use of one route to visualize and operate on the larynx. Additionally, the introduction of the needle through the working channel of the

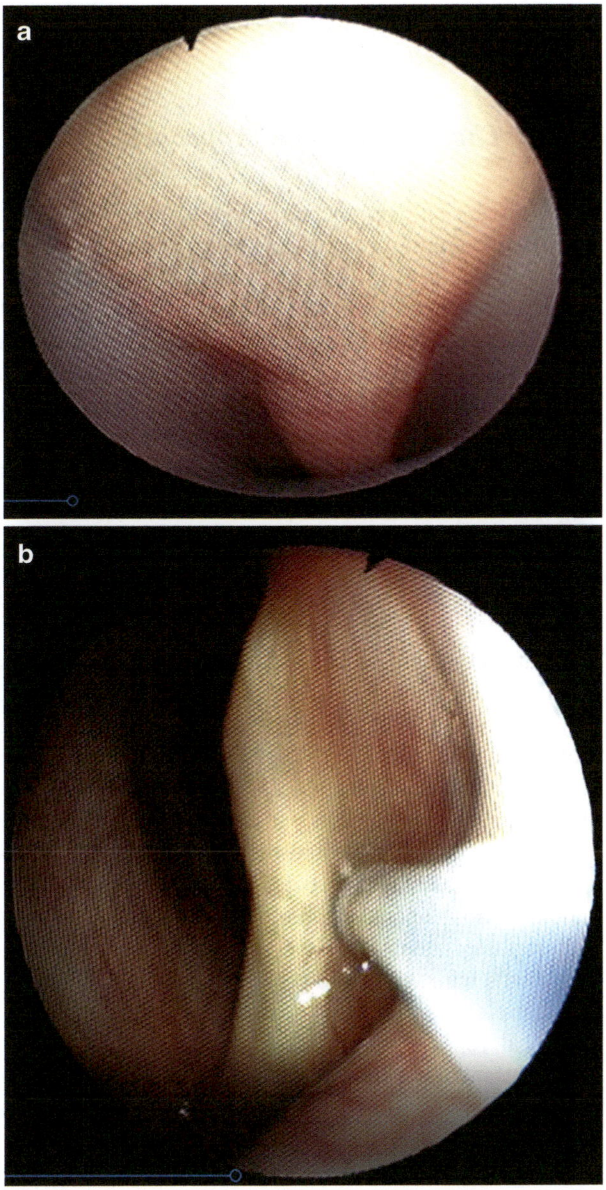

Fig. 7.3 The endoscope at the base of tongue directed toward the laryngeal inlet (**a**). The tip of the flexible needle inserted lateral to the vocal process (**b**)

endoscope avoids any risk of injury to the mucosal lining of the oropharynx, hypopharynx, and larynx, which may occur inadvertently while using sharp curved instruments or needles introduced orally. Of particular importance, this approach does not require an assistant, particularly in patients undergoing vocal fold steroid injections. The transoral flexible endoscopic approach also may be used in office-based laser therapy, particularly in patients with severe septal deviation or patients using multiple anticoagulants. The "non-touch" technique allows both patient safety and minimal discomfort. A main limitation to this approach is patient tolerance particularly in those with hyperactive gag reflex.

7.2.2 *The Transcervical Approach*

The transcervical approach is a viable and safe alternative to the peroral approach. It is used commonly for a variety of office-based laryngeal surgical procedures, such as injection laryngoplasty in patients with glottic insufficiency, vocal fold steroid injection in patients with inflammatory laryngeal disorders or scar, and botulinum toxin injection in patients with laryngeal movement disorders [4, 5]. The transcervical approach can be performed via three different routes: the cricothyroid membrane route, the transthyroid route, and the thyrohyoid membrane route (Illustrations 7.1, 7.2, and 7.3). A common limitation to the transcervical approach using any of these three routes is the need for an assistant to hold and navigate the flexible endoscope during the procedure.

7.2.2.1 The Transcervical-Cricothyroid Membrane Approach

The transcervical approach via the cricothyroid membrane is one of the most commonly used approaches in office-based laryngeal injections. It was advocated by Blitzer et al. in 1988 for injection of botulinum toxin in patients with laryngeal movement disorders [25]. The same approach has been adopted for treatment of patients with vocal fold paresis/paralysis and benign vocal fold lesions [4–6, 26–28]. In their review of 236 patients who underwent injection laryngoplasty, Sulica et al. reported that 47% had their injections done via the cricothyroid membrane approach. The authors reported a success rate of 99%, very comparable to that of patients whose operations had been performed under general anesthesia [26]. Hsu et al. reported the use of the cricothyroid approach in vocal fold steroid injection in 24 patients with vocal fold polyp. The procedure was completed successfully in 22, and complete remission was achieved in 59% of the cases [27]. In another study, Woo et al. reported vocal fold steroid injection in 51 patients with exudative lesions of the vocal folds and/or scar. Using the cricothyroid approach, complete or partial remission was obtained in 34.8% and 49.6% of the cases, respectively [28].

Despite the popularity of the cricothyroid membrane approach, a main limitation is the inability of the surgeon to visualize the tip of the needle before injecting and

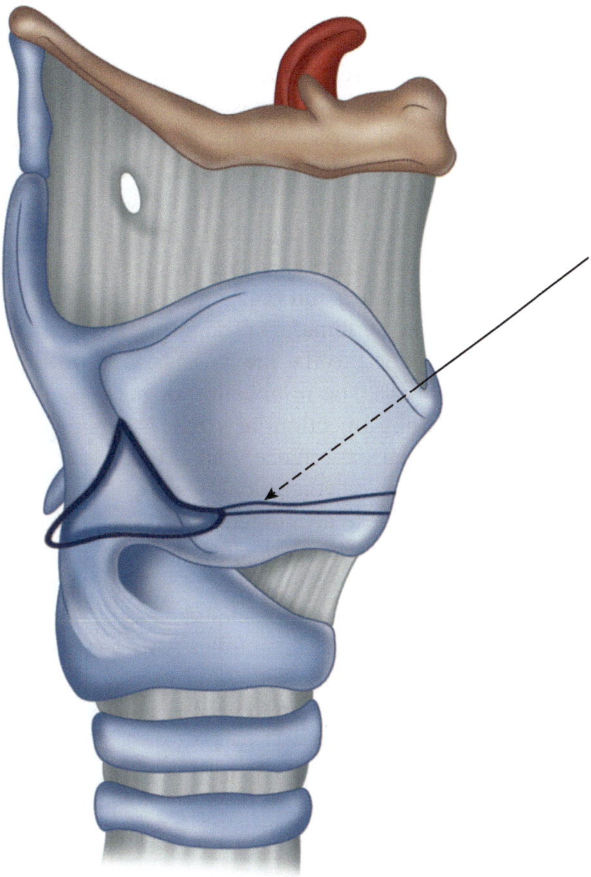

Illustration 7.1 Transcervical thyrohyoid approach

the limited control in gauging the depth of the needle entry. To that end, the surgeon should take into account the different angulations of the needle at its entry site during the procedure. In an anatomical study comparing two cricothyroid approaches to the mid-membranous portion of the vocal folds, Panossian et al. reported a significant difference in the insertion angle between the infrathyroid approach and the supracricoid approach (22.2 + 6.9 vs. 33.0 + 5.2, respectively). Moreover, the mean insertion depth was less in the infrathyroid approach vs. the supracricoid approach (11.3 + 1.8 mm vs. 18.2 + 2.4 mm, respectively) [29]. The surgeon also should take into consideration anatomic variations across genders. In the abovementioned anatomic study, the mean distance from the midline to the target site without the need for angulation was higher in males than females (5.7 ± 0.7 mm vs. 4.8 ± 0.8 mm, respectively) [29]. In a study by Jin et al. looking at anatomic references for the cricothyroid approach using three-dimensionally reconstructed computed tomography, the authors also noted differences in angulation and depth of penetration across genders. The depth of penetration, measured by the distance from the surface of

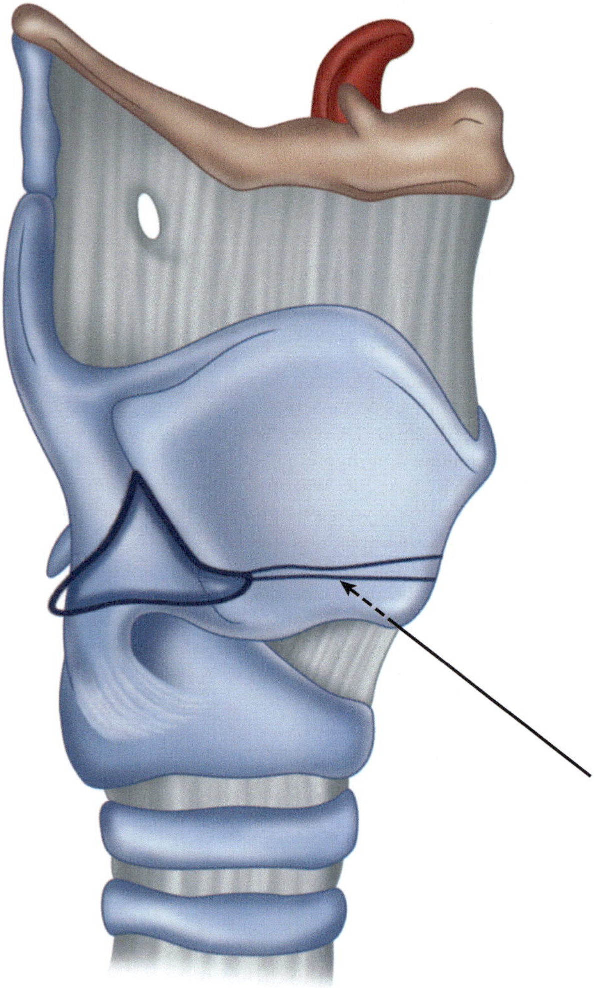

Illustration 7.2 Trans-cervical cricothyroid approach

injection (7 mm from midline) to the target site of injection (posterior one third of the vocal fold), was greater in men than in women (15.75 mm vs. 13.91 mm, respectively). Similarly, the angle of penetration in the medial direction was more acute in women than men (12.71° vs. 10.57°, respectively) [30]. Mau and Courey also found gender-related anatomic differences in their cadaveric dissection of human larynges [31]. The authors demonstrated that males undergoing injection laryngoplasty required almost 50% more filling substance than females.

Surgical technique: After having applied topical anesthesia to the larynx and pharynx, and while the patient is seated with the head relaxed in the neutral position, the cricothyroid membrane is identified, and a 23- or 25-guage needle is intro-

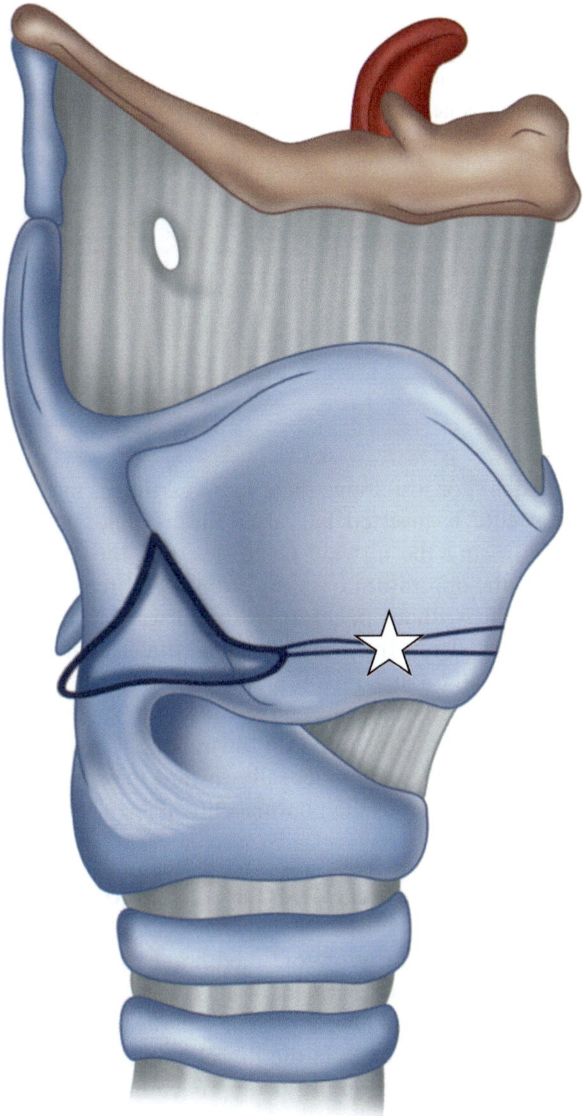

Illustration 7.3 Trans-cervical transthyroid approach: site of entry

duced gently through the skin and subcutaneous tissue, while a flexible endoscope is positioned above the level of the vocal folds to provide visualization. Some very experienced physicians perform this procedure without visualization (Fig. 7.4). The needle may be straight or bent at its base depending on the surgeon's preference. The entry site may be in the midline or up to about 7-mm off the midline. If the needle is introduced at midline, it will enter the lumen and must be directed right or left and postero-laterally toward the site of injection. The needle can be introduced either just underneath the free edge of the thyroid lamina (the "infrathyroid

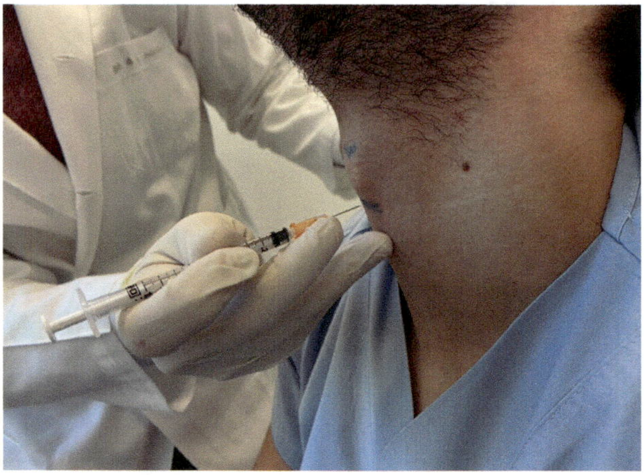

Fig. 7.4 Percutaneous cricothyroid approach. The needle is inserted through the cricothyroid membrane. Note that the angle at the entry site can vary based on whether the entry is adjacent to the cricoid cartilage (supracricoid) or thyroid cartilage (infrathyroid). The entry may be in the midline or lateral to the midline

approach") or just above the cricoid cartilage (the "supracricoid approach") [29]. If the needle is inserted lateral to the midline, it can enter the target site without transgressing the airway. Once inserted, the needle either penetrates the airway toward the opposite site for injection or is directed cephalically and laterally into the vocal fold without penetrating the airway. In that case, some surgeons bend the needle 45° 1 cm from the tip to facilitate its entry into the vocal fold muscle. In patients undergoing injection laryngoplasty, the needle should be directed toward the medial belly thyroarytenoid muscle or just lateral to it. In patients undergoing vocal fold steroid injection for the treatment of benign lesions of the vocal folds, the needle is directed submucosally toward the superficial layer of the lamina propria where deposition of the pharmaceutical agent is intended.

7.2.2.2 The Transcervical-Thyrohyoid Membrane Approach

The transcervical-thyrohyoid membrane approach was described initially by Getz et al. in 2005 in the treatment of a 52-year-old man with recurrent respiratory papillomatosis. In view of the patient's intolerance to the peroral approach, cidofovir injections were made via the thyrohyoid membrane [32]. In 2006, Amin reported the clinical application of this approach in ten patients undergoing injection laryngoplasty and showed marked improvement in VHI-10 score with minimal patient discomfort (average 2.1 on a scale of 1–10). The authors reiterated on the main advantage of the thyrohyoid approach, namely, the combination of good visualization and improved patient tolerance [33]. Since its inception, the thyrohyoid membrane approach has been advocated as an alternative to the cricothyroid membrane approach in patients undergoing injection laryngoplasty, vocal fold steroid injection, and botulinum toxin injection. Woo et al. investigated the effectiveness of injection laryngoplasty using the thyrohyoid membrane approach in comparison to the cricothyroid membrane approach in 64 patients with glottic insufficiency. All patients underwent a comprehensive voice evaluation that included laryngeal video-stroboscopic examination, acoustic analysis, perceptual evaluation, and self-report questionnaire. The results were comparable in both groups, and significant improvement was noted in all voice outcome measures [34]. In a review by Sulica et al. on current practice in injection laryngoplasty, 21% of their office procedures were performed using the thyrohyoid membrane approach. The results were comparable to those who were operated upon under general anesthesia [26]. The thyrohyoid membrane approach also has been advocated for vocal fold steroid injection. Woo et al. used the thyrohyoid membrane approach to treat 41 patients with various benign vocal fold lesions. All patients had successful vocal fold injection with 0.15–0.20 ml of triamcinolone acetonide (40 mg/ml) [28].

Despite the advantages of the thyrohyoid membrane approach, namely, adequate visualization of the laryngeal lumen with flexible laryngoscopy and good patient tolerance, this approach has its limitations, the most important of which is limited access to the most anterior portions of the vocal folds [35, 36]. According to a study by Rees et al., 13% of 55 injection laryngoplasty performed using the thyrohyoid membrane approach had to be aborted because of "inability to achieve an appropriate injection angle" [37]. Another limitation to this approach is the difficulty in introducing the needle through a calcified thyrohyoid membrane commonly encountered in elderly patients. These limitations have prompted the need for modifications to this approach. Achkar et al. described bending the needle in order to circumvent the limited access of a straight needle to the anterior one third of the vocal fold. Two 45-degree bends, one placed at the hub of the needle and the other 1–1.5 cm from the tip, allow the surgeon to gain better access to the anterior glottis as well as the false vocal folds. Another value to this modification is the ability to gauge the depth of injection. The bend 1 cm away from the tip allows the surgeon to estimate with some accuracy how deep the injection is made. A major drawback is the difficulty in maneuvering the bended needle through the skin and subcutaneous tissue while directing the needle to the site of injection [38]. Based on the author experience (ALH and RTS), bending the needle 45° at the mid-length of the needle instead of bending it at the hub allows better handling of the needle at the insertion while improving access to the anterior one third of the vocal fold. Another modification to the thyrohyoid membrane approach was reported by Clary et al. The authors described the use of an 18-gauge needle as an introducer through which a 25-gauge needle is used to perform the injection. The 18-gauge needle is introduced through the thyrohyoid membrane at the level of the thyroid notch. The authors reported their experience in 21 patients with glottic insufficiency who had undergone injection laryngoplasty using the laryngeal introducer technique and reported good patient tolerance and favorable voice outcome [39]. The procedure was completed successfully by 71.4% of the physicians. Moreover, close to 90% of the patients expressed their willingness to repeat the procedure. The main advantages of using the introducer included the ease of insertion, the need to puncture the thyrohyoid membrane only once, and the increased accessibility to the anterior aspect of the vocal folds by curving the needle. This approach also helps overcome the problem of thyrohyoid membrane calcification by using a thicker and less pliable needle. The author (RTS) also has addressed this issue using a spinal needle with the obturator in place during the insertion.

Surgical technique: After having anesthetized the larynx and pharynx, and while the patient is seated and the neck extended, the skin and subcutaneous tissues at the thyrohyoid notch are identified and infiltrated with topical anesthetic (0.5 cc of 1% lidocaine mixed with 1:100,000 epinephrine). Some surgeons do not use topical skin anesthesia, although anesthesia of the laryngeal mucosa is necessary. A flexible nasopharyngoscope is introduced in the nose/nasopharynx and held behind the soft palate while a 22- to 25-guage, 1.5-inch-long needle is inserted just above the thyroid notch into the thyrohyoid membrane and laryngeal lumen. The needle is then directed downward and posteriorly (Fig. 7.5). In some cases, it may need to be bent in order to gain access especially anteriorly, for the injection. The needle should penetrate the pre-epiglottic space at the petiole into the laryngeal lumen and then be directed laterally toward the site of injection. In patients with vocal fold paresis/paralysis undergoing injection laryngoplasty, the needle is directed posteriorly and laterally into the posterior one third of the vocal fold (Fig. 7.6, Videos 7.1 and 7.2). In patients with spasmodic dysphonia undergoing bilateral botulinum injections, the neurotoxin is placed in the mid-third of the vocal fold, lateral to the vocal ligament in the medial belly of the thyroarytenoid muscle. Similarly, in patients undergoing vocal fold steroid injection for androphonia, the needle is inserted at the mid-third of the vocal fold (Fig. 7.7, Video 7.3). In patients with benign vocal fold lesions or scar, the needle is inserted in the lamina propria near the free edge of the vocal fold (Fig. 7.8). In patients with vocal process granuloma, the needle for botulinum toxin injection is directed posteriorly into the inter-arytenoid muscle (ALH), (Fig. 7.9) or laterally for injection into the lateral cricoarytenoid (LCA) muscle (RTS). LCA injection generally can be performed more easily through the cricothyroid membrane than the thyrohyoid membrane; and the author (RTS) used laryngeal electromyographic guidance for these injections.

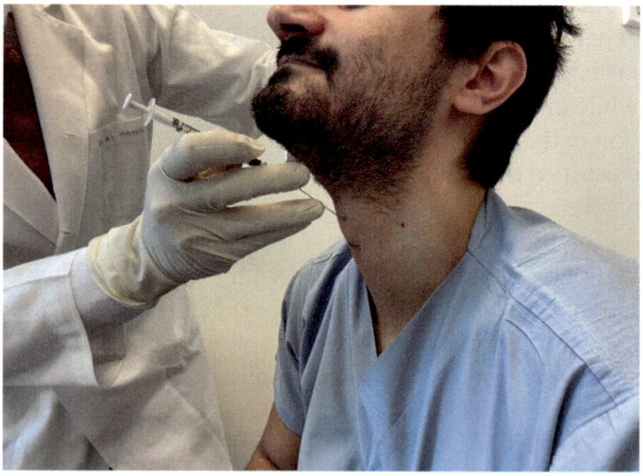

Fig. 7.5 Percutaneous thyrohyoid approach using a 23 G × $2^{3/8''}$. The site of entry is at the thyroid notch. Note the angulation of the needle. The needle can be bent 10–20° at its hub to facilitate the approach

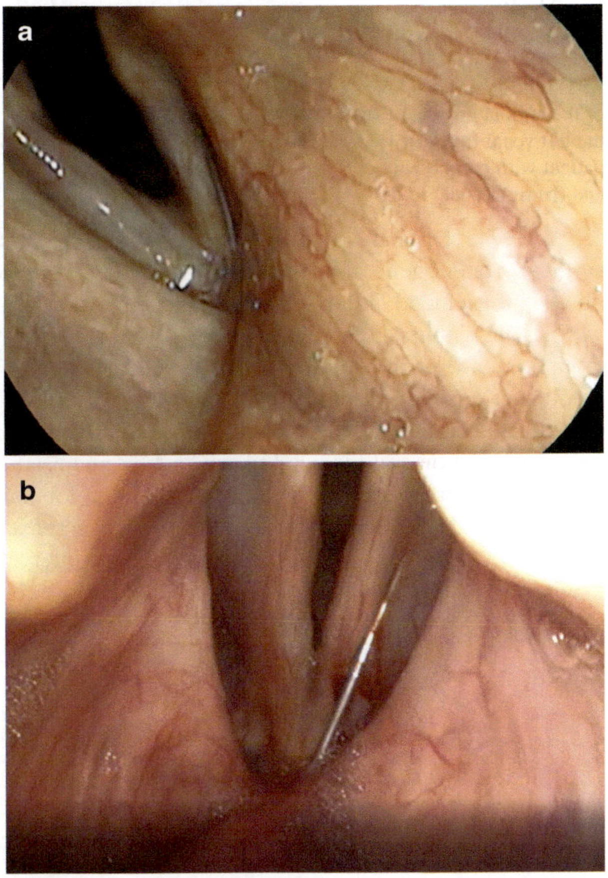

Fig. 7.6 Percutaneous thyrohyoid membrane approach injection laryngoplasty. (**a**) Posterior injection of the filling substance, (**b**) more anterior injection of the filling substance

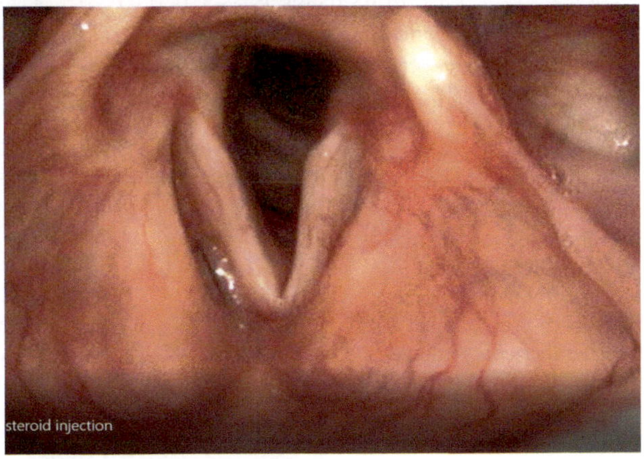

Fig. 7.7 Percutaneous thyrohyoid injection of steroid at mid-third of the right thyroarytenoid muscle

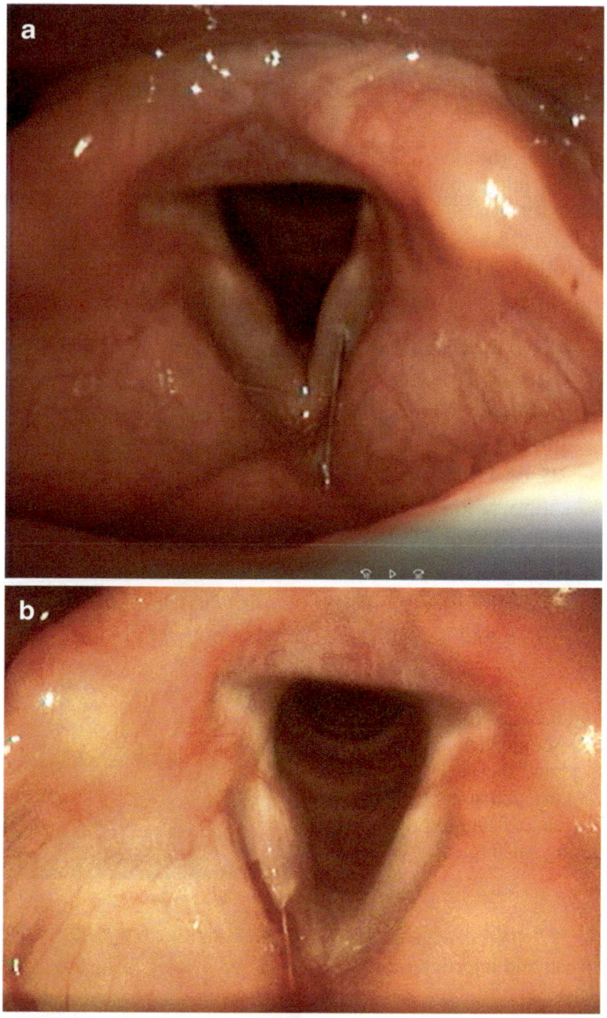

Fig. 7.8 Percutaneous thyrohyoid injection of Dexamethasone 0.1 mg/cc within the superficial layer of the lamina propria of (**a**) the left vocal fold in a patient with bamboo nodes and (**b**) right vocal fold

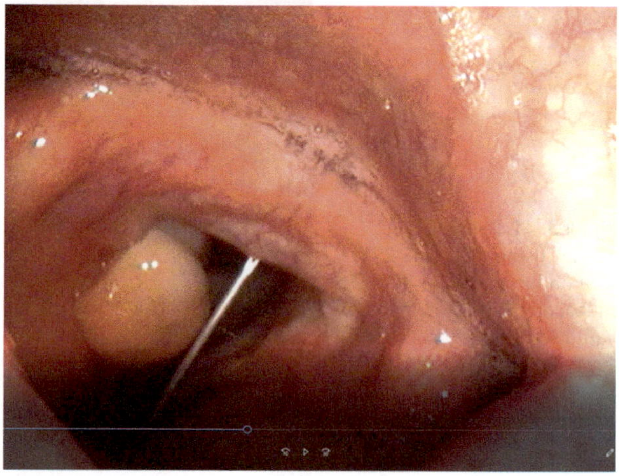

Fig. 7.9 Percutaneous injection of botulinum toxin into the interarytenoid muscle in a patient with right vocal process granuloma. Some surgeons prefer to inject the lateral cricoarytenoid muscle; The thyroarytenoid muscle is targeted by many surgeons as well

7.2.2.3 The Transcervical-Transthyroid Cartilage Approach

Another option for office-based laryngeal surgery is the transthyroid approach. It is used mostly for injection laryngoplasty for the treatment of vocal fold paresis/paralysis and/or glottic insufficiency due to other causes such as presbylarynx and less frequently for vocal fold injection of pharmaceutical agents. The main advantage of this approach is that the needle remains submucosal without entering the laryngeal lumen. Moreover, the distance travelled from the point of skin penetration to the site of injection is shorter than the distance covered using the cricothyroid or thyrohyoid membrane approach. However, a major limitation to the transthyroid approach is calcification of the thyroid cartilage which may prohibit the introduction of the needle. In a study on the anatomical evolution of the thyroid cartilage using computerized tomography, Glikson et al. reported increased calcification of the thyroid cartilage with aging. The degree of calcification varies across gender and is a continuum throughout the years of puberty and adulthood [40]. Age-associated changes have been reviewed in detail by Sataloff et al. [41], and it is helpful for surgeons to understand anatomic changes over the lifespan.

Surgical technique: After having administered topical anesthesia to the upper airway and while the patient is seated and the head in neutral position, the skin and subcutaneous tissues at the site of the thyroid ala may be infiltrated with 1% or 2% lidocaine mixed with 1:100,000 epinephrine. Some surgeons do not use local anesthesia to the skin. A 22- to 25-gauge needle is then inserted in a plane perpendicular to the thyroid lamina into the thyroid cartilage at the level of the vocal folds (Fig. 7.10). Mucosal puncture secondary to "past-pointing" should be avoided or detected by watching for any brisk movement while penetrating the thyroid lamina. The correct position of the needle is estimated best by inducing movement to the overlying vocal fold tissue visualized through a flexible laryngoscope, although some experienced surgeons perform this technique without laryngoscope monitoring. The flexible endoscope, when used, is positioned above the laryngeal inlet at

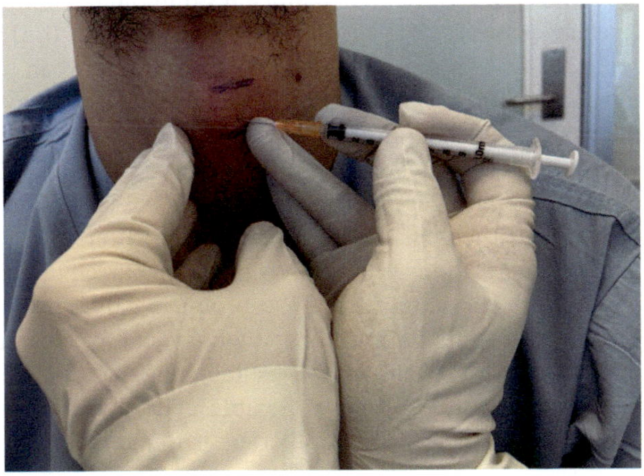

Fig. 7.10 Transthyroid cartilage approach. Note that the angle between the needle and the thyroid lamina is almost 90°. Note also that the entry site is few millimeters above the lower free edge of the thyroid lamina

the start of the procedure. The surgeon should avoid exerting excessive pressure while injecting. This may occur inadvertently if the tip of the needle gets obstructed with cartilage fragments during its insertion through the thyroid lamina.

7.2.3 The Transnasal Approach Using a Flexible Nasopharyngoscope with a Working Channel

The transnasal approach using a flexible nasopharyngoscope with a working channel has enabled otolaryngologists to diagnose and treat patients with numerous laryngeal disorders. The working channel allows the introduction of cup forceps or flexible "handles" for laryngeal tissue biopsy, as well as "flexible" needles for the purpose of various injections. The injected substances include augmentation material in patients with glottic insufficiency, steroids (or other medications), or cidofovir in patients with benign vocal fold lesions or recurrent respiratory papillomatosis and botulinum toxin in patients with laryngeal movement disorders. In 2005, Trask et al. reported their experience using the transnasal approach in 20 patients undergoing injection laryngoplasty in an office setting. The injection was successful in all the cases except one who needed a tracheotomy [42]. Similarly, Hamdan et al. reviewed the voice outcome of 16 patients with glottic insufficiency treated with transnasal injection laryngoplasty and reported complete or partial closure of the glottic gap with significant increase in the mean closed quotient using frame by frame analysis [43]. The transnasal approach also has been used for vocal fold steroid injection [43–47]. In a systematic review and meta-analysis that included 321 patients with vocal fold benign lesions or scar, Wang et al. reported the successful use of office-based steroid injection using the transnasal route. There was significant improvement in voice outcome measures, such as voice handicap index and maximum phonation time [44]. In another study on the long-term success rate and recurrence rate following office-based steroid injection using the transnasal route, the same authors reported significant symptom resolution in 74.6% of the cases with a recurrence rate of 17% at 12-month follow-up [45]. The transnasal endoscopic route has revolutionized office-based laser therapy in patients with benign, premalignant, and malignant laryngeal lesions. The ability to slide the laser glass fiber in the working channel of the endoscope has enabled otolaryngologists to treat laryngeal lesions that previously were inaccessible in an office setting. Koufman et al. reported their successful experience with 443 laryngotracheal cases who underwent unsedated office-based laser therapy using three different wavelengths with no major complications [48]. Zeitels et al. concurred about the effectiveness of office-based laryngeal surgery and the promising use of photo-angiolytic lasers in the treatment of epithelial and subepithelial vocal fold lesions [49]. Similar results were described by numerous authors establishing the feasibility, safety, and value of laser therapy using the transnasal flexible endoscope [50, 51]. A thorough review of unsedated, office-based laser therapy is found in Chap. 12.

Surgical technique: While the patient is seated and the head in its neutral position and after having administered topical anesthesia to the nose, pharynx, and larynx, the fiberoptic nasopharyngoscope with a working channel is introduced gently through the nose and passed through the nasopharynx, oropharynx, and hypopharynx into the laryngeal inlet until the vocal folds are visualized well. In patients undergoing injection laryngoplasty, a 19-guage flexible needle attached to a syringe filled with the injectable material is introduced thru the working channel of the flexible endoscope until the tip of the needle is visualized. At that time, the flexible endoscope is advanced, and the tip of the needle is directed toward the site of injection. In patients with vocal fold paresis/paralysis, the needle is directed toward the posterior one third of the vocal fold and inserted just anterior to the vocal process and lateral to the thyroarytenoid muscle (Fig. 7.11, Video 7.4). In patients with glottic insufficiency secondary to vocal fold atrophy or scar, the needle is directed toward the mid-third of the vocal fold or lateral to the site of scar where the filling material is injected. In patients with laryngeal papilloma, or benign lesions of the vocal folds, a 25-gauge flexible needle is directed toward the lesion where the pharmaceutical agent (steroids or nonsteroidal agent) is to be injected (Fig. 7.12, Video 7.5). A submucosal bleb at the site of injection is usually a sign that the injection has been successful. In patients undergoing laser therapy, the surgeon must ensure that the glass fiber is introduced while holding the flexible nasopharyngoscope straight with no bending. This is usually accomplished by introducing the glass fiber before the endoscope is inserted, keeping the tip of the fiber just inside the distal tip of the working channel while it is still in the nasal cavity. Otherwise, injury to the working channel may occur (Figs. 7.13 and 7.14).

In summary, office-based laryngeal surgery has become a mainstay treatment option in patients with voice disorders. Three different approaches can be used and these include the peroral, the transcervical, and the transnasal approaches. The choice of approach hinges on the surgeon's expertise, patient tolerance, anatomic variations, and the pathology being treated. A cooperative patient is key for the

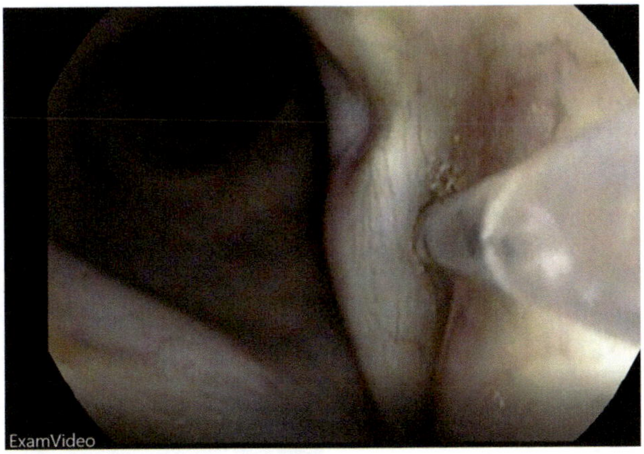

Fig. 7.11 Transnasal approach in injection laryngoplasty. Note the insertion point of the needle lateral to the vocal process

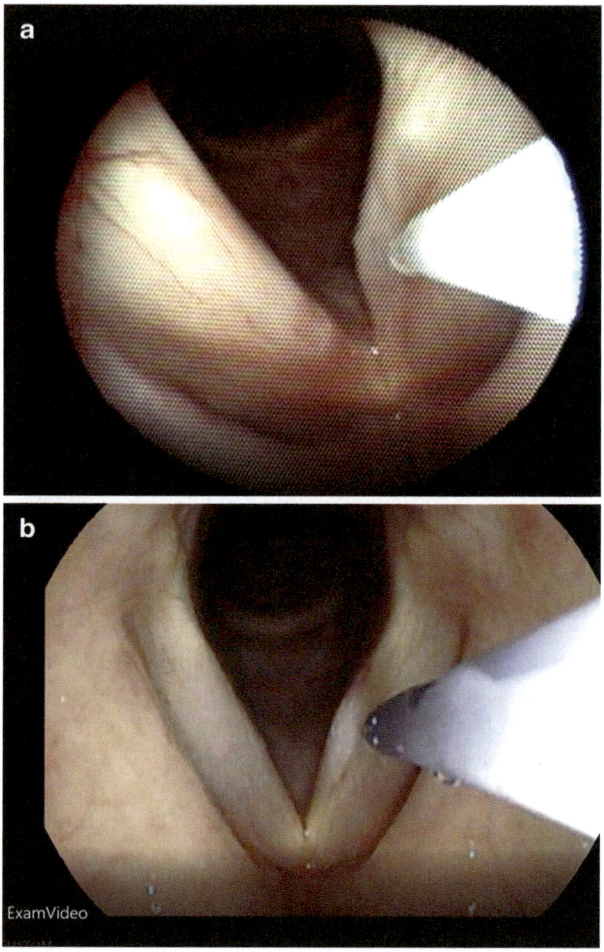

Fig. 7.12 Transnasal approach in vocal fold steroid injection in a patient with (**a**) left vocal fold nodule, (**b**) left vocal fold scar

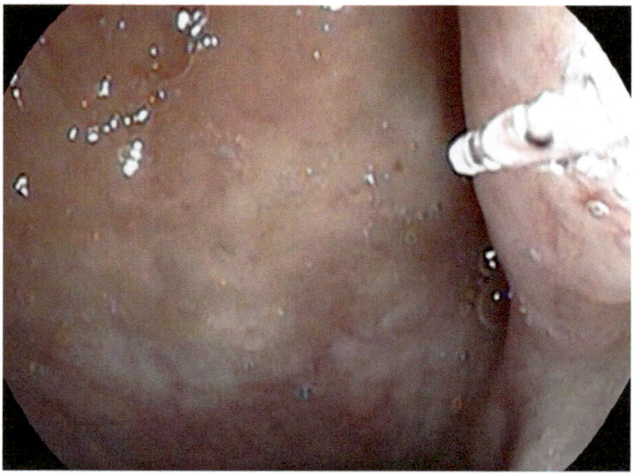

Fig. 7.13 Laser glass fiber seen at the tip of the flexible endoscope in the nasal cavity. Note that the laser tip is kept inside the working channel when the endoscope is approaching the laryngeal inlet

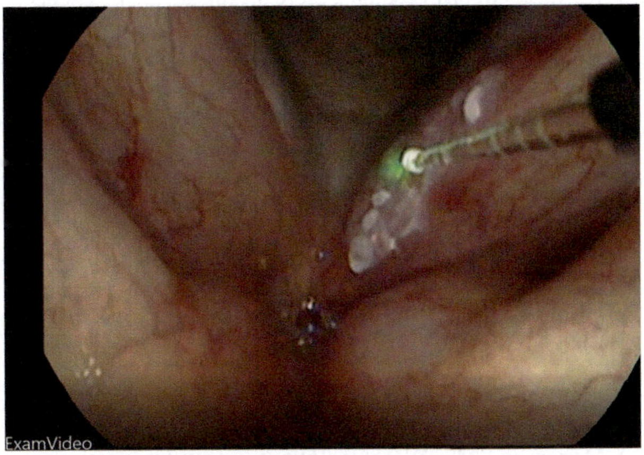

Fig. 7.14 An endoscopic view showing Blue Laser glass fiber in the treatment of a patient with left vocal fold leukoplakia

success of any office-based laryngeal procedure. Preoperative patient counseling, proper administration of topical anesthesia to the upper airway, and detailed description of the various steps of the approach to be used are crucial. Administration of an anxiolytic or sedative the night before the procedure and/or in the morning of the day of the procedure is optional. It is usually left at the discretion of the surgeon based on his assessment of the patient's level of tolerance.

References

1. Linder TE, Simmen D, Stool SE. Revolutionary inventions in the 20th century: the history of endoscopy. Arch Otolaryngol Head Neck Surg. 1997;123(11):1161–3.
2. Eller R, Ginsburg M, Lurie D, Heman-Ackah Y, Lyons K, Sataloff R. Flexible laryngoscopy: a comparison of fiber optic and distal chip technologies—part 2: laryngopharyngeal reflux. J Voice. 2009;23(3):389–95.
3. Bastian RW, Delsupehe KG. Indirect larynx and pharynx surgery: a replacement for direct laryngoscopy. Laryngoscope. 1996;106(10):1280–6.
4. Rosen CA, Amin MR, Sulica L, et al. Advances in office-based diagnosis and treatment in laryngology. Laryngoscope. 2009;119(Suppl 2):S185–212.
5. Wellenstein DJ, Schutte HW, Takes RP, et al. Office-based procedures for the diagnosis and treatment of laryngeal pathology. J Voice. 2018;32(4):502–13.
6. Woo P. Office-based laryngeal procedures. Otolaryngol Clin N Am. 2006;39(1):111–33.
7. Schimberg AS, Wellenstein DJ, van den Broek EM, et al. Office-based vs. operating room-performed laryngopharyngeal surgery: a review of cost differences. Eur Arch Otorhinolaryngol. 2019;276(11):2963–73.
8. Rees CJ, Postma GN, Koufman JA. Cost savings of unsedated office-based laser surgery for laryngeal papillomas. Ann Otol Rhinol Laryngol. 2007;116(1):45–8.
9. Shahshahan N, Panossian H, Sataloff RT. In-office resection of vocal fold polyp. Ear Nose Throat J. 2020;99(3):NP33–4.
10. Green H. Morbid growths within the larynx. In: Green H, editor. On the surgical treatment of polyps of the larynx and oedema of the glottis. New York: G. P. Putman; 1852. p. 56–65.
11. Kirstein A. Autoskopie des larynx und det trachea (laryngoscopia directa, Euthystopie, Besich Tigung ohme Spiegel). Arch Laryngol Rhinol. 1895;3:156–64.

12. Bruening W. Uber eine neue behandlungsmethode der rekurrensslahmung. Ver Deutsch Laryng. 1911;18:23:93–151.
13. Arnold GE. Vocal rehabilitation of paralytic dysphonia: I. Cartilage injection into a paralyzed vocal cord. Arch Otolaryngol. 1955;62(1):1–17.
14. Dedo HH, Urrea RD, Lawson L. Intracordal injection of Teflon® in the treatment of 135 patients with dysphonia. Ann Otol Rhinol Laryngol. 1973;82(5):661–7.
15. Halderman A, Bryson PC, Benninger M. Safety and length of benefit of restylane for office-based injection medialization. A retrospective review of one institution's experience. J Voice. 2014;28(5):631–5.
16. Lan MC, Hsu YB, Chang SY, et al. Office-based treatment of vocal fold polyp with flexible laryngosvideostroboscopic surgery. J Otolaryngol Head Neck Surg. 2010;39(1):90–5.
17. Omori K, Tsuji T, Shinohara K, Kojima H. Videoendoscopic laryngeal surgery. Ann Otol Rhinol Laryngol. 2000;109(2):149–55.
18. Tateya I, Omori K, Kojima H, Hirano S, Kaneko KI, Ito J. Steroid injection to vocal nodules using fiberoptic laryngeal surgery under topical anesthesia. Eur Arch Otorhinolarngol. 2004;261(9):489–92.
19. Mortensen M, Woo P. Office steroid injections of the larynx. Laryngoscope. 2006;116(10):1735–9.
20. Ford CN, Bless DM, Lowery JD. Indirect laryngoscopic approach for injection of botulinum toxin in spasmodic dysphonia. Otolaryngol Head Neck Surg. 1990;103(5):752–8.
21. Co J, Woo P. Serial office-based intralesional injection of cidofovir in adult onset recurrent respiratory papillomatosis. Ann Otol Rhinol Laryngol. 2004;113(11):859–62.
22. Medevnet.com/product. Medtronic Xomed, Inc. Address: 6743 Southpoint Dr. North C.
23. Sataloff Indirect Laryngeal Instrument Set. https://www.integrafile.com/file/general/1461595462.pdf.
24. Hamdan AL, Rizk M, Ayoub C, Ziade G. Injection laryngoplasty through a transoral approach using the Guedel oral airway. Acta Otorhinolaryngol Ital. 2017;37(5):444.
25. Blitzer A, Brin MF, Fahn S, Lovelace RE. Localized injections of botulinum toxin for the treatment of focal laryngeal dystonia (spastic dysphonia). Laryngoscope. 1988;98(2):193–7.
26. Sulica L, Rosen CA, Postma GN, et al. Current practice in injection augmentation of the vocal folds: indications, treatment principles, techniques, and complications. Laryngoscope. 2010;120(2):319–25.
27. Hsu YB, Lan MC, Chang SY. Percutaneous corticosteroid injection for vocal fold polyp. Arch Otolaryngol Head Neck Surg. 2009;135(8):776–80.
28. Woo JH, Kim DY, Kim JW, Oh EA, Lee SW. Efficacy of percutaneous vocal fold injections for benign laryngeal lesions: prospective multicenter study. Acta Otolaryngol. 2011;131(12):1326–32.
29. Panossian H, Pasick LJ, Sataloff RT. Anatomical study of two cricothyroid approaches to the cadaver larynx. J Voice. 2019;S0892-1997(19):30439–4.
30. Jin SM, Park CY, Lee JK, Ban JH, Lee SH, Lee KC. Transcutaneous injection laryngoplasty through the cricothyroid space in the sitting position: anatomical information and technique. Eur Arch Otolarhinolarngol. 2008;265(3):313–9.
31. Mau T, Courey MS. Influence of gender and injection site on vocal fold augmentation. Otolaryngol Head Neck Surg. 2008;138(2):221–5.
32. Getz AE, Scharf J, Amin MR. Thyrohyoid approach to cidofovir injection: a case study. J Voice. 2005;19(3):501–3.
33. Amin MR. Thyrohyoid approach for vocal fold augmentation. Ann Otol Rhinol Laryngol. 2006;115(9):699–702.
34. Woo SH, Son YI, Lee SH, Park JJ, Pyeong Kim J. Comparative analysis on the efficiency of the injection laryngoplasty technique using calcium hydroxyapatite (CaHA): the thyrohyoid approach versus the cricothyroid approach. J Voice. 2013;27(2):236–41.
35. Zeitler DM, Amin MR. The thyrohyoid approach to in-office injection augmentation of the vocal fold. Curr Opin Otolaryngol Head Neck Surg. 2007;15(6):412–6.

36. Pearson W, Hutchinson CT, Noordzij JP. Accessing the vocal folds by transcutaneous injection. Clin Anat. 2010;23(3):270–6.
37. Rees CJ, Mouadeb DA, Belafsky PC. Thyrohyoid vocal fold augmentation with calcium hydroxyapatite. Otolaryngol Head Neck Surg. 2008;138(6):743–6.
38. Achkar J, Song P, Andrus J, Franco R Jr. Double-bend needle modification for transthyrohyoid vocal fold injection. Laryngoscope. 2012;122(4):865–7.
39. Clary MS, Milam BM, Courey MS. Office-based vocal fold injection with the laryngeal introducer technique. Laryngoscope. 2014;124(9):2114–7.
40. Glikson E, Sagiv D, Eyal A, Wolf M, Primov-Fever A. The anatomical evolution of the thyroid cartilage from childhood to adulthood: a computed tomography evaluation. Laryngoscope. 2017;127(10):E354–8.
41. Sataloff RT, Kost KM, Linville SE. The effects of age on the voice. In: Sataloff RT, editor. Professional voice: the science and art of clinical care. 4th ed. San Diego: Plural Publishing; 2017. p. 585–604.
42. Trask DK, Shellenberger DL, Hoffman HT. Transnasal, endoscopic vocal fold augmentation. Laryngoscope. 2005;115(12):2262–5.
43. Hamdan AL, Ziade G, Jaffal H, Skaff G. Transnasal injection laryngoplasty. Ann Otol Rhinol Laryngol. 2015;124(6):474–9.
44. Wang CT, Liao LJ, Cheng PW, et al. Intralesional steroid injection for benign vocal fold disorders: a systematic review and meta-analysis. Laryngoscope. 2013;123(1):197–203.
45. Wang CT, Lai MS, Cheng PW. Long-term surveillance following intralesional steroid injection for benign vocal fold lesions. JAMA Otolaryngol Head Neck Surg. 2017;143(6):589–94.
46. Tateya I. Laryngeal steroid injection. Curr Opin Otolaryngol Head Neck Surg. 2009; 17(6):424–6.
47. Shoffel-Havakuk H, Sadoughi B, Sulica L, Johns MM III. In-office procedures for the treatment of benign vocal fold lesions in the awake patient: a contemporary review. Laryngoscope. 2019;129(9):2131–8.
48. Koufman JA, Rees CJ, Frazier WD, et al. Office-based laryngeal laser surgery: a review of 443 cases using three wavelengths. Otolaryngol Head Neck Surg. 2007;137(1):146–51.
49. Zeitels SM, Burns JA. Office-based laryngeal laser surgery with local anesthesia. Curr Opin Otolaryngol Head Neck Surg. 2007;15(3):141–7.
50. Hamdan AL, Khalifee E, Ghanem A. Application of thulium laser as office-based procedure in patients with vocal fold polyps. J Voice. 2020;34(1):140–4.
51. Centric A, Hu A, Heman-Ackah YD, Divi V, Sataloff RT. Office-based pulsed-dye laser surgery for laryngeal lesions: a retrospective review. J Voice. 2014;28(2):262.e9–262.e12.

Chapter 8
Office-Based Injection Laryngoplasty

8.1 Introduction

Injection laryngoplasty was introduced by Bruening in 1911 and later revisited by Arnold for the management of patients with unilateral vocal fold paralysis [1, 2]. The rationale of injection laryngoplasty is to push the vocal fold medially to improve glottic closure and improve phonation and swallowing. Phonatory symptoms such as breathiness, loss of volume, and inability to cough effectively that often arise because of incomplete closure of the vocal folds improve following successful injection. As the larynx plays a role in controlling the amount of air exhaled and alveolar expansion, complaints of dyspnea and shortness of breath also are attenuated. Moreover, the laryngeal "sphincter-like closure" improves during swallowing postinjection, improving dysphagia and aspiration [3]. Since its inception more than 100 years ago, the indications for injection laryngoplasty have expanded to include other causes of glottic insufficiency. Patients with vocal fold paresis, atrophy, bowing, elected cases of scar and/or sulcus vocalis, and other causes of glottic insufficiency benefit from this procedure. However, disturbed sound quality from derangement in the layered structure of the vocal fold edges may persist because injection laryngoplasty does not address the suppleness of the vocal fold directly [3, 4].

The change in clinical indications for injection laryngoplasty has led to refinements in the surgical technique and material injected. In addition to the traditional peroral approach, several other approaches have been described, the most common of which is the transcervical approach, via the thyroid cartilage referred to as transthyroid (TT), via the thyrohyoid membrane (TH), or via the cricothyroid membrane (CT) and the transnasal fiberoptic approach using a flexible endoscope with a working channel. The choice of approach depends on the patient's tolerance and anatomic variations, physician's expertise, the viscosity and volume of the material to

A.-l. Hamdan et al., *Office-Based Laryngeal Surgery*,
https://doi.org/10.1007/978-3-030-91936-8_8

be injected, and last but not least the availability of resources [4–6]. A detailed description of the operative approaches and surgical techniques is available in Chap. 7 of this book. In parallel with the evolution in the surgical approaches and techniques, different types of injectate substances have been introduced, each with its advantages and limitations. In 1955, Arnold used cartilage and bone dust with the purpose of circumventing the adverse effects of paraffin reported initially by Bruening [1]. More than a decade later, Teflon paste (Teflon particles mixed with glycerine) was introduced as another filling substance. It was used for more than two decades but was abandoned in the 1980s due to its limited success particularly in patients with vocal fold atrophy and/or scar and its local and distant complications, especially Teflon granuloma. The failures were ascribed to over injection and/or wrong placement of the injectate within the vocal fold which led to alteration in the vibratory behavior of the vocal fold. Additionally, postinjection complications such as extrusion and inflammation at the site of injection were reported by many [7–10]. Inflammation in the form of Teflon granuloma appeared in some patients years after injection and was difficult to treat. The limitations in the use of Teflon led the search for alternative substances, such as collagen, fat, hyaluronic acid, and calcium hydroxylapatite (CaHA) [3, 11]. The main challenges in finding the ideal filling substance were biocompatibility, availability, ease of harvesting, and cost. The choice of injection material also varied with the desired duration of effect. Injection laryngoplasty may be temporary if recovery within 1 year is anticipated or maybe long-lasting for patients with transection to the recurrent laryngeal nerve.

This chapter reviews the timing for injection laryngoplasty, the surgical outcomes, and complications reported with the use of different substances. The impact of age, gender, and other patient-related factors are stressed.

8.2 When to Perform Injection Laryngoplasty?

Injection laryngoplasty is one of many options offered to patients with vocal fold paresis or paralysis. Traditionally, affected patients are observed for a period of 6 months to 1 year before any permanent surgical intervention is contemplated. During the observation period, the surgeon watches for laryngeal and electromyographic signs of spontaneous recovery and/ or compensation that may affect the position of the paralyzed and contralateral vocal fold [3, 12]. If symptoms are troublesome, early injection medialization may be appropriate using materials that resorb within weeks to months. Given that vocal fold paralysis is not "an all or none" phenomenon, as stated by Woodson in her review on the evolving concepts of laryngeal paralysis, the position of the vocal fold following paralysis changes [12]. The dynamic change in position is ascribed to the persistent synchronous innervation of the thyroarytenoid muscle. Laryngeal electromyographic studies by Blitzer et al. [13] and by Sataloff et al. [14] assert that the thyroarytenoid muscle of a "paralyzed" vocal fold usually is active and not silent. Nevertheless, the laryngeal synkinesis is not always a "good synkinesis" that helps restore the vocal fold to its phonatory position. In many instances, the synkinesis is only responsible for maintaining the bulk of the paralyzed vocal fold [12–14], and it can even impair vocal fold motion.

Based on the above, physicians are reluctant to perform permanent medialization procedures early after the injury, except in selected patients in whom recurrent laryngeal nerve resection or transection has been documented. Alternatively, patients are started on voice therapy that aims at eliminating hyperfunctional compensation and optimizing glottic closure. The increased understanding of the link between body kinetics and laryngeal behavior has hastened recovery by enabling voice therapists and speech-language pathologists use body gestures in their treatment. A major limitation of voice therapy is the need for long-term patient commitment and compliance [15, 16]. The outcome of voice function exercises hinges on patient's collaboration and perseverance. Over the last two decades, injection laryngoplasty has gained popularity to be used in conjunction with voice therapy and sometimes as an alternative to voice therapy, particularly in patients who fail to commit to treatment. Injection laryngoplasty often offers immediate relief of phonatory and swallowing disturbances in affected patients. More widespread use of injection laryngoplasty as the first line of therapy in affected patients has been based on the assumption that early intervention may obviate the need for permanent medicalization [17, 18], although this concept remains controversial. The impact of temporary injection laryngoplasty on the long-term need for permanent medicalization has been an issue of debate in the literature. In 2011, Yung et al. reported a lower rate of permanent medicalization in patients with vocal fold paralysis who underwent injection laryngoplasty in comparison to those who did not. The lower rate of permanent medialization has been attributed to vibro-tactile feedback from the opposite mobile vocal fold. This feedback hypothetically promotes or enhances reinnervation. Hence, putting the vocal fold in phonatory position by temporary medicalization may allow a more "favorable" synkinetic reinnervation and recovery. This explanation remains hypothetical given the lack of electromyographic evidence to support it. A second hypothesis put forward by the authors is that fibrosis at the site of the injectate may be partially responsible for the adducted position of the vocal folds on long-term follow-up. The augmentation materials used in their study were Cymetra (LifeCell, Branchburg, NJ), Restylane (Medicis, Aesthetics, Scottsdale, AZ), and Radiesse voice gel (Merz Aesthetics, San Mateo, CA) [17]. This last hypothesis is supported partially by the study of Milstein et al. on the long-term effect of Cymetra in injection laryngoplasty [19] and also by a histologic study on a rabbit model documenting fibroblast recruitment and the ingrowth of connective tissue at the site of hyaluronic acid injection, leading to an endogenous kind of augmentation [20]. The findings of Yung et al. were supported by Prendes et al. in 2012. The authors noted that patients with unilateral vocal fold paralysis who had undergone injection laryngoplasty ($n = 14$) had less need for medialization laryngoplasty (ML) in comparison to a control group ($n = 24$) with unilateral vocal fold paralysis who were just observed (29% vs. 75%, respectively). Those who underwent injection laryngoplasty had significant improvement in 11/18 of the laryngoscopic criteria and in almost half of the CAPE-V parameters [18]. However, in

2016, Francis et al. conducted a retrospective study on a cohort of 633 patients with unilateral vocal fold paralysis and showed that early injection laryngoplasty did not reduce the need for laryngeal framework surgery long term. Stepwise multivariate logistic regression analyses were used by the authors to determine the odds of needing laryngeal framework surgery in patients who had undergone injection laryngoplasty [21]. Similarly, Merea et al., in their investigation of 135 patients who underwent medicalization laryngoplasty, half of whom had prior injection laryngoplasty, reported no effect of previous injection laryngoplasty or the time interval between the injection and medicalization on the outcome of medicalization laryngoplasty. Moreover, the amount of injectate used had no impact on the revision rate [22]. In a meta-analysis that included 275 patients with UVFP, Vila et al. explored whether performing vocal fold injection laryngoplasty within 6 months following vocal fold paralysis decreased the need for thyroplasty. The result of the analysis showed that the overall pooled relative risk of thyroplasty in those who had undergone injection (4.5 months as mean time from diagnosis) was 0.25, i.e., those who had no injection were four times more likely to undergo thyroplasty. The authors alluded to the benefit of early injection in patients with unilateral vocal fold paralysis and concluded that otolaryngologists should advocate injection laryngoplasty within 6 months from the time of [23].

In summary, patients with unilateral vocal fold paralysis or glottic insufficiency are offered various treatment options. These include observation for signs of recovery and/or compensatory movement, voice and swallowing therapy, and injection laryngoplasty. Early injection usually is advocated despite the lack of consensus on its benefit in obviating the need for permanent medicalization surgery. Medialization with laryngeal framework surgery usually is reserved for patients with persistently symptomatic glottic insufficiency, at least 6–12 months after the time of nerve injury.

8.3 Voice Outcome Following Injection Laryngoplasty

There are a growing number of reports on the short and long-term outcome of injection laryngoplasty in patients with vocal fold paresis/paralysis and/or glottic insufficiency. In 1999 Berke et al. conducted a retrospective study looking at the outcome of injection laryngoplasty in 35 patients with Parkinson's s disease and hypophonia. Using a telephone survey, the authors reported a success rate of 75%. Nevertheless, one out of five needed repeated injections after 15 days to optimize the benefit. The injections were done using collagen that was injected percutaneously under fiberoptic guidance [24]. In 2005, Milstein et al. investigated the longevity of micronized Alloderm (Cymetra) in injection laryngoplasty in 20 patients with unilateral vocal fold paralysis. At a mean follow-up of 11.2 months, the authors noted significant improvement in glottal closure, vocal fold bowing, and voice quality. These were accompanied by improvement in quality of life which was long-lasting in three fourths of the study group [19]. In 2007, Luu et al. reviewed their experience with 1290 injection laryngoplasties using cross-linked dermal bovine collagen and reported a success rate of 83.9%. Two hundred patients of their study group had either worsening or no change in voice quality. Patients were assessed 2–3 months following the injection using a self-reported questionnaire and laryngeal videostroboscopy [25]. In 2008, Kimura et al. reported subjective and objective improvement 3 months post-surgery in155 out of 275 patients. The patients were evaluated using GRBAS, acoustic analysis, and aerodynamic measurements [26]. In another study, Min et al. investigated the long-term results of Artecoll (polymethyl methacrylate microspheres mixed with bovine collagen) injection laryngoplasty in 96 patients with unilateral vocal fold paralysis and reported significant improvement in the subjective grading of voice quality and in patient-related score of hoarseness. Additionally, there was an increase in maximum phonation time (MPT) and a decrease in jitter, shimmer, and noise-to-harmonic ratio. The postinjection improvement lasted 12 months [27]. Similarly, Dursun et al. in 2008 examined the long-term results of injection laryngoplasty in a subgroup of patients with glottic bowing and/or sulcus vocalis and noted improvement in dysphonia, roughness, and breathiness and a significant increase in MPT, and a decrease in jitter. Patients were followed up between 1 and 7 years [28]. In 2008, Sulica et al. conducted a multi-institutional review of 460 injections laryngoplasty, half of which (51%) were performed on awake patients, and they reported a success rate of 99%. The most common indications for injection laryngoplasty were paralysis (54%), paresis (21%), and atrophy (15%). The most common filling materials used in the office setting were methylcellulose in 35% and bovine collagen in 28%. In conclusion, the authors noted the high success rate of office-based procedures and their fast adoption in clinical practice [6]. In 2009, Gillespie et al. reviewed the outcome of 39 patients who had undergone injection laryngoplasty using calcium hydroxylapatite (CaHA) and reported improvement in the mean VHI score (61.2 ± 24 vs. 35.9 ± 26.3,). The mean follow-up period was 17.8 ± 13.6 months [29]. In 2011, Carroll and Rosen reviewed the long-term effectiveness of CaHA using the VHI-10 questionnaire as a primary outcome measure and reported an average length of benefit of 18.6 months (range 8–36 months) [30]. In 2012, Choi et al. reported improvement in 44 of 59 patients with unilateral vocal fold paralysis who underwent injection laryngoplasty using Artecoll (polymethyl methacrylate microspheres mixed with bovine collagen) [31]. In 2013, Wen et al. investigated the outcomes of injection laryngoplasty in 60 patients who had undergone vocal fold augmentation using either cross-linked porcine collagen ($n = 33$) or hyaluronic acid ($n = 27$) and reported significant improvement in MPT and self-reported voice outcome with a mean symptom-free duration of 10.9 months in the former group and 14.4 months in the latter. The authors noted no significant difference between those who were injected with porcine collagen and those injected with hyaluronic acid [32]. In 2013, Birkent et al. reviewed 35 cases of percutaneous injection laryngoplasty and reported improvement in all 3 components of the VHI, CAPE-V, as well as GRBAS perceptual evaluation except for roughness. The authors noted the effectiveness of injection laryngoplasty in the management of glottal insufficiency and in meeting patient's expectations at 2 months follow-up [33]. That same year, Jamal et al. investigated the outcome of 100 cases of glottal incompetence who had undergone injection laryngoplasty and reported a success rate of 96%. The injections were performed percutaneously using bovine collagen. The most common etiology of glottal incompetence was vocal fold paralysis in 76%, followed by atrophy in 13% and paresis in 5% of the cases [34]. In 2013, Woo et al. conducted a comparative study on 64 patients who had undergone injection laryngoplasty using either the CT membrane approach (n = 30) or the TH membrane approach (TH) and reported comparable outcomes with both approaches. The authors concluded that the TH membrane approach is a good alternative to CT membrane approach in the management of patients with unilateral vocal fold paralysis [35]. In 2014, Powell et al. assessed the self-reported symptoms and perceptual evaluation of 57 patients with glottic insufficiency who had undergone injection laryngoplasty and reported a decrease improvement in the median voice performance questionnaire score (42 preoperative vs. 21 postoperative). Additionally, there was an improvement in the grade of dysphonia and other perceptual rating parameters. Patients were evaluated before and 2 weeks after the injection [36]. In 2014, Halderman et al. reported their experience with 64 patients who underwent 82 injection laryngoplasties using Restylane. The overall success rate was 94%, and the mean duration of benefit of the injection was 12.2 weeks [37]. In 2015, Sardesai et al. reported the voice outcome of 35 patients who had undergone awake office-based injection laryngoplasty and noted a change in the mean of VHI and CAPE-V by 19.9 and 15.5, respectively, in male and 24.0 and 15.8, respectively, in females [38]. In 2017, McLaughlin et al. reviewed 53 patients with unilateral vocal fold paralysis, 19 of whom underwent injection laryngoplasty using a temporary agent, 8 had injection laryngoplasty followed by permanent medicalization, and 20 had permanent medicalization. Of the total group, six had only conservative (nonsurgical) management. There was no significant difference in normal glottal gap area (NGGA) and CAPE-V scores among the three subgroups who had an intervention. All subgroups had improvement in NGGA and CAPE-V scores at the last follow-up which ranged between 19.4 and 28 months [39]. Sielska-Badurek et al., in 2017, reported a comprehensive voice evaluation of 14 patients who underwent injection laryngoplasty using CaHA and showed complete glottic closure with improvement in all voice quality parameters. These included vocal loudness, MPT, acoustic parameters, and the GRBAS subjective evaluation [40]. In 2018, Hu et al. investigated the outcomes of office-based autologous fat injection laryngoplasty in 23 patients under the age of 50 years with glottic insufficiency and reported significant improvement in VHI-10, grade of dysphonia, breathiness, noise-to-harmonic ratio, and jitter at 6 months [41]. In 2018, Maccarini et al. reported their experience with transnasal fiberendoscopic injection laryngoplasty using centrifuged autologous fat in 22 patients with unilateral vocal fold paralysis and reported significant improvement in all but 1 of their study group. The patients were evaluated using laryngeal videostroboscopy, maximum phonation time, and perceptually 1 week and 6 months after the injection [42]. Similarly, in 2018, Hamdan et al. reported their experience using the same approach in 46 patients with glottic insufficiency. Using hyaluronic acid as an injectate, the authors noted significant improvement in the mean VHI-10 score, as well as in the perceptual evaluation parameters. There was also an increase in the closed quotient from 0.19 preinjection to 0.46

postinjection [43]. In a study on the safety of injection laryngoplasty while taking antithrombotic therapy, Sato et al. reported optimal results in 17 patients who underwent 47 injection laryngoplasty. Only three cases of bleeding were observed [44]. In 2019, Bertroche et al. studied the longevity of injection laryngoplasty using hyaluronic acid and reported a mean duration of 10.6 months. The latter was defined as the interval time between the injection and the date when improvement started fading. There was improvement in the mean VRQOL (49.2 preinjection vs. 68.2 postinjection) [45]. In 2020, Jeong et al. investigated the value of voice therapy (VT) following injection laryngoplasty. The study showed that those who had VT had significantly more reduction in shimmer, jitter and noise-to-harmonic ratio, and prolongation in maximum phonation time more than those who did not. The authors advocated voice therapy in patients undergoing injection laryngoplasty [46]. Novakovic et al. expanded the indication of injection laryngoplasty to include muscle tension dysphonia. Interestingly, the authors noted a decrease in VHI-10 score even in patients with no glottis insufficiency at the time of diagnosis [47]. Last but not least, Wang et al. conducted a systematic review on the use of hyaluronic acid in injection laryngoplasty and reported significant improvement in both objective and subjective voice measures. The authors noted prolongation of the maximum phonation time, improvement in glottic closure, and perceptual voice parameters. The duration of improvement varied across different studies [48].

Injection laryngoplasty has also been shown to improve dysphagia and aspiration. Numerous authors reported significant improvement in swallowing following medialization procedures in patients with unilateral vocal fold paralysis. In 2018, Zuniga et al. studied the impact of injection laryngoplasty on swallowing in 21 patients with vocal fold immobility and reported significant improvement in the median eating assessment score and the functional oral intake scale score. The authors reiterated the effectiveness of injection laryngoplasty in reducing the risk of aspiration [49]. Anis and Memon assessed the impact of injection laryngoplasty on swallowing in 21 patients and reported improvement in 76% of those who had dysphagia before injection. The decrease in the mean score of EAT-10 was significant (17.0 preoperative vs. 4.2 postoperative, respectively) [50]. In another study, Han et al. investigated the impact of injection laryngoplasty on functional oral intake in six patients with long-standing history of aspiration. The authors reported an increase in mean inspiratory and expiratory pressure and an increase in mean peak cough flow. The authors concluded that injection laryngoplasty is an effective adjunctive treatment modality for patients with glottis insufficiency [51]. These findings concur with those of Chen et al. in 2018 who advocated early injection laryngoplasty in patients with vocal fold immobility secondary to thoracic aortic repair. The study, which included 35 patients, showed that those who had early injection had fewer pulmonary complications than those who had late injections (20% vs. 50%, respectively) and shorter length of stay (13 days vs. 20 days, respectively) [52]. In 2020, Choi et al. investigated the outcome of additional injection laryngoplasty in 76 patients with unilateral vocal fold paralysis who had undergone previously the same procedure. The authors reported significant improvement in aspiration. Moreover, there was a significant improvement in the overall grade of dysphonia and roughness, as well as in VHI-30 score [53]. In 2020, Pan and Sadoughi in their systematic review on the effect of injection laryngoplasty on aspiration reported improvement in penetration aspiration scores and diet intake in the majority of the studies. Nonetheless, the authors noted the lack of a control group in all the studies reviewed and the need for more robust investigations to draw evidence-based conclusions [54].

In summary, the short- and long-term results of injection laryngoplasty performed in patients with unilateral vocal fold paralysis or glottic insufficiency are satisfactory. There is a significant improvement in self-reported phonatory symptoms as well as in subjective and objective voice assessment. There is also a significant improvement in swallowing symptoms such as dysphagia and aspiration. The duration of improvement varies with the type of augmentation material used.

8.4 Factors Affecting the Outcome of Office-Based Injection Laryngoplasty

8.4.1 Effect of Age on the Outcome of Office-Based Injection Laryngoplasty

Age has a significant impact on musculoskeletal structures. With aging, there is a decrease in muscle mass and density and an increase in fibrosis and intramuscular lipid deposition [55]. The decrease in muscle density is attributed to alteration in neuromuscular synaptic architecture and decrease in microcirculation [56]. As a musculoskeletal structure, the larynx is equally affected by aging [57]. Davids et al. reviewed the current trends of dysphonia in patients above the age of 65 years and reported a prevalence of 58%, with vocal fold atrophy being the most common cause [58]. Similarly, Marino and Johns stressed the multifaceted etiology of dysphonia in the elderly patient, the psychosocial associated challenges, and the need for a multidisciplinary approach to manage the aging voice [59]. The change in voice quality with aging is attributed to both morphologic and histologic changes. In their review of muscle function with aging, Thomas et al. reviewed the metabolic, neurologic, and hormonal changes responsible for remodeling of the thyroarytenoid muscle and the decline in its function [57]. Ziade et al. reported significant differences in the computerized tomographic (CT) attenuation (using Hounsfield units (HU)) of the thyroarytenoid (TA) muscles in subjects above the age of 65 years in comparison to subjects below the age of 65 years (right TA 31.2 ± 11.9 HU vs. 20.8 ± 14.4 HU, respectively, left TA 29.6 ± 99 HU vs. 22.8 ± 15.0 HU, respectively) [60]. Note that the study design consisted of a hybrid imaging modality, namely, PET/CT in which the average CT density (measured in HU) and regional tissue activity concentration (maximal standard uptake) of the TA muscles were measured. Their results concur with those of Wehrli et al. who also reported a decrease in CT attenuation with aging. In their review of 213 subjects, the authors noted attenuation in the metabolism of the muscles, adipose tissues, and skin [61]. The lamina propria of the vocal fold is also subject to many histologic changes in its cellular and extracellular constituents. There is an increase in collagen deposition, a decrease in elastic fiber concentration, and alteration in hyaluronic acid distribution associated with increase in age. Sataloff et al. have provided a thorough review on the effects of age on voice [62].

These age-induced structural vocal fold changes need to be considered in patients undergoing injection laryngoplasty. Many studies in the literature investigated the predictive role of age on the outcome of vocal fold augmentation, with no clear consensus. In 2012, Choi et al. reviewed the demographic variables of 59 patients with unilateral vocal fold paralysis who had undergone injection laryngoplasty and reported that those who improved were significantly younger than those who did not. All patients were injected with Artecoll (polymethyl methacrylate microspheres plus bovine collagen) using the transcutaneous approach and were evaluated using GRBAS perceptual rating and laryngeal videostroboscopy [31]. In 2015, Sardesai et al. reviewed a series of 35 patients who underwent awake injection laryngoplasty and reported no association between age, gender, and the outcome of injection. What was noticeable in that study was that patients with high VHI scores before injection had a better outcome than those with low VHI scores, alluding to a ceiling effect [38]. Similarly, in a radiologic study looking at the volumetric measures of the vocal folds in patients undergoing injection laryngoplasty, Hamdan et al. reported that the difference in the mean volume of paralyzed and nonparalyzed vocal fold was higher in subjects above the age of 65 years in comparison to those below the age of 65 years (152.04 ± 90.77 mm3 vs. 194.46 ± 155.82 mm3, respectively). The authors highlighted the need to account for the age-related larger discrepancy in vocal fold volume in patients undergoing injection laryngoplasty [63].

8.4.2 *Effect of Gender on the Outcome of Office-Based Injection Laryngoplasty*

Gender is an important variable that needs to be considered in patients undergoing injection laryngoplasty. Laryngeal structural and histological differences between males and females have been described in the literature. Males in comparison to females have longer vocal folds (15.4 mm vs.11.1 mm, respectively), greater thyroid cartilage height (42.3 mm vs. 32.5 mm, respectively), and longer thyroid lamina [64]. Zeitler and Amin reported that men had a longer distance between the thyroid notch and tip of the vocal process (27.4 vs. 19.7 mm, respectively) and a longer distance between the thyroid notch and mid-vocal fold (21.8 vs.15.5 mm, respectively) in comparison to women [4]. In another radiologic study, a significant difference in vocal fold volume in men compared to women was noted (389.761 ± 180.210 vs. 257.550 ± 108.982 mm3, respectively). The study was conducted on 21 subjects using computerized tomography [63]. There are also histologic differences in the vocal folds of men and women. In a study by Butler et al. on gender differences in hyaluronic acid (HA) distribution in 25 vocal folds analyzed at autopsy, the authors noted less HA in the superficial layer of the lamina propria and a higher concentration in the deep layer in females compared to males [65]. These structural and histologic changes may contribute the higher prevalence of dysphonia in females compared to males. In an epidemiologic study looking at the prevalence of voice disorders in the normal population, Roy et al. reported a higher prevalence in women and subjects aged 40–59 years. Sex and age increased the odds of having chronic voice disorders in their random sample which included 1326 adults [66].

Based on the above, gender as a variable must also be considered in patients undergoing injection laryngoplasty. The site and amount of injectate during injection laryngoplasty differ across genders. In 2008, Mau and Courey investigated gender effect on the amount of injectate in cadaveric larynges that were evaluated before and after injection using high-resolution computerized tomography. The authors found that males required on average 50–60% more filling substance than females. The difference in the mean of injectate was significant in both lateral injections (0.62 ml in males and 0.41 ml in females) and medial injections (0.23 ml in males and 0.14 ml in females). The larger amount of injectate needed in males vs. females was ascribed to the known anatomic differences in laryngeal dimensions across genders [64]. The implication of these findings on the surgical outcome of patients undergoing injection laryngoplasty remains controversial. In 2013, Jamal et al. reviewed their experience with 100 cases of injection laryngoplasty, and they reported no change in voice quality or worsening in 4 cases, all of whom were women. Notably, these accounted for 10% of the women who had undergone this procedure [34]. However, in a study by Wen et al. of 60 patients who underwent injection laryngoplasty using either cross-linked porcine collagen ($n = 33$) or hyaluronic acid ($n = 27$), the authors noted no significant difference in outcome between genders. Patients were evaluated using the VHI-10 score and maximum phonation time at 1, 3, and 6 months following treatment [32]. In a study by Lin et al. that included 73 patients with unilateral vocal fold paralysis, the authors noted that female patients had better Jita (absolute jitter, microsec) than male patients 12 months after lipoinjection. The authors alluded to the importance of gender in addition to age as a prognostic indicator of the success of this procedure [67].

8.4.3 Other Patient-Related Factors in Injection Laryngoplasty

Other very important patient-related factors that may affect the outcome of injection laryngoplasty are the size of the posterior gap and the position of the vocal fold at the time of injection. Patients with a large glottal gap are less likely to improve fully following medicalization procedures than patients with a small glottal gap. This is attributed to the fact that vocal fold movement is not limited to the horizontal plane. The vocal process moves medial and downward during phonation and lateral and upward during breathing. When the gap is large at the time of the injection, this means that the paralyzed vocal fold is also higher than the nonparalyzed vocal fold creating a vertical discrepancy between the two vocal folds. Injection laryngoplasty addresses only the axial position of the vocal fold and not its vertical position [12], at least in most cases. In a review on glottal gap size in predicting the need for permanent laryngoplasty, Fang et al. reported that patients with a large glottal gap were more in need of permanent laryngoplasty than those who had a small glottal gap [68]. Similarly, in a study by Choi et al. of 59 patients with unilateral vocal fold paralysis who had undergone injection laryngoplasty, the authors found a significant association between the outcome of injection laryngoplasty and the size of the posterior glottal gap [31].

8.4.4 Technical Factors: Site of Injection, Amount to Be Injected, and Injection Force Mechanics

Injection laryngoplasty is a procedure that aims to reposition the lateralized vocal fold in the midline. As the injection does not address directly the vibratory behavior of the vocal fold, the injectate material is placed usually as lateral as possible in the paraglottic space adjacent to the thyroid cartilage inner perichondrium, to help minimize its effect on the vibratory margin. For some materials in selected cases, the injection may be placed just lateral to the vocalis muscle. The exact positioning of the injectate material dictates the amount that needs to be injected. In 2008, Mau and Courey reported that a larger amount of injectate is needed to medialize the vocal fold if the injection is made lateral to the thyroarytenoid muscle in comparison to injections made in the medial belly of the thyroarytenoid muscle. The lateral-medial volume ratio in males and females was 2.7 and 2.9, respectively [64]. The authors also noted the effect of the injectate on the position of the arytenoid cartilages. The movement, which was described as rotatory and passive, was more obvious when the injection was placed laterally. The clinical implication of these findings is that the site of injection and the amount injected need to be individualized according to the position of the vocal fold and the cause of glottic incompetence. In a patient with a large gap secondary to unilateral vocal fold paralysis, the injection should be placed laterally, and a large amount of injectate is usually needed. In patients with vocal fold scar or atrophy, the injection can be placed more medially within or just lateral to the medial belly of the thyroarytenoid muscle (vocalis), and less injectate material is needed. This is more challenging because of the proximity of the injected substance to the vibratory surface of the vocal fold.

Injection force is another technical issue to consider while performing injection laryngoplasty. The injection force required to achieve vocal fold augmentation is extremely important in achieving the desired results. Important variables to consider are the size of the needle, its length, and its configuration. Pearson et al. compared the injection forces using various needles and filling substances at different temperatures [69]. Using swine larynges affixed to a stabilizing crossbeam, the authors tested the injection forces at a compressive load of 40 mm/minute, using different needles with or without denting. The results showed the highest steady-state force (44.55 N) and the lowest stiffness rate (19.75 N/mm) while using the peroral needle. Similarly, the stiffness was affected with higher values reported using the 27-gauge percutaneous needle vs. the 25-gauge needle and the peroral needle. The orientation of the needle, whether straight or bent, also had an effect. The straight needle had a higher maximum load than a bent needle. Moreover, the maximum load increased with increasing length and decreasing gauge of the needle. For instance, a 27-gauge had a higher load than a 25-gauge needle. In clinical practice, the results of this investigation indicate that the easiest way is to inject a viscous material thru a large gauge needle that is straight and not bent. The authors noted also that increasing the temperature of the injectate reduces the material resistive forces at least at the onset of the injection. In conclusion, the authors stressed the importance of needle stability in injection laryngoplasty, which is accomplished partially by the use of different needle types and orientations [69]. Lisi et al. stressed the differences between the viscosity of materials used for medial (vibratory margin) injection vs. lateral injection. Although low viscosity materials are ideal for medial injections, more evidence-based research is needed to establish the ideal properties for materials used in lateral injection laryngoplasty. Proper positioning of the injectate and its maintenance are also crucial predictors of the long-term success [70].

In summary, injection medialization laryngoplasty involves injecting the vocal fold with a filling material that aims to restore glottic closure. The improvement noted following injection is ascribed to the mass effect of the injectate displacing the vocal fold medially. The filling material is placed either laterally or medially within the thyroarytenoid muscle, depending on the material and cause and severity of glottic insufficiency. The outcome of this procedure depends on surgery-related factors, type of augmentation material used, and patient-related factors. Age, gender, and glottic configuration are important variables to consider for predicting surgical outcome of injection laryngoplasty. It is also important to note that injection laryngoplasty does not address the impairment of pliability of the vibratory membrane seen in patients with vocal fold scar, but improving glottic closure may provide better voice by improving the ability of the contralateral vocal fold to compensate for unilateral stiffness.

8.5 Complications of Injection Laryngoplasty

Complications following injection laryngoplasty are rare. The most common are deposition of the injectate within the superficial layer of the lamina propria, vocal fold bolus or abscess formation, hypersensitivity reactions, and bleeding. An important predisposing factor for bleeding is the use of anticoagulants, although their etiologic role in the development of bleeding remains controversial [44, 71]. Patients with complications following injection laryngoplasty usually present with symptoms that may include globus sensation, throat clearing, dysphonia, dysphagia, shortness of breath, and stridor among others. These symptoms are usually managed conservatively under close observation, with or without the prescription of anti-inflammatory medications and/or antibiotics. When a long-acting augmentation material has been used, surgical intervention and excision of the injectate endoscopically through a lateral cordotomy incision or externally through the thyroid cartilage may be necessary. If left untreated, patients can develop vocal fold scar, and bleeding and other adverse events may lead to tethering of the vocal fold cover to the underlying vocal fold ligament.

The prevalence of complications following injection laryngoplasty varies mostly with the type of filling substance used for augmentation and the surgeons' expertise. This section reviews complications of injection laryngoplasty using collagen, fat, calcium hydroxylapatite, and hyaluronic acid.

8.5.1 Complications of Injection Laryngoplasty Using Collagen

Following its success in dermatology as a filling material that redefines skin contour and scar tissue, collagen gained popularity in laryngology as a safe alternative to previously used substances such as paraffin and Teflon [3]. Its abundant availability in dermal tissue, ease of preparation/injection, and long-lasting effect has paved the way for its adoption among many otolaryngologists. Its natural presence as a main constituent of the vocal fold lamina propria also made it appealing. In patients with vocal fold scar, collagen injection acts by promoting the proliferation of collagenase and remodeling the scar tissue, in addition to its mass effect. Despite the many advantages of collagen use in injection laryngoplasty, one main limitation used to be recipient hypersensitivity. This was associated with xenograft proteins within the injectate when bovine or porcine collagen was used. Although its occurrence is rare, the potential severe collagen-induced hypersensitivity can be life-threatening. This led to a decline in its use until purified, human forms were developed. By harvesting collagen from the patient's dermal tissue and reinjecting it into the vocal fold, foreign body reaction decreased, and tissue tolerance improved [3]. The enhanced tissue tolerance was associated with improvement in subjective and objective voice parameters following injection [72]. To further reduce the limitations of allograft collagen use, namely, donor site morbidity and time needed to harvest the grafted material, purified forms derived from cadaveric skin dermal tissue were introduced, the most common of which was Cymetra (Cymetra; Life Cell Corporation, Brandenburg) [73]. Unfortunately, manufacture of that excellent product has been discontinued.

Despite its availability and many advantages, collagen injection still had complications, particularly when injected in the superficial layer of the lamina propria.

Based on an animal study by Courey, homologous collagen compounds are best injected in the medial part of the thyroarytenoid muscle just deep to the vocal ligament to avert impairment of vocal fold vibration [74]. In a clinical study of 39 patients who had undergone injection laryngoplasty for the treatment of glottal incompetence using collagen, Remacle et al. cautioned about the adverse effect of superficial injection and the resultant permanent stiffening of the vocal fold. Their study group was evaluated using laryngeal stroboscopic examination, acoustic analysis, and aerodynamic measures [75]. Berke et al., in their review of 35 patients with Parkinson's disease and hypophonia who underwent percutaneous injection laryngoplasty, reported two cases of superficial injections that resulted in the formation of collagen nodules [24]. In 2004, Anderson and Sataloff reported two unusual cases of injection laryngoplasty using collagen. Both patients developed submucosal deposits that hindered the malleability of the vocal fold cover and resulted in dysphonia. Microsurgical dissection of the injectate resulted in improvement in voice quality. The authors highlighted the common complications of collagen injection in the vocal folds among which are hypersensitivity reactions, the formation of an abscess at the site of injection, and possibly injection-induced collagen vascular disease [76]. Similarly, Sulica et al. reviewed 460 injection laryngoplasty mostly performed on patients with paralysis, paresis, vocal fold atrophy, and scar and reported a complication rate of 3% for in-office injections in comparison to 2% under general anesthesia. The most commonly used materials for augmentation were methylcellulose in 35% of the cases and bovine collagen in 28% of the cases [6]. In another review of 100 patients who had undergone percutaneous injection laryngoplasty using collagen as an augmentation material, Jamal et al. reported a complication rate of 4%. All four patients had an inadvertent superficial injection that resulted in blanching of the upper surface of the vocal fold and a decrease in mucosal wave amplitude. The patients were managed conservatively for 6 months with no subsequent adverse phonatory sequelae. No other complications such as bleeding or hypersensitivity reactions were reported [34].

8.5.2 Complications of Injection Laryngoplasty Using Fat

Fat is a substance commonly used in injection laryngoplasty. The similarity of its viscoelastic properties to those of the lamina propria and its abundant availability and ease to harvest have fostered its popularity over the last four decades [77–80]. In 2013, DeFatta et al. reviewed their experience in laryngeal lipotransfer in 89 patients with glottic insufficiency and reported significant improvement in vocal fold closure and vibration. The fat was injected laterally in patients with impaired vocal fold motion and/or implanted medially through a submucosal tunnel in patients with vibratory margin pathology. The authors stressed the need for long-term effect and repeated injections in selected cases [81]. Based on a systematic review by Truzzi et al., fat grafts in injection laryngoplasty usually are harvested from the lower abdomen by liposuction and processed by manual selection and washing using saline, lactated ringer, insulin solution, methylprednisolone, dexamethasone, or other corticosteroid solution, with successful results [82]. Nonetheless, a major limitation to its usage is its unpredictable resorption rate which makes it hard to decide on the amount that needs to be injected. The resorption rate depends on the size of the fat cells harvested and the "health" of the surrounding ground substance. Fat graft survival and the fate of adipose-derived stem cells (ASCs) contained within the fat grafts depend also on the microenvironment of the recipient bed [83]. By promoting the release of vascular endothelial growth factors and fibroblast growth factors, adipose-derived stem cells can help promote the survival of fat cells following transplantation, with the subsequent remodeling of the vocal fold constituents.

Most of the literature on the longevity and complications of fat injection laryngoplasty is derived from studies on patients operated under suspension microlaryngoscopy. In 2002, McCulloch et al. reported a success rate of 70% and 55% at 2- and 4-year follow-up. Their study group had improvement in the mean grade of dysphonia and breathiness at a mean period of 52 days. No complications were reported [84]. A year later, Laccourreye et al. reported a success rate of 91.1% at 3 months and 63.1% at 12 months [85]. Their study group consisted of 80 patients, 3 of whom developed hematoma at the site of injection, 1 had extrusion, and another had dyspnea. Late complications included intracordal cyst formation in three cases. Similarly, Umeno et al. in 2005 reported sustainability of intracordal fat injection for more than 2 years following injection. The study was conducted on 41 patients with unilateral vocal fold paralysis who had fat injection laryngoplasty under suspension microlaryngeal surgery. The authors reported one case of fat extrusion and two cases of mild airway obstruction that subsided with no need for intervention [86]. Fang et al., in 2010, reported sustainability of fat injection laryngoplasty up to 1 year. The study conducted on 33 patients with unilateral vocal fold paralysis showed a marked increase in maximum phonation time and s/z ratio, as well as a decrease in jitter. No complications were noted in their study group [87]. In 2018, Maccarini et al. reported the safety of fat as an injection material in 22 patients who underwent flexible intranasal endoscopic injection. The patients were evaluated 1 week and 6 months after the injection, and no complications were reported [42].

8.5.3 Complications Following Injection Laryngoplasty Using Calcium Hydroxylapatite

Calcium hydroxylapatite (CaHA) is a mixture of 25–45 micrometer calcium microspheres and carboxymethylcellulose gel-type carrier. It has gained popularity among otolaryngologists as a long-term filling substance in injection laryngoplasty. Its long-term effect is attributed to the fact that microspheres maintain their volume at the injected site long after resorption of the calcium particles. With the increase in its usage in the operating room or office setting, there have been an increasing number of reported complications with symptoms of globus, cough, neck pain, dysphonia, and dyspnea [29, 88–90]. In 2008, Chheda et al. reported five cases who had undergone revision microsurgery for removal of the implanted CaHA. The authors ascribed the complication of superficial injection and/or over-medicalization that resulted in voice impairment [88]. In 2009, Gillespie et al. reviewed the complication rate of CaHA injection laryngoplasty in 39 patients and reported worsening of the VHI score in 43% of those with vocal fold soft tissue defects and 7% of those with vocal fold paralysis. In total, eight patients had complications, the most common of which were superficial injections. Only one patient developed respiratory distress which necessitated the removal of injectate [29]. In another review by Carroll and Rosen on the longevity of CaHA in the treatment of patients with glottal insufficiency, the authors noted three complications, including superficial injection in one and infraglottic deposition in two [30]. In 2012, DeFatta et al. reported 16 patients who had complications following CaHA injection laryngoplasty. The major ones included granuloma formation in two cases and adynamic or decreased mucosal waves in four and six cases, respectively. The injected implants were removed surgically under general anesthesia using a lateral cordotomy incision. Minor complications included inflammation and edema with mild impairment in mucosal waves. The authors stressed the adverse effects of CaHA on phonation secondary to inflammatory reactions and possible extrusion [89]. Similarly, Lee et al. reviewed their experience of 955 injection laryngoplasty using CaHA and reported superficial injections in eight cases. The authors stressed the importance of early recognition of this complication and the need to aspirate the material once blanching of the vocal fold is seen intraoperatively. Failure to drain the lobulated material using the tip of the needle and persistence of dysphonia with a decrease in mucosal waves on laryngeal videostroboscopy should prompt surgical intervention, namely, incising the overlying vocal fold cover. Acute and delayed onset of dyspnea occurred in 0.3% and 0.2% of the cases, respectively [90].

8.5.4 Complications of Hyaluronic Acid as a Filling Material in Injection Laryngoplasty

Since its availability in a purified and engineered commercial form, hyaluronic acid (HA) has gained popularity as a safe augmentation material in injection laryngoplasty. The increase in its usage is ascribed to its biocompatibility, favorable viscoelastic properties, slow absorption rate, and resistance to migration [91, 92]. The incidence of adverse reactions in injection laryngoplasty using HA is rare. The clinical presentation may be subtle with ill-defined symptoms such as globus and sore throat or life-threatening with symptoms of airway obstruction. Hertegård et al. reported three cases of adverse reactions to hyaluronic acid injection characterized by inflammation at the site of injection. The main reported symptoms were dysphonia and cough [93, 94]. In 2010, Song et al. reviewed the voice outcome of HA injection laryngoplasty in 27 patients with vocal fold immobility and reported 1 case of superficial injection. The patient had worsening of his voice quality which necessitated surgical removal of the collection under suspension microlaryngoscopy [95]. In 2012, Rudolf and Sibylle reported a patient who developed dyspnea 3 days after having undergone injection laryngoplasty using HA. On laryngeal examination, there was evidence of edema of the false vocal fold and aryepiglottic fold [96]. Their study group consisted of 19 patients who were assessed at three-time intervals, 6 weeks, 6 months, and 12 months following HA injection laryngoplasty. It is noticeable that 42% of their study group had a decrease in voice quality at 6 weeks follow-up [96]. Halderman et al. reviewed 64 patients who underwent HA injection laryngoplasty and reported 5 cases of adverse events, 2 of whom had superficial injections and 1 had dyspnea and shortness of breath [37]. Shamanna et al. reported a 53-year-old woman who developed mucosal ulceration and necrosis at the site of injection attributed to a compartment syndrome-like reaction [97]. Dominguez et al. reported seven cases of inflammatory reactions at the site of HA injection laryngoplasty. The study group consisted of 186 patients who had undergone 245 procedures. The most commonly described symptoms were dysphonia, odynophagia, and dyspnea. On laryngeal examination, patients had a decrease in vocal fold cover pliability. Although all patients received adequate treatment, the VHI-10 score did not normalize in all cases [98]. In a review of 63 patients with glottal insufficiency who had undergone HA injection laryngoplasty, Hamdan et al. reported three cases of adverse reactions who presented with symptoms of globus sensation, dysphagia, throat pain, and shortness of breath 48–72 hours after the injection. Two patients had severe edema of the arytenoid, false vocal fold, and aryepiglottic fold. All three patients were managed successfully using conservative therapy, namely, systemic steroids and antibiotics under close observation (Figs. 8.1 and 8.2) [99].

The adverse reactions to HA are not very surprising. Perazzo et al., in their histologic study using a rabbit model, showed inflammatory response around the injectate in all 22 cases, although the inflammation was mild and not time-dependent

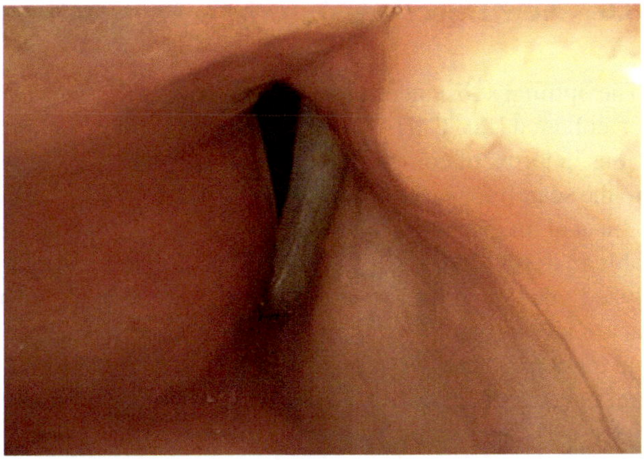

Fig. 8.1 A 54-year old woman who presented with dyspnea and throat discomfort 2 days following injection laryngoplasty using Hyaluronic acid. Patient had history of right cordotomy as a treatment of bilateral vocal fold paralysis. Note the edema, redness and fullness of the right false vocal fold

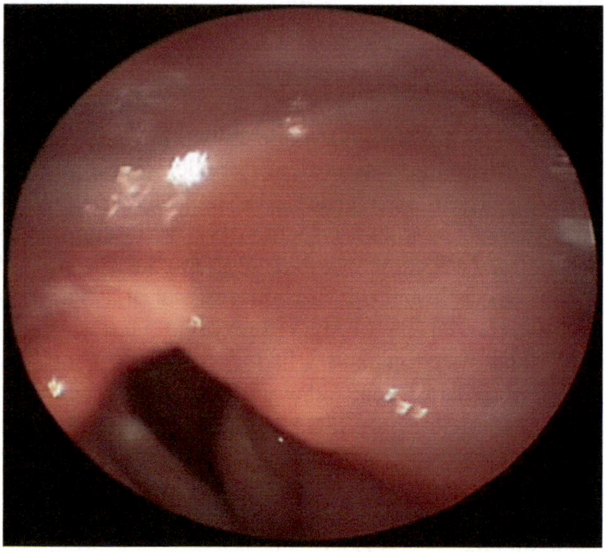

Fig. 8.2 A laryngeal endoscopic view of a 23-year-old woman who presented 2 days following vocal fold injection using hyaluronic acid with globus sensation, dysphagia and dyspnea. The figure shows edema of the left false vocal fold, aryepiglottic fold and true vocal fold

[100]. The adverse reactions to HA can be attributed to several factors; one is local hypersensitivity to impurities in the product introduced during manufacturing, namely, bacterial proteins. The unilaterality of the inflammatory reaction, the lack of cell-specific histologic response at the site of inflammation, the normal immunoglobulin level in affected patients, and last but not least the longevity of the reaction (many months in certain cases) argue against this theory [37, 98]. Other possible causes include contamination and vascular compression, although tissue necrosis is seen rarely. Selecting the size of the HA cross-linked particle, using short needles to help reduce the force of injection, and avoidance of overfilling are crucial factors in reducing vascular compression at the site of injection.

8.6 New Injection Materials: Prospective and Safety

The optimal substance for injection laryngoplasty has yet to be determined. The use of collagen, fat, CaHA, hyaluronic acid, and other synthetic materials has limitations in terms of compatibility, resorption rate, availability, and/or cost. This has led to the search for safer, more biocompatible, and less expensive alternatives. In 2004, Lee et al. investigated the tolerance and durability of auricular cartilage as an injectable material. In a study on nine dogs, minced cartilage was injected into the paralyzed vocal fold and re-examined at several time intervals. The authors reported acute inflammatory reactions early postinjection and marked volume augmentation up to 12 months [101]. Lim et al., inspired by the longevity of cartilage injection in animal studies, investigated the surgical outcome in 14 patients with unilateral vocal fold paralysis who were injected using the peroral approach under general anesthesia. The authors noted significant voice improvement up to 1 year with no major complications reported [102]. Hong et al. reported the use of plasma gel as an augmentation material in injection laryngoplasty in a rabbit model. The vocal folds (right side) of 12 rabbits were injected with 0.005 ml of plasma and later examined at 2, 4, and weeks following the injection. On histologic examination, the authors showed less inflammation and foreign body reaction in comparison to vocal folds that were injected with Artecoll (polymethyl methacrylate microspheres mixed with bovine collagen) or hyaluronic acid. However, there were no quantitative differences in the extent of collagen deposition and neovascularization. At 8 weeks following the injection, there was significant absorption of the plasma gel in two of four rabbits [103]. Similarly, Woo et al. reported a clinical study on 11 patients with unilateral vocal fold paralysis who underwent autologous plasma gel injection and showed improvement in self-reported quality of voice as well as acoustic (shimmer, jitter) and aerodynamic measure (MPT) at 2 months following treatment. The authors reiterated the rate of absorption of plasma gel which necessitated reinjection in patients [104]. De Souza et al. evaluated the medialization effect of bacterial cellulose and associated tissue response. Using a rabbit model, the authors noted minimal inflammation and retainment of the material up to 4 months [105]. Sataloff reviewed the literature on autologous fascia injection [106]. This material works well. Recently, the author (RTS, unpublished data) has used homograft fascia lata with similar success, avoiding the need for a donor site incision. Beginning 2019, he also developed a new procedure involving homograft fascia sheet implant, but this has been performed only through direct microlaryngoscopy, so far.

References

1. Bruening W. Uber eine neue Behanlungsmethode der Rekurrenslahmung. Ver Deutsch Laryng. 1991:18–23.
2. Arnold GE. Vocal rehabilitation of paralytic dysphonia: I. cartilage injection into a paralyzed vocal cord. Arch Otolaryngol. 1955;62(1):1–17.
3. Courey MS. Injection laryngoplasty. Otolaryngol Clin N Am. 2004;37(1):121–38.
4. Zeitler DM, Amin MR. The thyrohyoid approach to in-office injection augmentation of the vocal fold. Curr Opin Otolaryngol Head Neck Surg. 2007;15(6):412–6.
5. Rosen CA, Amin MR, Sulica L, et al. Advances in office-based diagnosis and treatment in laryngology. Laryngoscope. 2009;119(S2):S185–212.
6. Sulica L, Rosen CA, Postma GN, et al. Current practice in injection augmentation of the vocal folds: indications, treatment principles, techniques, and complications. Laryngoscope. 2010;120(2):319–25.
7. Reich AR, Lerman JW. Teflon laryngoplasty: an acoustical and perceptual study. J Speech Hear Disord. 1978;43(4):496–505.
8. Montgomery WW. Laryngeal paralysis Teflon® injection. Ann Otol Rhinol Laryngol. 1979;88(5):647–57.
9. Ellis JC, Mccaffrey TV, Desanto LW, Reiman HV. Migration of Teflon after vocal cord injection. Otolaryngol Head Neck Surg. 1987;96(1):63–6.
10. Dedo HH, Carlsouou B. Histologic evaluation of Teflon granulomas of human vocal cords: a light and electron microscopic study. Acta Otolaryngol. 1982;93(1–6):475–84.

11. Matton G, Anseeuw A, De Keyser F. The history of injectable biomaterials and the biology of collagen. Aesthet Plast Surg. 1985;9(2):133–40.
12. Woodson G. Evolving concepts of laryngeal paralysis. J Laryngol Otol. 2008;122(5):437–41.
13. Blitzer A, Jahn AF, Keidar A. Semon's law revisited: an electromyographic analysis of laryngeal synkinesis. Ann Otol Rhinol Laryngol. 1996;105(10):764–9.
14. Sataloff RT, Praneetvatakul P, Heuer RJ, et al. Laryngeal electromyography: clinical application. J Voice. 2010;24(2):228–34.
15. Behlau M, Oliveira G. Vocal hygiene for the voice professional. Curr Opin Otolaryngol Head Neck Surg. 2009;17(3):149–54.
16. Rosen B, Horman M, Sataloff RT. Voice therapy. In: Sataloff RT, editor. Professional voice: the science and art of clinical care. 4th ed. San Diego, CA: Plural Publishing; 2017. p. 1171–94.
17. Yung KC, Likhterov I, Courey MS. Effect of temporary vocal fold injection medialization on the rate of permanent medialization laryngoplasty in unilateral vocal fold paralysis patients. Laryngoscope. 2011;121(10):2191–4.
18. Prendes BL, Yung KC, Likhterov I, Schneider SL, Al-Jurf SA, Courey MS. Long-term effects of injection laryngoplasty with a temporary agent on voice quality and vocal fold position. Laryngoscope. 2012;122(10):2227–33.
19. Milstein CF, Akst LM, Hicks MD, Abelson TI, Strome M. Long-term effects of micronized Alloderm injection for unilateral vocal fold paralysis. Laryngoscope. 2005;115(9):1691–6.
20. Borzacchiello A, Mayol L, Gärskog O, Dahlqvist Å, Ambrosio L. Evaluation of injection augmentation treatment of hyaluronic acid based materials on rabbit vocal folds viscoelasticity. J Mater Sci Mater Med. 2005;16(6):553–7.
21. Francis DO, Williamson K, Hovis K, et al. Effect of injection augmentation on need for framework surgery in unilateral vocal fold paralysis. Laryngoscope. 2016;126(1):128–34.
22. Merea VS, Husain S, Sulica L. Medialization laryngoplasty after injection augmentation. J Voice. 2018;32(2):249–55.
23. Vila PM, Bhatt NK, Paniello RC. Early-injection laryngoplasty may lower risk of thyroplasty: a systematic review and meta-analysis. Laryngoscope. 2018;128(4):935–40.
24. Berke GS, Gerratt B, Kreiman J, Jackson K. Treatment of Parkinson hypophonia with percutaneous collagen augmentation. Laryngoscope. 1999;109(8):1295–9.
25. Luu Q, Tsai V, Mangunta V, Berke GS, Chhetri DK. Safety of percutaneous injection of bovine dermal crosslinked collagen for glottic insufficiency. Otolaryngol Head Neck Surg. 2007;136(3):445–9.
26. Kimura M, Nito T, Sakakibara KI, Tayama N, Niimi S. Clinical experience with collagen injection of the vocal fold: a study of 155 patients. Auris Nasus Larynx. 2008;35(1):67–75.
27. Min JY, Hong SD, Kim K, Son YI. Long-term results of Artecoll injection laryngoplasty for patients with unilateral vocal fold motion impairment: safety and clinical efficacy. Arch Otolaryngol Head Neck Surg. 2008;134(5):490–6.
28. Dursun G, Boynukalin S, Ozgursoy OB, Coruh I. Long-term results of different treatment modalities for glottic insufficiency. Am J Otolaryngol. 2008;29(1):7–12.
29. Gillespie MB, Dozier TS, Day TA, Martin-Harris B, Nguyen SA. Effectiveness of calcium hydroxylapatite paste in vocal rehabilitation. Ann Otol Rhinol Laryngol. 2009;118(8):546–51.
30. Carroll TL, Rosen CA. Long-term results of calcium hydroxylapatite for vocal fold augmentation. Laryngoscope. 2011;121(2):313–9.
31. Choi J, Son YI, So YK, Byun H, Lee EK, Yun YS. Posterior glottic gap and age as factors predicting voice outcome of injection laryngoplasty in patients with unilateral vocal fold paralysis. J Laryngol Otol. 2012;126(3):260–6.
32. Wen MH, Cheng PW, Liao LJ, Chou HW, Wang CT. Treatment outcomes of injection laryngoplasty using cross-linked porcine collagen and hyaluronic acid. Otolaryngol Head Neck Surg. 2013;149(6):900–6.
33. Birkent H, Sardesai M, Hu A, Merati AL. Prospective study of voice outcomes and patient tolerance of in-office percutaneous injection laryngoplasty. Laryngoscope. 20131;123(7):1759–62.

34. Jamal N, Mundi J, Chhetri DK. Higher risk of superficial injection during injection laryngoplasty in women. Am J Otolaryngol. 2014;35(2):159–63.
35. Woo SH, Son YI, Lee SH, Park JJ, Pyeong Kim J. Comparative analysis on the efficiency of the injection laryngoplasty technique using calcium hydroxyapatite (CaHA): the thyrohyoid approach versus the cricothyroid approach. J Voice. 2013;27(2):236–41.
36. Powell J, Carding P, Birdi R, Wilson JA. Injection laryngoplasty in the outpatient clinic under local anaesthetic: a case series of sixty-eight patients. Clin Otolaryngol. 2014;39(4):224–7.
37. Halderman AA, Bryson PC, Benninger MS, Chota R. Safety and length of benefit of restylane for office-based injection medialization—a retrospective review of one institution's experience. J Voice. 2014;28(5):631–5.
38. Sardesai MG, Merati AL, Hu A, Birkent H. Impact of patient-related factors on the outcomes of office-based injection laryngoplasty. Laryngoscope. 2016;126(8):1806–9.
39. McLaughlin CW, Swendseid B, Courey MS, Schneider S, Gartner-Schmidt JL, Yung KC. Long-term outcomes in unilateral vocal fold paralysis patients. Laryngoscope. 2018;128(2):430–6.
40. Sielska-Badurek EM, Sobol M, Jędra K, Rzepakowska A, Osuch-Wojcikiewicz E, Niemczyk K. Injection laryngoplasty as miniinvasive office-based surgery in patients with unilateral vocal fold paralysis–voice quality outcomes. Wideochir Inne Tech Maloinwazyjne. 2017;12(3):277–84.
41. Hu HC, Hung YT, Lin SY, Tung TH, Chang SY. Office-based autologous fat injection laryngoplasty for glottic insufficiency in patients under 50 years old. J Voice. 2019;33(5):747–50.
42. Maccarini AR, Stacchini M, Mozzanica F, et al. Efficacy of trans-nasal fiberendoscopic injection laryngoplasty with centrifuged autologous fat in the treatment of glottic insufficiency due to unilateral vocal fold paralysis. Acta Otorhinolaryngol Ital. 2018;38(3):204–13.
43. Hamdan AL, Rizk M, Khalife E, Ziade G, Kasti M. Voice outcome measures after flexible endoscopic injection laryngoplasty. World J Otorhinolaryngol Head Neck Surg. 2018;4(2):130–4.
44. Sato T, Nito T, Ueha R, Goto T, Yamasoba T. Investigation of the safety of injection laryngoplasty under antithrombotic therapy. ORL J Otorhinolaryngol Relat Spec. 2019;81(4):215–23.
45. Bertroche JT, Radder M, Kallogjeri D, Paniello RC, Bradley JP. Patient-defined duration of benefit from juvederm (hyaluronic acid) used in injection laryngoplasty. Laryngoscope. 2019;129(12):2744–7.
46. Jeong GE, Lee DH, Lee YS, et al. Treatment efficacy of voice therapy following injection laryngoplasty for unilateral vocal fold paralysis. J Voice. 2020:S0892-1997(20)30188-0.
47. Novakovic D, Nguyen DD, Chacon A, Madill C. Injection laryngoplasty as adjunct treatment method for muscle tension dysphonia: preliminary findings. Laryngoscope. 2020;130(4):980–5.
48. Wang CC, Wu SH, Tu YK, Lin WJ, Liu SA. Hyaluronic acid injection Laryngoplasty for unilateral vocal fold paralysis—a systematic review and meta-analysis. Cell. 2020;9(11):2417.
49. Zuniga S, Ebersole B, Jamal N. Improved swallow outcomes after injection laryngoplasty in unilateral vocal fold immobility. Ear Nose Throat J. 2018;97(8):250–6.
50. Anis MM, Memon Z. Injection medialization laryngoplasty improves dysphagia in patients with unilateral vocal fold immobility. World J Otorhinolaryngol Head Neck Surg. 2018;4(2):126–9.
51. Han YJ, Jang YJ, Park GY, Joo YH, Im S. Role of injection laryngoplasty in preventing post-stroke aspiration pneumonia, case series report. Medicine (Baltimore). 2020 Feb;99(7):e19220.
52. Chen DW, Price MD, LeMaire SA, Coselli JS, Liou NE, Ongkasuwan J. Early versus late inpatient awake transcervical injection laryngoplasty after thoracic aortic repair. Laryngoscope. 2018;128(1):144–7.
53. Choi N, Won S, Jin H, Kim HJ, Park W, Son YI. Additional injection laryngoplasty for patients with unilateral vocal fold paralysis. Laryngoscope. 2020;130(12):2863–8.

54. Pan S, Sadoughi B. Effectiveness of injection laryngoplasty for aspiration in acute iatrogenic vocal fold paralysis: a systematic review. Laryngoscope. 2020; https://doi.org/10.1002/lary.29326.
55. Frontera WR, Hughes VA, Fielding RA, Fiatarone MA, Evans WJ, Roubenoff R. Aging of skeletal muscle: a 12-yr longitudinal study. J Appl Physiol. 2000;88(4):1321–6.
56. Nair KS. Aging muscle. Am J Clin Nutr. 2005;81(5):953–63.
57. Thomas LB, Harrison AL, Stemple JC. Aging thyroarytenoid and limb skeletal muscle: lessons in contrast. J Voice. 2008;22(4):430–50.
58. Davids T, Klein AM, Johns MM III. Current dysphonia trends in patients over the age of 65: is vocal atrophy becoming more prevalent? Laryngoscope. 2012;122(2):332–5.
59. Marino JP, Johns MM III. The epidemiology of dysphonia in the aging population. Curr Opin Otolaryngol Head Neck Surg. 2014;22(6):455–9.
60. Ziade G, Semaan S, Fakhri G, El Natout T, Hamdan AL. Thyroarytenoid muscle uptake and attenuation in PET/CT in elderly. Eur Arch Otorhinolaryngol. 2016;273(12):4385–9.
61. Wehrli NE, Bural G, Houseni M, Alkhawaldeh K, Alavi A, Torigian DA. Determination of age-related changes in structure and function of skin, adipose tissue, and skeletal muscle with computed tomography, magnetic resonance imaging, and positron emission tomography. Semin Nucl Med. 2007;37(3):195–205.
62. Sataloff RT, Kost KM, Linville SE. The effects of age on the voice. In: Sataloff RT, editor. Professional voice: the science and art of clinical care. 4th ed. San Diego, CA: Plural Publ; 2017. p. 585–604.
63. Hamdan AL, Khalifee E, Al Arab N, Asmar K, Hourani R. Volumetric measures of the paralyzed vocal fold using computerized tomography; its clinical implication. Logoped Phoniatr Vocol. 2020:1–5. https://doi.org/10.1080/14015439.2020.1753809.
64. Mau T, Courey MS. Influence of gender and injection site on vocal fold augmentation. Otolaryngol Head Neck Surg. 2008;138(2):221–5.
65. Butler JE, Hammond TH, Gray SD. Gender-related differences of hyaluronic acid distribution in the human vocal fold. Laryngoscope. 2001;111(5):907–11.
66. Roy N, Merrill RM, Gray SD, Smith EM. Voice disorders in the general population: prevalence, risk factors, and occupational impact. Laryngoscope. 2005;115(11):1988–95.
67. Lin WY, Chang WD, Ko LW, Tsou YA, Chen SH. Impact of patient-related factors on successful autologous fat injection laryngoplasty in thyroid surgical treated related unilateral vocal fold paralysis-observational study. Medicine (Baltimore). 2020;99(1):e18579.
68. Fang TJ, Pei YC, Li HY, Wong AM, Chiang HC. Glottal gap as an early predictor for permanent laryngoplasty in unilateral vocal fold paralysis. Laryngoscope. 2014;124(9):2125–30.
69. Pearson JJ, Ortiz AS, Montelongo S, Montelongo S, Simpson B, Guda T, Dion GR. Quantification of injection force mechanics during injection laryngoplasty. Laryngoscope. 2019;129(5):1060–6.
70. Lisi C, Hawkshaw MJ, Sataloff RT. Viscosity of materials for laryngeal injection: a review of current knowledge and clinical implications. J Voice. 2013;27(1):119–23.
71. Dang JH, Liou NE, Ongkasuwan J. Anticoagulation and antiplatelet therapy in awake transcervical injection laryngoplasty. Laryngoscope. 2017;127(8):1850–4.
72. Sakai N, Takizawa M, Furuta Y, Kumagai M, Anadolu YR, Inuyama Y. Histological study of atelocollagen infused into the human vocal cords. Auris Nasus Larynx. 1991;18(1):61–5.
73. "CYMETRA® Micronized AlloDerm® Tissue". WoundReference. https://woundreference.com/app/topic?id=cymetra-micronized-alloderm-tissue. 2018; Accessed Mar 2021.
74. Courey MS. Homologous collagen substances for vocal fold augmentation. Laryngoscope. 2001;111(5):747–58.
75. Remacle M, Marbaix E, Bertrand B, Hamoir M, van den Eeckhaut J. Correction of glottic insufficiency by collagen injection. Ann Otol Rhinol Laryngol. 1990;99(6):438–44.
76. Anderson TD, Sataloff RT. Complications of collagen injection of the vocal fold: report of several unusual cases and review of the literature. J Voice. 2004;18(3):392–7.

77. Mikaelian DO, Lowry LD, Sataloff RT. Lipoinjection for unilateral vocal cord paralysis. Laryngoscope. 1991;101(5):465–8.
78. Elbadan HE, Hussein WK, Elmaghraby RM. Transcervical fat injection laryngoplasty for unilateral vocal fold paralysis: an easy way to do the job. Eur Arch Otorhinolaryngol. 2017;274(12):4161–7.
79. Hsiung MW, Woo P, Minasian A, Schaefer MJ. Fat augmentation for glottic insufficiency. Laryngoscope. 2000;110(6):1026–33.
80. Shindo ML, Zaretsky LS, Rice DH. Autologous fat injection for unilateral vocal fold paralysis. Ann Otol Rhinol Laryngol. 1996;105(8):602–6.
81. DeFatta RA, DeFatta RJ, Sataloff RT. Laryngeal lipotransfer: review of a 14-year experience. J Voice. 2013;27(4):512–5.
82. Truzzi GM, Pauna HF, Bette P, Gusmao RJ, Crespo AN, Semenzati GO. Methods of fat tissue processing for human vocal fold injection: a systematic review. J Voice. 2017;31(2):244.e17–21.
83. Rinker BD, Vyas KS. Do stem cells have an effect when we fat graft? Ann Plast Surg. 2016;76(S4):S359–63.
84. McCulloch TM, Andrews BT, Hoffman HT, Graham SM, Karnell MP, Minnick C. Long-term follow-up of fat injection laryngoplasty for unilateral vocal cord paralysis. Laryngoscope. 2002;112(7):1235–8.
85. Laccourreye O, Papon JF, Kania R, Crevier-Buchman L, Brasnu D, Hans S. Intracordal injection of autologous fat in patients with unilateral laryngeal nerve paralysis: long-term results from the patient's perspective. Laryngoscope. 2003;113(3):541–5. (SAME AS 79).
86. Umeno H, Shirouzu H, Chitose SI, Nakashima T. Analysis of voice function following autologous fat injection for vocal fold paralysis. Otolaryngol Head Neck Surg. 2005;132(1):103–7.
87. Fang TJ, Li HY, Gliklich RE, Chen YH, Wang PC, Chuang HF. Outcomes of fat injection laryngoplasty in unilateral vocal cord paralysis. Arch Otolaryngol Head Neck Surg. 2010;136(5):457–62.
88. Chheda NN, Rosen CA, Belafsky PC, Simpson CB, Postma GN. Revision laryngeal surgery for the suboptimal injection of calcium hydroxylapatite. Laryngoscope. 2008;118(12):2260–3.
89. DeFatta RA, Chowdhury FR, Sataloff RT. Complications of injection laryngoplasty using calcium hydroxylapatite. J Voice. 2012;26(5):614–8.
90. Lee M, Lee DY, Kwon TK. Safety of office-based percutaneous injection laryngoplasty with calcium hydroxylapatite. Laryngoscope. 2019;129(10):2361–5.
91. Wang C, Wu S, Tu Y, Liu S. Hyaluronic acid injection laryngoplasty for unilateral vocal fold paralysis- a systematic review and meta-analysis. Cell. 2020;9(11):2417.
92. King JM, Simpson CB. Modern injection augmentation for glottic insufficiency. Curr Opin Otolaryngol Head Neck Surg. 2007;15(3):153–8.
93. Hertegård S, Hallén L, Laurent C, et al. Cross-linked hyaluronan versus collagen for injection treatment of glottal insufficiency: 2-year follow-up. Acta Otolaryngol. 2004;124(10):1208–14.
94. Hertegård S, Hallén L, Laurent C, et al. Cross-linked hyaluronan used as augmentation substance for treatment of glottal insufficiency: safety aspects and vocal fold function. Laryngoscope. 2002;112(12):2211–9.
95. Song PC, Sung CK, Franco RA Jr. Voice outcomes after endoscopic injection laryngoplasty with hyaluronic acid stabilized gel. Laryngoscope. 2010;120 Suppl 4:S199.
96. Rudolf R, Sibylle B. Laryngoplasty with hyaluronic acid in patients with unilateral vocal fold paralysis. J Voice. 2012;26(6):785–91.
97. Shamanna SG, Bosch JD. Injection laryngoplasty: a serious reaction to hyaluronic acid. J Otolaryngol Head Neck Surg. 2011;40(5):E39–42.
98. Dominguez LM, Tibbetts KM, Simpson CB. Inflammatory reaction to hyaluronic acid: a newly described complication in vocal fold augmentation. Laryngoscope. 2017;127(2):445–9.
99. Hamdan AL, Khalifee E. Adverse reaction to restylane: a review of 63 cases of injection laryngoplasty. Ear Nose Throat J. 2019;98(4):212–6.

100. Perazzo PS, de Campos DA, Lancellotti CL. Histological behavior of the vocal fold after hyaluronic acid injection. J Voice. 2009;23(1):95–8.
101. Lee BJ, Wang SG, Goh EK, Chon KM, Lee CH. Intracordal injection of autologous auricular cartilage in the paralyzed canine vocal fold. Otolaryngol Head Neck Surg. 2004;131(1):34–43.
102. Lim YS, Lee YS, Lee JC, et al. Intracordal auricular cartilage injection for unilateral vocal fold paralysis. J Biomed Mater Res B Appl Biomater. 2015;103(1):47–51.
103. Hong SJ, Lee SH, Jin SM, et al. Plasma gel as a new augmentation material for injection laryngoplasty in rabbit model: histologic analysis. Otolaryngol Head Neck Surg. 2013;149(4):596–602.
104. Woo SH, Kim JP, Park JJ, Chung PS, Lee SH, Jeong HS. Autologous platelet-poor plasma gel for injection laryngoplasty. Yonsei Med J. 2013;54(6):1516.
105. de Souza FC, Olival-Costa H, da Silva L, Pontes PA, Lancellotti CL. Bacterial cellulose as laryngeal medialization material: an experimental study. J Voice. 2011;25(6):765–9.
106. Sataloff RT. Voice surgery. In: Sataloff RT, editor. Professional voice: the science and art of clinical care. 4th ed. San Diego, CA: Plural Publishing; 2017. p. 1371–478.

Chapter 9
Office-Based Laryngeal Botulinum Toxin Injection

Abdul-latif Hamdan, Robert Thayer Sataloff, Ghiath Alnouri, and Mary J. Hawkshaw

9.1 Introduction

Botulinum toxin (BT) is a neurotoxin produced by fermentation of *Clostridium botulinum*. In 1973, Scott et al. introduced BT for medical therapy of strabismus [1]. Since then, BT injection has emerged as a therapeutic modality for other neuromuscular disorders. Botulinum toxin acts by inhibiting the release of acetylcholine at the neuromuscular junction of the targeted muscle leading to temporary chemical denervation and reduction in excessive and/or uncontrolled muscle activity [2]. The heavy chain of the toxin allows binding of the toxin to neurons and penetration of synapses, whereas the light chain is responsible for blocking of calcium-mediated release of acetylcholine [3, 4]. The clinical benefit of BT starts 1–3 days following the injection and usually lasts 3–6 months. The effect is attenuated by resprouting of the terminal axons and the formation of new motor endplates. Resistance to treatment secondary to antibodies production is a concern, and it has been suggested that

Supplementary Information The online version contains supplementary material available at [https://doi.org/10.1007/978-3-030-91936-8_9].

A.-l. Hamdan (✉)
Otolaryngology, Head & Neck Surgery, American University of Beirut Medical Center, Beirut, Lebanon

Department of Otolaryngology Head and Neck Surgery, Drexel University College of Medicine, Philadelphia, PA, USA
e-mail: ah77@aub.edu.lb

R. T. Sataloff · M. J. Hawkshaw
Otolaryngology – Head and Neck Surgery, Drexel University, Philadelphia, PA, USA

G. Alnouri
Department of Otolaryngology – Head and Neck Surgery, Drexel University College of Medicine, Philadelphia, PA, USA

A.-l. Hamdan et al., *Office-Based Laryngeal Surgery*,
https://doi.org/10.1007/978-3-030-91936-8_9

antibody formation may be triggered by BT injections given repeatedly over short intervals and/or when large doses are used. Other factors responsible for immunogenicity include the manufacturing and formulation of the toxin. For that reason, switching to an alternate type of toxin, such as BT-B in cases of resistance to BT-A, might be a solution [4]. Although antibody formation usually is thought to be a concern after 300 mouse units (mu) have been given (total over time), the author (RTS) has seen antibodies develop after as few as 50 mu; and rarely patients have antibodies prior to their first therapeutic injection, presumably due to exposure through food. When a long-term effect is desired (in the absence of antibodies against BT), repeated injections are needed.

There are eight serotypes of botulinum toxin (A to G), the most common of which is type A [5, 6]. In an evidence-based review on the safety and therapeutic effect of Botox, Hallett et al. asserted the efficacious use of different commercial formulations (abobotulinumtoxin A, onabotulinumtoxin A, incobotulinumtoxin A, and rimabotulinumtoxin B) in the treatment of blepharospasm, oromandibular dystonia, torticollis, hemifacial spasm, and focal limb dystonia [6]. Their findings concur with those of Hughes in his report on clinical practice of Botox injection published in 1994 [3]. The author noted the high success rate of Botox injections in comparison to other treatment methods traditionally used in patients with dystonia. For instance, injections of Botox into the trapezius and sternocleidomastoid muscles in patients with spasmodic torticollis were found to be successful in 70–80% of the cases. Similarly, by injecting Botox at various sites of the orbicularis muscle, improvement in patients with blepharospasm was reported in 90% of the cases [3]. Notably, the effect of Botox injection is not only local but also central. A "nonclassical" effect on the central nervous system has been suggested by many authors [7, 8]. It includes alteration in the cortical network, change in brainstem interneuronal pathways, and reform in spinal synaptic transmission [9–11].

Given the success of Botox in the treatment of various forms of focal dystonia, the indications for its use have expanded to include laryngeal movement disorders, namely, spasmodic dysphonia, essential voice tremor, paradoxical vocal fold movement disorders or "induced laryngeal obstruction," laryngeal tics, muscle tension dysphonia, and others. This chapter reviews the application of Botox injections in the management of laryngeal movement disorders. The site and dose of injection, as well as associated adverse effects, are discussed.

9.2 Office-Based Botulinum Toxin Injection in Patients with Spasmodic Dysphonia

Spasmodic dysphonia (SD) is a central neurologic disorder that affects voice and speech. Women are affected more than men with a female to male ratio of 7:1. The peak onset is during the fourth decade of life, and a positive family history is present in 10–12% of the cases [12, 13]. DTY6 (dystonia gene 6) families seem to play a major role, and deletion of three nucleotides in the DYT1 gene has been shown to be responsible for early-onset focal dystonia [14]. Other predisposing factors include prior history of upper respiratory tract infection and/or stress [12] although causal relationship between these factors and dystonic remain controversial. One out of five patients with SD reports a major stressful life event, a fact that has masked the true etiology of SD for decades. The pathophysiology of SD is multifactorial and includes decreased or loss of motor cortex inhibition, increased plasticity, and abnormal sensory input. Affected individuals have reduced inhibition of the laryngeal adductor reflexes with abnormal sensory gating, all of which leads to disturbance in motor output [15, 16].

Spasmodic dysphonia is a disabling communication disorder that has a profound impact on quality of life. In a review of 60 patients with adductor focal laryngeal dystonia, Stewart et al. reported a VHI-10 score of 21.3 [17]. Affected patients often report difficulty in speech initiation, uncontrolled voice breaks, and marked effort to speak. However, primary vocalization may not be disturbed. Unlike patients with muscle tension dysphonia, in patients with SD singing, yawning, laughing, and crying often are not affected [18], especially early in the disease. Other maneuvers referred to as "sensory tricks" such as chewing also inhibit some of the speech and phonatory symptoms [19]. In adductor SD, the voice breaks are associated with a feeling of choking and strangulation while speaking, particularly when reading all-voiced passages such as "Albert Eat Eggs Every Easter Early in the AM," or when asked to count from 80 to 89. In patients with abductor SD, the voice has breathy breaks associated particularly with prolongation of voiceless sounds such as /p/, /t/, /h/ and /ch/. Voice symptoms also are elicited when patients are asked to count from 60 to 69 or to read a sentence such as "She sells seashells by the seashore."

Voice tremor is reported in up to one-third of affected patients [12, 18–21] or more. In a review of the demographic data of 718 patients with SD, Patel et al. reported voice tremor in 54.4% of ADSD patients and 32.1% of ABSD patients [22]. Notably, other forms of dystonia such as blepharospasm and cervical dystonia were found in 1.4% and 2.3% of the cases, respectively [22]. Unlike patients with essential voice tremor, patients with SD have no laryngeal tremor at rest and lack pharyngeal and extra-laryngeal muscle tremor. Perceptual evaluation using the GRBAS scale has limited value in patients with SD. As a substitute, the I(I)-NFVO rating scale where the first "I" stands for overall impression, second "I" for the impression of intelligibility, "N" for noise, "F" for fluency, and "V" for voicing is used commonly [23]. Similarly, acoustic analysis using the multidimensional voice program is of limited use in view of the aperiodicity of the vocal signal, variations in voice onset, and high frequency of voice breaks in affected patients. As an alternative, the auditory model-based pitch extractor (AMPEX) has been adopted by some as a robust model that helps characterize and differentiate substitute voices from normal voices [24].

The diagnosis of SD is not limited to perceptual evaluation but relies heavily on laryngeal examination. Task-specific abnormal movements of laryngeal structures usually are seen on flexible nasopharyngoscopy. In cases of adductor SD (ADSD), there is episodic excessive adduction of the vocal folds during phonation, whereas in patients with abductor SD (ABSD), there is excessive abduction with intermittent incomplete closure of the vocal folds during phonation. The distinction between ADSD and ABSD is not always clear. In many cases, the two entities may coexist, and the clinical demarcation between the two is blurred [25]. Either or both may coexist with tremor, and this combination is called dystonia tremor. It is also important to note the coexistence of compensatory supraglottic muscle tension and/or vocal fold paresis/paralysis in many cases. The use of laryngeal electromyography (EMG) is very useful in excluding other neurologic conditions. Patients with SD typically display a time delay (0.5–1 second) between onset electrical activity of the muscle tested and the onset of phonation [26]. More information on laryngeal EMG findings in patients with SD is available to the reader elsewhere [20].

Treatment of SD is multifaceted. It includes voice/speech therapy, psychotherapy, pharmacotherapy, surgery, and neuromuscular blockade [20]. Voice/speech therapy aims at unloading the laryngeal tension commonly observed in patients with SD, thus reducing symptoms of voice strain and fatigue. The author (RTS) describes successful use of singing to treat SD patients. By attenuating voice spasms during singing and by bridging the singing voice to the speaking voice, affected patients may show marked improvement. Medical treatment using benzodiazepines or phenytoin and psychotherapy to relieve associated stress have been recommended either in isolation or in combination with voice/speech therapy. Surgery has evolved over the last few decades as an alternative especially in recalcitrant cases. Since the introduction of recurrent laryngeal nerve (RLN) sectioning by Dedo in 1976 [27], several surgical options were described among which are RLN crushing by Biller et al. [28], RLN avulsion by Netterville et al. [29], selective section/excision of the thyroarytenoid branch of the recurrent laryngeal nerve by Iwamura [30], and selective denervation/reinnervation of the thyroarytenoid muscle by Mendelsohn and Berke [31]. Other surgical options include endoscopic thyroarytenoid myectomy using cold steel instruments [32], transoral laser thyroarytenoid myoneurectomy [33, 34], radiofrequency thyroarytenoid myothermy [35], and laryngeal framework surgery such as thyroplasty type II with the insertion of a spreading bridge to reduce the forceful closure of the vocal folds and/or thyroplasty type III for relaxation of the anterior commissure [36].

Despite the evolution of surgical techniques in the treatment of SD, the long-term results and high recurrence rates following surgery (recurrent laryngeal nerve section) were discouraging. This spurred efforts to find an alternative treatment. The successful use of neurotoxin in the management of focal dystonia in other parts of the body inspired its widespread usage in patients with SD. Eskander et al. conducted a cross-sectional study looking at the practice in the treatment of ADSD in the Canadian Society of Otolaryngology-Head and Neck Surgery and reported laryngeal BT injections as the most common treatment. The injections were done mostly through the cricothyroid membrane under EMG guidance [37]. Similarly, in the United States, laryngeal BT injection is the most common treatment option in patients with SD. Based on the National Institutes of Health consensus statement, botulinum toxin is a safe and effective treatment of SD among other conditions, when given by health care professionals [38]. Its safety and efficacy depend partially on the low antigenicity of the botulinum toxin used [20]. In a review of more than 900 patients with SD treated with laryngeal BT injections, Blitzer et al. reported improvement in 90% of patients with ADSD and two-thirds of patients with ABSD [20]. In 2006, Srirompotong et al. reported their experience in the treatment of 37 patients with SD, 25 of whom had undergone BT injection, and reported improvement in 76.8% of the cases at the final stage of treatment. The treatment effect lasted 13.6 weeks on average [39]. Kendall and Leonard investigated the effect of interarytenoid Botox injection in combination with TA muscle injection in the treatment of SD-associated voice tremor. The authors reported better results in those who had both IA and TA injections in comparison to those who had only TA injections. In addition, there was an improvement in most acoustic parameters except for cycle-to-cycle variation in frequency [40]. In 2018, Patel et al. reviewed 548 patients with ADSD, laryngeal tremor, and ADSD with laryngeal tremor, who had undergone 12,771 laryngeal BT injections. The percentage of maximal benefit following BT injection was 88.1% for patients with ADSD and 83.4% for patients with ADSD and lateral tremor. The authors emphasized the effectiveness of onabotulinum toxin A injections into the TA/LCA muscle complex in affected patients (Video 9.1) [41].

The improvement in voice quality following BT injection in patients with SD is attributed to both a local and central effect. BT injection into the intrinsic and extrinsic laryngeal muscles has been shown to result in favorable alteration in laryngeal airflow. Finnegan et al. investigated the effect of BT injection on laryngeal airflow in patients with SD with voice tremor and reported an increase in the mean airflow and a decrease in the coefficient of airflow variation. The latter is indicative of improved stability of laryngeal muscle activity and breathing [42]. Ali et al. investigated BT-induced alterations in CNS activity in patients with ADSD and reported a significant increase in speech-related sensory response in heteromodal sensory areas. The increase in sensory response was commensurate with clinical improvement in voice breaks and percentage aperiodicity. The regional cerebral blood flow (RCBF) was assessed using positron-emission tomography before and after administration of botulinum [43]. The clinical improvement correlated significantly with attenuation in RCBF in motor-associated regions and augmentation in RCBF in unimodal and heteromodal sensory regions associated with oro-motor control.

The outcome of botulinum toxin injection in patients with SD depends on several factors, the most important of which is the dose injected. The effect is believed to be faster when higher doses are used. In a national survey on the use of BT injection in the treatment of SD by experts in the United States, most treating physicians performed bilateral injections with a starting dose of 1.25 IU in ADSD and unilateral injections with a starting dose of 5 IU in ABDSD. The survey included 70 laryngologists who answered a 58-item online survey [44]. Based on the above survey, laryngeal EMG is used by physicians in 87% of patients with ADSD and 67% of patients with ABSD [44]. Other muscles injected include the cricothyroid muscle. The dose varies markedly between patients and with the type of botulinum toxin used and its potency [20]. Another important determinant of the outcome of

BT injection is the ability to target the muscles affected the most. In a review on the clinical application of laryngeal EMG, Sataloff et al. emphasized the added value of laryngeal EMG in targeting the affected muscles and in differentiating between the different forms of SD [45]. In a study of 214 patients with laryngeal dystonia, Klotz et al. showed that difficulty in achieving the desired result was attributed to failure to inject the muscles affected the most. Using fine-wire electromyography, the authors noted that the TA muscle was predominantly affected in ADSD, whereas both the TA and lateral cricoarytenoid muscles are predominantly affected in tremor SD [46]. Maronian et al. reviewed their experience with 81 patients with tremor laryngeal dystonia treated with Botox injection; they used fine-wire electromyography and reported clinical improvement in most patients. The thyroarytenoid muscles and lateral cricoarytenoid muscle were injected in 52% and 48%, respectively. The authors discussed the efficacy of LCA Botox injection in the treatment of these patients [47]. Other factors to be considered in predicting the voice outcome of BT injection are patients' characteristics. Nonbiological factors may contribute significantly to the success or failure of therapy. In a study of 36 patients with ADSD treated with BT injection, Rutt et al. reported that preprocedure education, body position, and stress experienced during the procedure are important factors that can influence the results in 87%, 33%, and 30% of the cases, respectively. The authors stressed the role of patient education before the procedure in improving patient experience and outcome [48]. History of prior surgical treatment is also an important determinant. In a review of 16 patients with ADSD who had undergone nerve section and later BT injection (n-181), Sulica et al. reported less satisfactory results in comparison to patients who were treated primarily with chemodenervation. Nevertheless, there was a significant improvement in voice quality that peaked in 10 days following the injection and lasted 14 weeks, on average [49].

The use of BT in the treatment of SD carries risks and expected adverse effects of which patients should be aware. Preoperative education and counseling are essential for improvement of patients' experience and tolerance of the adverse effects of laryngeal BT injections. Complications reported following BT in the TA muscle in patients with ADSD include breathiness, aspiration of clear fluids, dysphagia, and throat pain. Another rare complication is temporary bilateral vocal fold paralysis. In a review of 352 patients with ADSD who had undergone botulinum toxin injection, Venkatesan et al. reported bilateral abductor paralysis in eight patients, one of whom needed a tracheotomy. The vocal fold paralysis was ascribed to diffusion of the neurotoxin into the posterior cricoarytenoid muscle [50].

SD is a laryngeal movement disorder that can be treated successfully with BT injections. Targeting the affected muscle under EMG guidance helps optimize the outcome. History of prior treatment, site of injection, and dose of BT are important determinants of the success of injection. Patient counseling and education are crucial. Side effects such as breathiness and dysphagia need to be discussed with the patient before intervening.

9.3 Office-Based Botulinum Toxin Injection in Patients with Essential Voice Tremor

Essential voice tremor (EVT) is a neurologic disorder characterized by periodic fluctuation in loudness and pitch that impairs normal communication. Based on the International Parkinson and Movement Disorder Society, EVT is a clinical variant of essential tremor that affects the larynx and pharynx during speech and quiet respiration [51]. The structures commonly affected are the soft palate, base of tongue, lateral pharyngeal wall, false vocal folds, and true vocal folds. Other structures such as the strap muscles and respiratory muscles also may be involved [51]. Essential voice tremor affects women (75–93% of the cases) more often than men, with a mean age of onset at 60 years. Positive family history is reported in 38–42% of the cases [52]. In a clinical study of 34 patients with EVT, Sulica et al. noted a positive family history in 30–50% of the cases [53].

The diagnosis of EVT is challenging because less than one-third of affected patients have tremor of the extremities. This explains the delay in diagnosis of up to 7 years from the time of initial presentation [53]. The diagnosis of EVT relies on subjective and objective evaluation. Visualization of vocal folds and vocal tract kinetic behavior is key for diagnosis [54]. *On examination, tremor is not limited to the intrinsic laryngeal muscles but involves the extrinsic laryngeal muscles as well* [55]. The use of phonatory tasks such as phonating /a/, sustaining the */s/ or whistling may be useful in differentiating EVT from laryngeal dystonia. A delay between voice tremor and laryngeal muscle tremulous activity is observed in many cases.* Bové et al. developed and validated the vocal tract scaling system (VTSS), an assessment tool that helps evaluate EVT and determine treatment efficacy with a high predictive value. The VTSS accounts for various sites of tremor along the vocal tract, including the palate, base of tongue, pharyngeal wall, false vocal folds, and true vocal folds. Both the intra-rater and inter-rater variability are reported to be excellent, with the latter being at least 0.914 [56]. Acoustic/spectral analysis also has been used in diagnosing EVT. Paige et al. investigated the frequency of EVT in 160 patients using computerized peak detection method and reported a median frequency between 4 and 5 Hz, with a normative frequency range of 3.8 to 5.5 Hz [57]. Gamboa et al. in their acoustic analysis of 28 patients with essential tremor found higher jitter and lower harmonic-to-noise ratio values of the vowel /a/ and low intensity and frequency variability while reading a sentence [58]. The acoustic patterns of EVT were also investigated by Lester et al. who showed abnormal fundamental frequency and intensity modulation [59].

The treatment of EVT involves several modalities. Patients often are started on pharmacotherapy using beta-blockers such as propranolol or anticonvulsant barbiturates such as primidone. Nida et al. investigated the effect of primidone in patients with EVT and reported improvement in 14 of 26 patients. However, more than two-thirds experienced side effects, leading to cessation of therapy in half the cases [60]. Justicz et al. reported the effectiveness of propranolol in 18 patients treated with

60–80 mg per day for 2–4 weeks. The authors noted an average change in VRQOL of 9.31 and significant improvement in VRQOL (greater than 10) in 6 of the 18 patients [61]. *Another common treatment is neurotoxin injections. BT injections are offered as the first line of therapy and to patients who are refractory to medical treatment* [62]. In the above study by Justicz et al., 15 patients who were treated subsequently with BT injection reported improvement in their perceptual assessment and VRQOL score. Eighty-nine percent had bilateral injections into the TA/LAC complex, and the average dose used was 3.18 units [61]. In a longitudinal study on the use of BT in the treatment of EVT, Warrick et al. reported a decrease in the frequency and amplitude of tremor during the first week postinjection. Patients also had a decrease in voice effort that was commensurate with a decrease in laryngeal hyperactivity and airway resistance. All patients had bilateral injections into the TA muscle and were evaluated before injection and 2–16 weeks after [63]. The same authors investigated the efficacy of unilateral vs. bilateral BT vocal fold injections in a group of patients with EVT. Using laryngeal EMG guidance, patients were injected with either 2.5 IU bilaterally or 15 IU unilaterally. The authors noted a reduction in tremor and vocal effort that coincided with a decrease in laryngeal resistance in three of the ten patients who had bilateral injections and in two of the nine who had a unilateral injection [64].

Given that EVT is not limited to the true vocal folds, there are many studies on the benefit of BT injections in muscles other than the TA/LCA complex. In 2000, Hertegård et al. reviewed the voice outcome of 15 patients with EVT who had BT injection in the TA, cricothyroid, and thyrohyoid muscles and reported successful treatment in 50–65% of the cases. There was a significant decrease in fundamental frequency variation during sustained vowel production, which corresponded to a subjective decrease in voice tremor [65]. Nelson et al. reported their experience with BT injection in the TA and laryngeal strap muscles in 21 patients with laryngeal tremor, two-thirds of whom had both vertical and horizontal tremor. Using VHI-10 and CAPE evaluation, the authors reported subjective voice improvement in 96% of cases (100% in those who had both TA and strap muscles injection). The mean of improvement per injection was 70%. It is important to note that 62% of their study group had spasmodic dysphonia as well [66]. In another retrospective analysis of 16 patients with EVT, 15 of whom had horizontal laryngeal tremor and 13 of whom had vertical laryngeal tremor, Gurey et al. reported improvement in tremor amplitude following bilateral BT injection into the thyroarytenoid muscles. Patients with vertical tremor had additional BT injections into the strap muscles that were successful [67].

The role of injection laryngoplasty in in the treatment of EVT remains controversial. Van Doren et al. reported improvement in VHI-10 score and subglottal pressure in three of six patients with EVT and vocal fold atrophy who had undergone injection laryngoplasty. Overall, there was improvement in vocal fold function and patient satisfaction in two-third of the cases. The authors discussed the value of vocal fold augmentation in patients with EVT and comorbid vocal fold atrophy or glottal insufficiency from other causes [68]. However, in a comparative study on the utility of injection laryngoplasty in patients with EVT who had undergone BT injection, Estes et al. reported no significant advantage except for an increase in loudness on perceptual evaluation. Patients had had an increase in airflow following BT which then decreased after vocal fold augmentation. The study was conducted on seven patients who had voice assessment using laryngeal videostroboscopy, acoustic and airflow measures, and perceptual and self-reported assessment [69]. Another promising treatment option in patients with EVT who are refractory to medical treatment and/or BT injection is deep brain stimulation [70, 71]. In a report on five patients with essential tremor, which included a case of essential tremor of the vocal tract, Ruckart et al. reported a significant decrease in VHI-10 score in that patient from 33 to 1 following deep brain stimulation [70]. BT injection may be useful in optimizing the voice following surgery. Future studies on the use of laryngeal BT injections for improving the voice in selected patients' post-deep brain stimulation are needed.

In summary, BT injection is a safe and effective treatment for patients with EVT. The dose of BT should be tailored according to the patients' condition and site of tremor. Various intrinsic and extrinsic laryngeal muscle groups may be targeted. The treatment plan needs to be individualized with extreme care to minimize adverse events.

9.4 Laryngeal Botulinum Toxin Injection in Patients with Vocal Process Granuloma

Vocal process granulomas are benign exophytic lesions usually of the posterior glottis [72]. They were described by Jackson in 1928 as "contact ulcers "of the vocal processes as a result of injury to the overlying mucosa [73]. The injury is perpetuated by endogenous and exogenous factors leading to inflammation of the perichondrium and underling cartilages [74]. Phonotrauma and laryngopharyngeal reflux disease are the main culprits. Phonotrauma can be in the form of a hard glottal attacks, voice abuse, excessively low pitched voice, excessive throat clearing, and coughing [75–77]. The "hammer and anvil" effect between the vocal processes is thought to be the mechanical basis for the formation of these lesions [78]. Exposure of the vocal processes and interarytenoid mucosal lining to the gastric refluxate material is also a detrimental predisposing factor. The resultant irritation and aberrant sensation lead to a traumatic laryngeal behavior that perpetuates the mucosal injury. The vocal process proliferative lesions often raise the suspicion of an invasive carcinoma that is masked by an overlying reactive process [79]. Vocal process granuloma also may result from traumatic laryngeal manipulation and/or prolonged intubation. In 1932, Clausen was the first to report intubation granuloma [80]. When the contact pressure of the tube wall exceeds the mucosa capillary perfusion pressure, ischemia and inflammation occur leading to necrosis and mass formation. The size of the endotracheal tube and the duration of intubation are important factors [81, 82]. Another less recognized cause of vocal process granuloma formation is glottic insufficiency. In a study of 34 patients with vocal process granuloma, Carroll et al. reported glottic insufficiency in 53% of the cases. The authors alluded to the potential benefit of vocal fold augmentation in patients who are refractory to conventional medical therapy [83].

The clinical presentation of vocal process granuloma varies markedly. While some patients may be asymptomatic, others may present with life-threatening airway obstruction. The most commonly reported symptoms are globus sensation, excessive throat clearing, cough, change in voice quality, voice fatigue, and voice discomfort. Other reported symptoms include odynophagia and otalgia [72, 83]. In rare cases when the lesion is obstructive, patients may complain of shortness of breath and dyspnea [83]. The diagnosis of vocal process granuloma is based on visualization of the lesion on direct or indirect laryngoscopy. The lesion may look exophytic, nodular, hemorrhagic, or ulcerative. A grading system has been suggested by Farwell et al. that stratifies vocal process granuloma into four categories based on the size of the lesion and its appearance [84]. In grade 1 the lesion is limited to the vocal process, sessile, and nonulcerative. Grade 2 lesions are limited to the vocal process but are pedunculated and or ulcerative. Grade 3 granulomas extend beyond the vocal process; and grade 4 is diagnosed when the granuloma crosses the midline when the vocal folds are fully abducted.

The treatment of vocal process granuloma is daunting because of the diversity in clinical presentation and etiology. Several treatment options are described in the literature, with no clear guidelines on how to manage these lesions. In a systematic review of treatment of vocal process granuloma that included 19 studies (8 nonrandomized and 11 retrospective), Karkos et al. reported anti-reflux therapy, speech and language therapy (SALP), and intake of steroids as the most common treatments often used in combination [85]. The large number of treatment alternatives reflects the lack of success with any single modality of treatment. Anti-reflux therapy consists primarily of lifestyle behavioral changes, intake of proton pump inhibitors, antihistamine antagonists, and in rare cases fundoplication [86]. In a retrospective review of 66 patients with vocal process granuloma, 20 of whom were diagnosed with GERD, De Lima Pontes et al. reported resolution of the lesion following anti-reflux treatment in 75% of the cases [87]. In another study by Wani et al. which included 21 patients with vocal process granuloma, the authors reported complete regression in 14 of 18 patients who tolerated PPI treatment and partial regression in 4 [88]. Speech and language therapy (SALT) also has been shown to be efficacious in the treatment of patients with vocal process granuloma. It consists primarily of voice education and voice exercises that aim at reducing the hardness of the glottal attack and other manifestations of laryngeal hyperfunction. Bloch et al. in their study of 17 patients with contact granuloma treated with voice therapy reported resorption of the lesion in 12 and regression in 4. The treatment consisted of relaxation exercises, auditory and kinesthetic feedback, and avoidance of stress/bad phonatory habits [89]. Similar results have been reported in other studies, with a regression rate of 87.5% of the cases [87]. The efficacy of SALT is improved when combined with anti-reflux therapy. Steroid injection has been shown to be effective as well. In a study by Wang et al. on the use of intralesional steroid injection in patients with vocal process granuloma, the authors reported a reduction in the size of the lesion by 76% or more with complete remission in 60% at 6 months [90].

Conservative therapy using anti-reflux medications and/or SALT is not always sufficient. In patients who are refractory to treatment, or those with large obstructive lesions, surgery is offered as an option. The surgery can be performed using either cold steel instruments or lasers. The overall success rate following surgical removal does not exceed 50% with a high recurrence rate reported. In a study by Ylitalo et al., the recurrence rate in a group of 36 patients who had multiple surgical treatments was 92% [91]. In another study of 23 patients with contact granuloma, Hirano et al. reported resolution in 100% of the cases after 3 interventions. Ten of the 23 patients had recurrence after a single intervention. All patients underwent fiberoptic laryngeal surgery with or without additional laser therapy or steroid injection [92]. Similarly, in a study of 26 patients who underwent a mean of 1.65 ± 1.16 in-office KTP laser treatment, Dominguez et al. reported complete resolution in 73.1% with a median follow-up time of 9.5 months [93]. The incomplete regression of the lesions and the high recurrence rate were attributed to the fact that surgery does not address the cause of contact granuloma.

Laryngeal BT injection has gained popularity over the last two decades as a safe and effective treatment of vocal process granuloma. Botulinum toxin targets the forceful adduction of the vocal folds that is responsible for the mucosal injury or its perpetuation in the posterior glottis. By inducing a temporary paresis of the adductor muscles, the traumatic contact between the vocal processes is inhibited, thus allowing the injured mucosa to heal. The botulinum toxin is usually injected into one of the adductor muscles, the thyroarytenoid muscles (TA), lateral cricoarytenoid muscles (LCA), or the interarytenoid muscles (IA). Nasri et al. was the first to report Botox injection into the thyroarytenoid muscle in six patients with vocal process granuloma [94]. Using the "point-touch technique" described by Green et al. [95], the authors reported complete resolution of contact granuloma in all patients. A total of 10–15 units of botulinum toxin per patient was injected through the cricothyroid membrane or thyroid cartilage. The authors ascribed their therapeutic success to a decrease in the forceful closure of the vocal folds during phonation. The only side effect reported was breathiness which lasted between 2 and 5 months [94]. In 1996, Orloff et al. reported the successful treatment of eight patients with vocal fold granuloma who had undergone at least one previous surgical excision. Four patients needed a second injection, and one needed a third injection. The minimum follow-up was 11 months, and none of the 8 patients had a recurrence. Seven of the eight patients experienced breathiness as a side effect of the treatment. The authors attributed regression of the lesion to neurotoxin-induced temporary paresis which minimized contact trauma and provided a time window for the granuloma to heal [96*]. In 2004, Pham et al. reported successful resolution of the laryngeal granuloma (reduction in size by 50% or more) following BT injection into the TA muscle in five of six patients, all of whom had previous surgical resection. Three of the six patients had laryngopharyngeal reflux disease. The patient that did not respond to BT injection had a large obstructive pyogenic granuloma that needed surgical removal. No side effects were noted except for breathiness ($n = 1$) which subsided

[97]. In 2007, Damrose and Damrose reviewed a case series of seven patients with refractory laryngeal granuloma who had undergone vocal fold BT injection (10–15 units) using the percutaneous approach. Five patients had previous surgical excision and three had prior voice therapy. On 2–7 weeks of follow-up, all patients had resolution of their lesions. Hoarseness was reported by all patients and dysphagia was reported by four patients [98].

The high prevalence of breathiness following TA muscle BT injection and other factors have prompted the search for an alternative adductor muscle as a new site of injection. Although the change in voice quality was temporary and self-limited, in professional voice users or subjects who rely heavily on their voice at work, this side effect may be devastating. Another incapacitating side effect of BT injection within the TA muscle is dysphagia. The increased risk of aspiration may require a change in dietary habits. In an attempt to avoid these side effects, numerous authors targeted other laryngeal adductor muscles such as the IA muscle and the LCA muscle. In 2013, Fink et al. reported the use of IA BT injection in eight patients with refractory vocal process granuloma. Five patients had complete resolution of their granuloma, and two patients had partial regression. It is worth noting that four of the eight patients had concomitant intralesional steroid injection. Half the patients experienced mild-to-moderate breathiness which did not affect their daily work. No patient had dysphagia or aspiration. The authors highlighted the value of IA Botox injection in reducing the forceful closure of the vocal processes, with limited effect on the anterior glottis. Moreover, the IA muscle can be identified and targeted percutaneously under direct vision with no need for laryngeal electromyography [99]. In 2015, Yilmaz et al. reported Botox injection into the TA and LCA muscle in 22 patients with different grades of laryngeal granuloma who were followed up for 6 months. The authors noted complete regression in 77% of the cases. The unresponsive cases were treated surgically with additional BT injection [100]. In 2014, Lee et al. conducted a multicenter investigation comparing the treatment outcome of contact granuloma and reported the highest efficacy in BT injection of the TA and LCA (74.2%). The study included 590 patients who were classified as having either primary or refractory contact granuloma [101]. In 2017, Pham et al. reviewed the medical records of 14 patients with vocal process granuloma and reported 2 cases who were treated with botulinum toxin injection within the lateral cricoarytenoid muscles. Both patients had regression in the size of their lesion from grade 3 to grade 1 following one single in-office injection into the LCA muscle thru the cricothyroid membrane under electromyographic guidance. Breathiness was a side effect that lasted only 5 days. The authors ascribed the decrease in the size of the lesion to weakening of the LCA muscle contraction responsible for the forceful closure of the posterior glottis, thereby decreasing the contact trauma at the tips of the vocal processes. The authors also stressed the need for proper patient's selection, i.e., those who demonstrate LCA-dominant closure pattern on endoscopy with forceful point contact at the tip of the vocal process [102]. In 2019, Hamdan et al. reported the efficacy of interarytenoid Botox injection in eight patients with vocal process granuloma who had been treated with PPI without improvement. There was a decrease in the size of the lesion in four of the eight patients and complete regression in one. The adverse events reported in their study group were breathiness, voice breaks, and aspiration (Video 9.2) [103].

In summary, the treatment of vocal process granuloma should be individualized. The diversity in etiology and the high recurrence rate make treatment very challenging. Although anti-reflux therapy and SALP are the most common treatment approaches, BT injection may be offered to patients as a first line therapy, generally in conjunction with voice therapy and anti-reflux therapy when appropriate. The dose of botulinum toxin and the muscle targeted for injection are based on the type of glottic closure and response to prior treatment.

9.5 Laryngeal Botulinum Toxin Injection in Patients with Vocal Fold Dysfunction

Vocal fold dysfunction is a condition characterized by adduction of the vocal folds during inspiration associated with symptoms of airway obstruction [104]. The term was introduced by Patterson et al. in 1974 [105], following which several anonyms have been reported. These include paradoxical vocal fold movement disorder (PVFM or PVFMD), irritable larynx, hysteric croup, and fictitious asthma, among others. In 2013, the European Society of Otolaryngology, in collaboration with the American College of Surgeons, proposed the term "induced laryngeal obstruction (ILO)" in reference to airway symptoms that occur following a trigger and regress with the cessation of that trigger. The triggers include environmental irritants, cough, exercise, perfume, and other stimuli [106]. Affected patients may invariably complain of intermittent stridor, dyspnea, throat or neck tightness, dysphonia, and difficulty in swallowing. Dyspnea and stridor occur in 73–99% of the cases, and dysphonia is reported in almost two-thirds of the cases [107–110]. The most common cause of dysphonia is the forceful adduction of the vocal folds during inspiratory, which leads to an increase in the collision force between the vocal folds during stridor and hence trauma. The diagnostic criteria commonly used on laryngeal examination are vocal fold inspiratory adduction and/or persistence of a posterior diamond-shaped chink during the attack. More often than not, the laryngeal obstruction is not limited to the glottis but also involves the supraglottic structures. Medialization of the false vocal folds, shortening of the distance between the interarytenoid region and petiole, and abnormal positioning of the epiglottis are observed commonly [111]. The intermittency of the airway symptoms and the normal laryngeal examination between the attacks have led to the use of other tests such as the provocative laryngeal endoscopic test and continuous laryngeal examination (CLE) [108, 112]. The former allows provocation of ILO using an artificial stimulus, whereas the latter facilitates continuous observation of the laryngeal structures throughout the challenge. CLE has allowed diagnosis in patients whose symptoms occur only during peak working capacity and who exhibit normal laryngeal behavior early during attacks [112]. The immediate visual feedback provided by CL has also revealed abnormal laryngeal behavior at more than one site. Other diagnostic tests used commonly in patients with ILO are pulmonary function test and laryngeal electromyography. Pulmonary function test shows truncation of the inspiratory phase of flow-volume loop, a diagnostic sign of extra-thoracic airway obstruction. A negative methacholine challenge test may support a diagnosis of ILO, whereas a positive one is diagnostic of asthma. The treating physician must be aware of the high prevalence of asthma as a coexisting morbidity in patients with ILO, a fact that may influence the diagnostic utility of methacholine challenge [113, 114]. Laryngeal electromyography is also a diagnostic test useful in differentiating ILO from asthma and from other forms of laryngeal dystonia or movement disorders. Affected patients usually display increased activity in the thyroarytenoid and lateral cricoarytenoid muscles during inspiration even when they are not symptomatic [115]. Several pathophysiologic mechanisms for ILO have been suggested, the most important of which are respiratory dystonia which affects the adductor laryngeal muscles and laryngopharyngeal reflux disease. Other suggested mechanisms include laryngeal hypersensitivity, mechanical predisposition, upregulation in the adductor laryngeal reflex, and psychogenic disorders. Autonomic nervous system dysfunction precipitated by emotional and physical distress also has been suggested as a cause of ILO, very similar to patients with laryngeal hyperfunction [116–121].

Given the multidimensional etiology of ILO, there is no clear consensus on the best management strategy. Numerous treatment modalities are adopted commonly either in isolation or in combination. These include the intake of proton pump inhibitors (PPI) for the control of laryngopharyngeal reflux, speech and voice therapy that focuses on the patient education and control of breathing (respiratory training), cognitive therapy with feedback laryngeal visualization, psychotherapy, and BT injection [122]. BT injection has gained acceptance over the last three decades as a conventional, safe, and cost-effective treatment option for ILO, as well as other forms of laryngeal dystonia and movement disorders [13]. In 1994, Grillone et al. reported the successful use of bilateral vocal fold botulinum injection in seven patients with "adductor laryngeal breathing dystonia." Successful treatment lasted 13.8 months on average but was associated with adverse events, namely, aspiration and change in voice quality [123]. In 2000, Altman et al. reviewed their experience in ten patients diagnosed with PVCM, five of whom were treated successfully with BT injection and two of whom received biofeedback therapy. The authors stressed the value of BT injection as a treatment modality in affected patients [124]. Similarly, Maillard et al. reported a case of ILO treated with BT in whom the injection had obviated the need for intubation and/or tracheotomy. The vital efficacy of Botox injection in the management of acute respiratory distress was highlighted [125]. In a review of 46 patients with PVFMD (another name for ILO), Marcinow et al. stressed the role of TA muscle BT injection in the treatment of patients not responsive to laryngeal control therapy. The authors stressed the sensitivity of post-exertion flexible laryngoscopy in the diagnosis of PVFMD [109]. In 2014, Baxter et al. evaluated the benefits of BT injection in asthmatic patients who suffered from abnormal vocal fold movement. The study was conducted on 11 patients who underwent a total of 24 injections and showed an increase in asthma control test score and improvement in the size of the upper airway using computerized tomography of the larynx [126]. Similarly, in 2015, Montojo et al. described a 13-year-old girl diagnosed with PVFM who underwent office-based laryngeal injection using BT type A. The patient had complete regression of her symptoms for 5 months [127]. The effectiveness of BT injection in patients with PVFMD also has been reported by deSilva et al. in their review of 13 patients who had 3.85 injections on average per patient. The authors noted a significant decrease in dyspnea severity index score and improvement/complete resolution of dyspnea in 84.6% of the cases [128]. In a retrospective chart review of 40 patients with PVFM, Vance et al. reported improvement in 90% of those who had BT injection, LPR treatment, and/or voice therapy. The authors stressed the effectiveness of BT treatment in affected patients [129].

9.6 Rare Application of Office-Based Botulinum Toxin Injection

9.6.1 Office-Based BT Injection in Patients with Muscle Tension Dysphonia

Muscle tension dysphonia (MTD) is a voice disorder characterized by excessive laryngeal activity. It is a common cause of dysphonia, accounting for one-third of patients presenting with a change in voice quality. MTD is considered primary in the absence of structural or neurologic disorders and secondary in the presence of underlying vocal fold pathology and/or glottic insufficiency [130, 131]. In a study of 100 patients above the age of 40 years, Belafsky et al. noted a higher prevalence of hyperkinetic laryngeal behavior in patients with vocal fold bowing in comparison to those with no vocal fold bowing (17 times more likely) [132]. Precipitating factors for MTD include underlying diseases such as gastroesophageal reflux disease, personality or psychological disorders, and phonotrauma [130]. Patients with MTD often report a change in voice quality described as inappropriate pitch and loudness, associated with neck pain or tightness, vocal fatigue, and sore throat. They are offered a variety of treatment options that include voice hygiene therapy, vocal function exercises, circum-laryngeal manual therapy, medical treatment for reflux disease, and phonosurgery in the presence of vocal fold lesions or structural or neurogenic abnormalities. An alternative rarely offered to patients who are refractory to voice therapy is BT injection (Video 9.3). Rosen and Murry reported a 52-year-old man who presented with severe dysphonia that was attributed to excessive hyperadduction of the false vocal folds during phonation. The voice was described as rough, raspy, and low in pitch. The patient had been treated with voice exercises and hygiene without success. Using the peroral approach, 20 units of BT per were injected into false vocal folds following which the patient had marked improvement in voice quality and resolution of false vocal fold adduction on examination [133].

The results of Rosen and Murry concur with those of Pacheco et al. who reviewed their experience with seven patients diagnosed with refractory muscle tension dysphonia who had false vocal fold Botox injection under general anesthesia. A total of 15 injections were performed with a dose that varied between 30 and 45 units. Of the six patients who were followed up, five had improvement in their voice-related quality of life score. The complications noted were breathiness in two patients and cough in three. The complications were transient and subsided in 1–2 weeks [134].

9.6.2 Office-Based Botulinum Toxin Injection in Patients with Phonetic Tics

Phonetic tic is a voice disorder characterized by abnormal laryngeal behavior that results in involuntary sounds such as grunting or throat clearing. Although the primary treatment of phonetic tics is pharmacologic, some patients are offered laryngeal BT injections as an alternative, although its effectiveness remains questionable [135]. In 2004, Porta et al. investigated the effect of vocal fold BT injection in 30 patients with Tourette's syndrome and reported improvement in voice tics in 93% of the cases, with complete resolution in 50% of the cases (n = 15 patients). Despite the fact the majority had hypophonia as an adverse effect of treatment, there was an improvement in overall quality of life and premonitory experiences. Patients were assessed on several occasions over 12 months [136]. The utility of BT (type A) injections also was assessed by Vincent et al. in their case series of two patients. The lowest effective dose used was 0.624 units, and repeated injections were needed to achieve complete resolution of the tic behavior. The author highlighted the successful use of neuromuscular blockade in patients with abnormal laryngeal behavior [137]. Similarly, Kholi and Blitzer reported a 26-year-old male with history of grunting and throat clearing who was treated successfully with laryngeal and facial BT injections. There was a subjective and objective improvement with a decrease in Yale Global Tic Severity Scale (YGTSS) [138]. Nevertheless, despite the above reports, the effectiveness of BT injection should be investigated further. In a review by Pandey et al. in 2018, the authors noted the uncertain effect of BT injections in the treatment of phonetic and motor tics. The authors also highlighted the high prevalence of adverse events following treatment [139].

9.6.3 Office-Based Botulinum Toxin Injection in Patients with Parkinson's Disease

Parkinson's disease is a slowly progressive, neurodegenerative disease characterized by a decrease/depletion of dopamine in the substantia nigra. Affected patients suffer from functional impairment secondary to muscle rigidity and tremor.

Hypokinesia and hyperkinesia are the extreme forms of muscle dysfunction commonly observed in these patients. Speech and voice disturbances are among the plethora of symptoms that prompt medical attention. The phonatory symptoms are ascribed often to restricted mobility of the intrinsic and extrinsic laryngeal muscles, both in the horizontal and vertical dimensions. The most commonly reported symptoms are dysphonia, voice tremor, pitch breaks, delayed onset of phonation, decreased volume, breathy voice, and difficulty in voice projection. Other symptoms include dysphagia and aspiration. On laryngeal examination, there is bowing of the vocal folds, glottic insufficiency, hypo-adduction during phonation, and hypo-abduction during inspiration. Abnormal laryngeal movement is observed in almost 50% of the cases [140]. A multidisciplinary approach is needed to optimize the voice outcome of affected patients. The treatment options commonly offered are medical therapy (levodopa), speech and swallowing therapy, medialization laryngoplasty (injection or thyroplasty), and deep brain stimulation [141–144]. Botulinum toxin injection is beneficial in selected cases. Sachdev et al. reported successful botulinum toxin injection into the posterior cricoarytenoid muscle in 53-year-old man with Parkinson's disease who also suffered from ABSD [145]. The authors attributed the ABSD to neurologic abnormalities in the basal ganglia. Further research on the clinical use of BT laryngeal injections in patients with Parkinson's disease is needed.

9.7 Technique of Office-Based Botulinum Toxin Injection

The procedure starts with identifying the patient, reviewing the patient's chart with confirmation of the diagnosis that requires BT injection, determining vocal fold mobility status on the day of the procedure (especially important in patients who have undergone BT injection previously), and reviewing history of prior treatment including sites and doses of previous injection, if any. The procedure is explained to the patient including expected time to onset of benefits; side effects such as allergic reaction, breathiness, aspiration, and dysphagia; and reasons for possible injection failure such as previously formed antibodies. A signed consent for the procedure is obtained after all patient questions and concerns have been addressed. The planned dose of BT and the muscles targeted for injection are confirmed verbally with the patient and staff. The dose of Botox should be tailored according to the patient's condition and site of the injection. BT can be injected through a flexible laryngoscope with a working channel as shown above, or through the cricothyroid membrane with EMG guidance, as discussed below. A single or multichannel diagnostic EMG machine can be used for EMG needle guidance. A portable, single-channel EMG device that provides only auditory information and single-channel recording was used in procedure illustrated below.

Step 1: BT bottle is checked for the expiration date, and the BT is mixed. The dose planned for the injection is drawn into a syringe (Fig. 9.1).

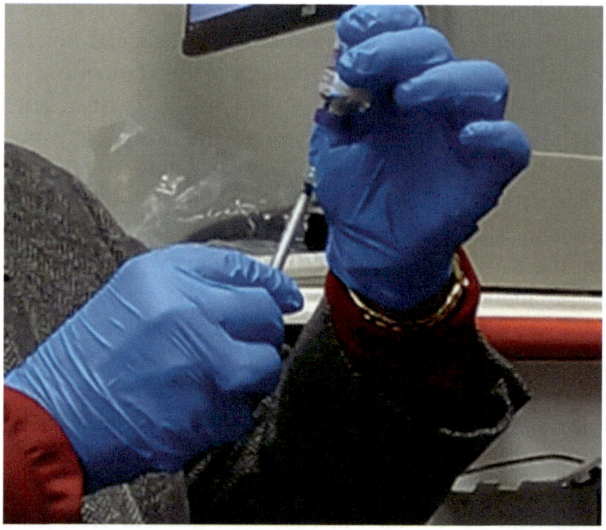

Fig. 9.1 BT injection preparation

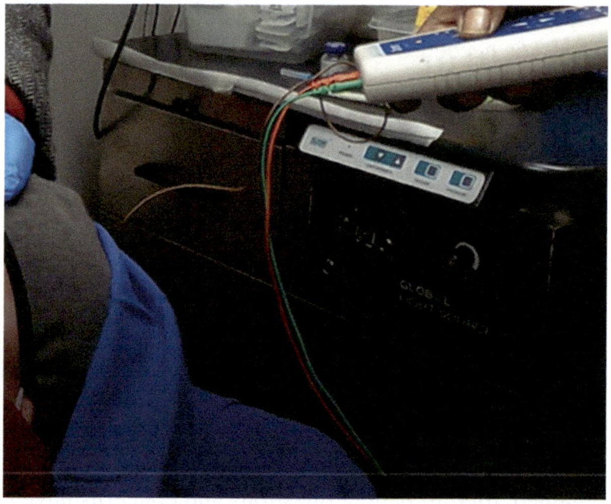

Fig. 9.2 EMG wires are connected

Step 2: The patient is placed in a supine position with the neck extended, after using a shoulder roll to improve exposure of the larynx. The procedure can be done with a facemask or tracheotomy in place. If the tracheotomy is high and the neck is short, it may be necessary to remove the tracheotomy tube to permit needle insertion at the correct angles.

Step 3: Surface electrodes are placed on the forehead, chest, or another part of the body away from the neck to ground the patient and help filter background electrical activity. Typically, surface electrodes consist of a metal disk with a diameter of 0.5–2.5 cm (Fig. 9.2).

Step 4: Laryngeal landmarks are palpated (laryngeal notch, laryngeal cartilage inferior border, cricoid cartilage, cricothyroid membrane) for accurate insertion of the electrode into the laryngeal muscles (Fig. 9.3).

Step 5: The neck is cleaned with alcohol pad.

Step 6: The needle electrode is inserted through the skin and into the target laryngeal muscle (Fig. 9.4).

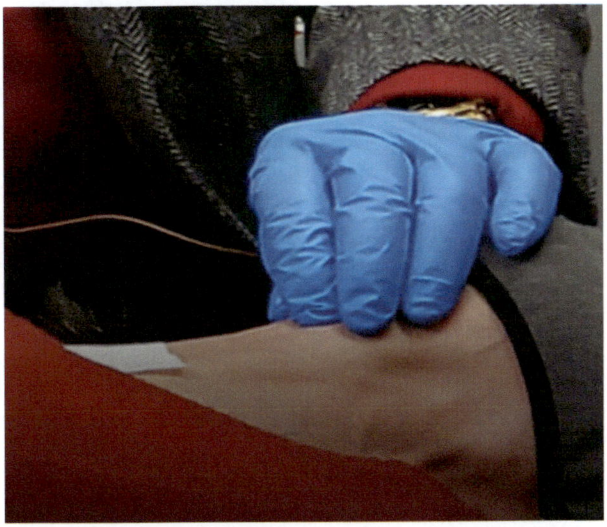

Fig. 9.3 Laryngeal landmarks palpation

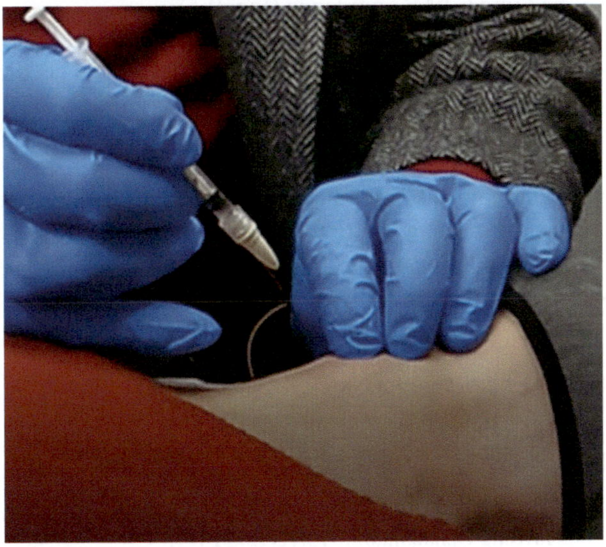

Fig. 9.4 Needle electrode insertion

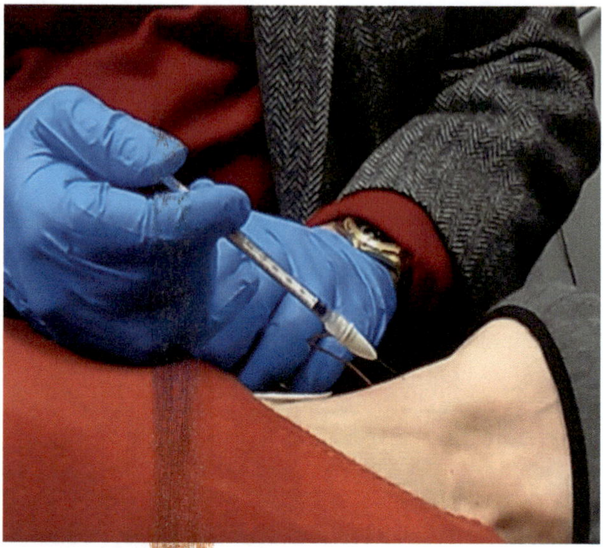

Fig. 9.5 BT is injected after identifying the intended muscle by vowel signal

Step 7: When the needle is positioned, the patient is asked to perform laryngeal maneuvers (phonatory, respiratory, or swallowing) that require activation of the muscle of interest and relative relaxation of other muscles of the larynx. When the needle is in the correct position, the auditory signal heard through the EMG device's speaker will be increased with the appropriate laryngeal maneuver (Video 9.4).

Step 8: BT is injected through needle electrode once the intended muscle is identified under EMG guidance (Fig. 9.5).

Step 9: Achieving the desired result is confirmed by hearing signal decrease in the laryngeal muscle targeted for the injection as needle tip is surrounded by liquid that separate it from muscle.

Safety Considerations

Current may leak from the electrodiagnostic system and lead to death or injury in a patient by causing ventricular fibrillation. To minimize the risk of this complication, every patient must be grounded, the current leakage from the instrument should not exceed 10 microamperes, and the procedure should be avoided in patients with a cardiac pacemaker.

References

1. Scott AB, Rosenbaum A, Collins CC. Pharmacologic weakening of extraocular muscles. Investig Ophthalmol. 1973;12(12):924–7.
2. Mayer NH, Esquenazi A. Muscle overactivity and movement dysfunction in the upper motoneuron syndrome. Phys Med Rehabil Clin N AM. 2003;14(4):855–83.

3. Hughes AJ. Botulinum toxin in clinical practice. Drugs. 1994;48(6):888–93.
4. Bellows S, Jankovic J. Immunogenicity associated with botulinum toxin treatment. Toxins (Basel). 2019;11(9):491.
5. Pfaff J, Neuenschwander M, Pribitkin E, Sataloff RT. Botulinum toxin in otolaryngology. In: Sataloff RT, editor. Professional voice: the science and art of clinical care. 4th ed. San Diego, CA: Plural Publishing; 2017. p. 1141–54.
6. Hallett M, Albanese A, Dressler D, et al. Evidence-based review and assessment of botulinum neurotoxin for the treatment of movement disorders. Toxicon. 2013;67:94–114.
7. Matak I, Lacković Z, Relja M. Botulinum toxin type A in motor nervous system: unexplained observations and new challenges. J Neural Transm. 2016;123(12):1415–21.
8. Mazzocchio R, Caleo M. More than at the neuromuscular synapse: actions of botulinum neurotoxin A in the central nervous system. Neuroscientist. 2015;21(1):44–61.
9. Bielamowicz S, Ludlow CL. Effects of botulinum toxin on pathophysiology in spasmodic dysphonia. Ann Otol Rhinol Laryngol. 2000;109(2):194–203.
10. Marchand-Pauvert V, Aymard C, Giboin LS, Dominici F, Rossi A, Mazzocchio. Beyond muscular effects: depression of spinal recurrent inhibition after botulinum neurotoxin A. J Physiol. 2013;591(4):1017–29.
11. Caleo M, Restani L. Direct central nervous system effects of botulinum neurotoxin. Toxicon. 2018;147:68–72.
12. Schweinfurth JM, Billante M, Courey MS. Risk factors and demographics in patients with spasmodic dysphonia. Laryngoscope. 2002;112(2):220–3.
13. Blitzer A, Brin MF. Laryngeal dystonia: a series with botulinum toxin therapy. Ann Otol Rhinol Laryngol. 1991;100(2):85–9.
14. Klein C, Brin MF, De Leon D, et al. De novo mutations (GAG deletion) in the DYT1 gene in two non-Jewish patients with early-onset dystonia. Hum Mol Genet. 1998;7(7):1133–6.
15. Hintze JM, Ludlow CL, Bansberg SF, Adler CH, Lott DG. Spasmodic dysphonia: a review. Part 1: pathogenic factors. Otolaryngol Head Neck Surg. 2017;157(4):551–7.
16. Hintze JM, Ludlow CL, Bansberg SF, Adler CH, Lott DG. Spasmodic dysphonia: a review. Part 2: characterization of pathophysiology. Otolaryngol Head Neck Surg. 2017;157(4):558–64.
17. Stewart CF, Sinclair CF, Kling IF, Diamond BE, Blitzer A. Adductor focal laryngeal dystonia: correlation between clinicians' ratings and subjects' perception of dysphonia. J Clin Mov Disord. 2017;4(1):20.
18. Kaye R, Blitzer A. Chemodenervation of the larynx. Toxins. 2017;9(11):356.
19. Sulica L. Contemporary management of spasmodic dysphonia. Curr Opin Otolaryngol Head Neck Surg. 2004;12(6):543–8.
20. Blitzer A, Brin MF, Stewart CF. Botulinum toxin management of spasmodic dysphonia (laryngeal dystonia): a 12-year experience in more than 900 patients. Laryngoscope. 1998;108(10):1435–41.
21. Jaworek AJ, Deems AD, Sataloff RT. Spasmodic dysphonia. In: Sataloff RT, editor. Professional voice: the science and art of clinical care. 4th ed. San Diego, CA: Plural Publishing; 2017. p. 1077–100.
22. Patel AB, Bansberg SF, Adler CH, Lott DG, Crujido L. The Mayo Clinic Arizona spasmodic dysphonia experience: a demographic analysis of 718 patients. Ann Otol Rhinol Laryngol. 2015;124(11):859–63.
23. Moerman M, Martens JP, Crevier-Buchman L, Woisard V, Dejonckere P. Perceptive evaluation of substitution voices: the I (I) NFVo rating scale. Rev Laryngol Otol Rhinol. 2005;126(5):323–5.
24. Moerman M, Martens JP, Dejonckere P. Multidimensional assessment of strongly irregular voices such as in substitution voicing and spasmodic dysphonia: a compilation of own research. Logoped Phoniatr Vocol. 2015;40(1):24–9.
25. Cannito MP, Johnson JP. Spastic dysphonia: a continuum disorder. J Commun Disord. 1981;14(3):215–23.

26. Guardiani E, Sadoughi B, Sulica L, Meyer TK, Blitzer A. Laryngeal electromyography. In: Rubin JS, Sataloff RT, Korovin GS, editors. Diagnosis and treatment of voice disorders. 4th ed. New York, NY: Plural Publishing; 1995. p. 289–303.
27. Dedo HH. Recurrent laryngeal nerve section for spastic dysphonia. Ann Otol Rhinol Laryngol. 1976;85(4):451–9.
28. Biller HF, Som ML, Lawson W. Laryngeal nerve crush for spastic dysphonia. Ann Otol Rhinol Laryngol. 1979;88(4):531–2.
29. Netterville JL, Stone RE, Zealear DL, Rainey C, Ossoff RH. Recurrent laryngeal nerve avulsion for treatment of spastic dysphonia. Ann Otol Rhinol Laryngol. 1991;100(1):10–4.
30. Iwamura S. Selective intralaryngeal excision of the thyroarytenoid branch of the recurrent laryngeal nerve for treatment of adductor spasmodic dysphonia and its long-term results. Presented at the Voice Foundation 21st Annual Symposium: Care of the Professional Voice; 1992; Philadelphia, PA.
31. Mendelsohn AH, Berke GS. Surgery or botulinum toxin for adductor spasmodic dysphonia: a comparative study. Ann Otol Rhinol Laryngol. 2012;121(4):231–8.
32. Nakamura K, Muta H, Watanabe Y, Mochizuki R, Yoshida T, Suzuki M. Surgical treatment for adductor spasmodic dysphonia–efficacy of bilateral thyroarytenoid myectomy under microlaryngoscopy. Acta Otolaryngol. 2008;128(12):1348–53.
33. Su CY, Lai CC, Wu PY, Huang HH. Transoral laser ventricular fold resection and thyroarytenoid myoneurectomy for adductor spasmodic dysphonia: long-term outcome. Laryngoscope. 2010;120(2):313–8.
34. Tsuji DH, Takahashi MT, Imamura R, Hachiya A, Sennes LU. Endoscopic laser thyroarytenoid myoneurectomy in patients with adductor spasmodic dysphonia: a pilot study on long-term outcome on voice quality. J Voice. 2012;26(5):666-e7–12.
35. Kim HS, Choi HS, Lim JY, Choi YL, Lim SE. Radiofrequency thyroarytenoid myothermy for treatment of adductor spasmodic dysphonia: how we do it. Clin Otolaryngol. 2008;33(6):621–5.
36. Isshiki N, Haji T, Yamamoto Y, Mahieu HF. Thyroplasty for adductor spasmodic dysphonia: further experiences. Laryngoscope. 2001;111(4):615–21.
37. Eskander A, Fung K, McBride S, Hogikyan N. Current practices in the management of adductor spasmodic dysphonia. J Otolaryngol Head Neck Surg. 2010;39(5):622–30.
38. Hall W. NIH Consensus Development Conference. Clinical use of botulinum toxin. National Institutes of Health Consensus Development Conference Statement. Arch Neurol. 1991;48(12):1294–8.
39. Srirompotong S, Saeseow P, Taweesaengsuksakul R, Kharmwar S, Srirompotong S. Botulinum toxin injection for treatment of spasmodic dysphonia: experience at Srinagarind hospital. J Med Assoc Thail. 2006;89(12):2077–80.
40. Kendall KA, Leonard RJ. Interarytenoid muscle botox injection for treatment of adductor spasmodic dysphonia with vocal tremor. J Voice. 2011;25(1):114–9.
41. Patel PN, Kabagambe EK, Starkweather JC, et al. Outcomes of onabotulinum toxin a treatment for adductor spasmodic dysphonia and laryngeal tremor. JAMA Otolaryngol Head Neck Surg. 2018;144(4):293–9.
42. Finnegan EM, Luschei ES, Gordon JD, Barkmeier JM, Hoffman HT. Increased stability of airflow following botulinum toxin injection. Laryngoscope. 1999;109(8):1300–6.
43. Ali SO, Thomassen M, Schulz GM, et al. Alterations in CNS activity induced by botulinum toxin treatment in spasmodic dysphonia: an H215O PET study. J Speech Lang Hear Res. 2006;49(5):1127–46.
44. Shoffel-Havakuk H, Rosow DE, Lava CX, Hapner ER, Johns MM III. Common practices in botulinum toxin injection for spasmodic dysphonia treatment: a national survey. Laryngoscope. 2019;129(7):1650–6.
45. Sataloff RT, Mandel S, Heman-Ackah YD. Laryngeal electromyography. In: Sataloff, editor. Professional voice: the science and art of clinical care. 4th ed. San Diego, CA: Plural Publishing; 2017. p. 459–88.

46. Klotz DA, Shahinfar A, Maronian NC, Robinson L, Waugh PF, Hillel AD. Findings of multiple muscle involvement in a study of 214 patients with laryngeal dystonia using fine-wire electromyography. Ann Otol Rhinol Laryngol. 2004;113(8):602–12.
47. Maronian NC, Robinson L, Waugh PF, Hillel AD. Tremor laryngeal dystonia: treatment of the lateral cricoarytenoid muscle. Ann Otol Rhinol Laryngol. 2004;113(5):349–55.
48. Rutt A, Kennelly KD, Martinez-Paredes JF. Patient experience contributing to outcomes of laryngeal botulinum toxin injection. J Voice. 2020:S0892-1997(20)30175-2.
49. Sulica L, Brin MF, Blitzer A, Stewart CF. Botulinum toxin management of adductor spasmodic dysphonia after failed recurrent laryngeal nerve section. Ann Otol Rhinol Laryngol. 2003;112(6):499–505.
50. Venkatesan NN, Johns MM, Hapner ER, DelGaudio JM. Abductor paralysis after botox injection for adductor spasmodic dysphonia. Laryngoscope. 2010;120(6):1177–80.
51. Bhatia KP, Bain P, Bajaj N, et al. Consensus Statement on the classification of tremors. From the task force on tremor of the International Parkinson and Movement Disorder Society. Mov Disord. 2018;33(1):75–87.
52. Barkmeier-Kraemer JM. Isolated voice tremor: a clinical variant of essential tremor or a distinct clinical phenotype? Tremor Other Hyperkinet Mov (NY). 2020:10.
53. Sulica L, Louis ED. Clinical characteristics of essential voice tremor: a study of 34 cases. Laryngoscope. 2010;120(3):516–28.
54. Moraes BT, Biase NG. Laryngoscopy evaluation protocol for the differentiation of essential and dystonic voice tremor. Braz J Otorhinolaryngol. 2016;82(1):88–96.
55. Dahl L, Lim JW, Mandel S, Gupta R, Sataloff RT. Neurologic disorders affecting the voice in performance. In: Sataloff RT, editor. Professional voice: the science and art of clinical care. 4th ed. San Diego, CA: Plural Publishing; 2017. p. 1031–58.
56. Bové M, Daamen N, Rosen C, Wang CC, Sulica L, Gartner-Schmidt J. Development and validation of the vocal tremor scoring system. Laryngoscope. 2006;116(9):1662–7.
57. Paige C, Hopewell BL, Gamsarian V, et al. Characterizing the normative voice tremor frequency in essential vocal tremor. JAMA Otolaryngol Head Neck Surg. 2018;144(12):1169–73.
58. Gamboa J, Jiménez-Jiménez FJ, Nieto A, et al. Acoustic voice analysis in patients with essential tremor. J Voice. 1998;12(4):444–52.
59. Lester RA, Barkmeier-Kraemer J, Story BH. Physiologic and acoustic patterns of essential vocal tremor. J Voice. 2013;27(4):422–32.
60. Nida A, Alston J, Schweinfurth J. Primidone therapy for essential vocal tremor. JAMA Otolaryngol Head Neck Surg. 2016;142(2):117–21.
61. Justicz N, Hapner ER, Josephs JS, Boone BC, Jinnah HA, Johns MM III. Comparative effectiveness of propranolol and botulinum for the treatment of essential voice tremor. Laryngoscope. 2016;126(1):113–7.
62. McGarey PO Jr, Simpson CB, Daniero JJ. Practice patterns and barriers in botulinum toxin injection for the treatment of voice disorders. J Voice. 2020:S0892-1997(20)30155-7.
63. Warrick P, Dromey C, Irish JC, Durkin L. The treatment of essential voice tremor with botulinum toxin A: a longitudinal case report. J Voice. 2000;14(3):410–21.
64. Warrick P, Dromey C, Irish JC, Durkin L, Pakiam A, Lang A. Botulinum toxin for essential tremor of the voice with multiple anatomical sites of tremor: a crossover design study of unilateral versus bilateral injection. Laryngoscope. 2000;110(8):1366–74.
65. Hertegård S, Granqvist S, Lindestad PÅ. Botulinum toxin injections for essential voice tremor. Ann Otol Rhinol Laryngol. 2000;109(2):204–9.
66. Nelson RC, Silva Merea V, Tierney WS, Milstein C, Benninger MS, Bryson PC. Laryngeal botulinum toxin injection for vocal tremor: utility of concurrent strap muscle injection. Laryngoscope. 2019;129(6):1433–7.
67. Gurey LE, Sinclair CF, Blitzer A. A new paradigm for the management of essential vocal tremor with botulinum toxin. Laryngoscope. 2013;123(10):2497–501.

68. Van Doren M, Faudoa E, Carroll TL. Treatment of patients with vocal fold atrophy and comorbid essential voice tremor: long-term injection augmentation outcomes after successful diagnostic vocal fold injection augmentation. J Voice. 2020;34(3):471–6.
69. Estes C, Sadoughi B, Coleman R, Sarva H, Mauer E, Sulica L. A prospective crossover trial of botulinum toxin chemodenervation versus injection augmentation for essential voice tremor. Laryngoscope. 2018;128(2):437–46.
70. Ruckart KW, Moya-Mendez ME, Nagatsuka M, Barry JL, Siddiqui MS, Madden LL. Comprehensive evaluation of voice-specific outcomes in patients with essential tremor before and after deep brain stimulation. J Voice. 2020:S0892-1997(20)30354-4.
71. Hägglund P, Sandström L, Blomstedt P, Karlsson F. Voice tremor in patients with essential tremor: effects of deep brain stimulation of caudal zona incerta. J Voice. 2016;30(2):228–33.
72. Hoffman HT, Overholt E, Karnell M, McCulloch TM. Vocal process granuloma. Head Neck. 2001;23(12):1061–74.
73. Jackson C. Contact ulcer of the larynx. Ann Otol Rhinol Laryngol. 1928;37:227–38.
74. McFerran DJ, Abdullah V, Gallimore AP, Pringle MB, Croft CB. Vocal process granulomata. J Laryngology Otol. 1994;108(3):216–20.
75. Ward PH, Zwitman D, Hanson D, Berci G. Contact ulcers and granulomas of the larynx: new insights into their etiology as a basis for more rational treatment. Otolaryngol Head Neck Surg. 1980;88(3):262–9.
76. Cherry J, Margulies SI. Contact ulcer of the larynx. Laryngoscope. 1968;78(11):1937–40.
77. Shoffel-Havakuk H, Halperin D, Yosef L, Feldberg E, Lahav Y. Lesions of the posterior glottis: clinical and pathologic considerations and treatment outcome. J Voice. 2014;28(2):263.e1–8.
78. Jackson C, Jackson CL. Contact ulcer of the larynx. Arch Otolaryngol. 1935;22(1):1–5.
79. Devaney KO, Rinaldo A, Ferlito A. Vocal process granuloma of the larynx—recognition, differential diagnosis and treatment. Oral Oncol. 2005;41(7):666–9.
80. Clausen RJ. Unusual sequela of tracheal intubation. Proc R Soc Med. 1932;25(10):1507.
81. Santos PM, Afrassiabi A, Weymuller EA Jr. Risk factors associated with prolonged intubation and laryngeal injury. Otolaryngol Head Neck Surg. 1994;111(4):453–9.
82. Chinachoti T, Pojai S, Sooksri N, Rungjindamai C. Risk factors of post-operative sore throat and hoarseness. J Med Assoc Thail. 2017;100(4):463–8.
83. Carroll TL, Gartner-Schmidt J, Statham MM, Rosen CA. Vocal process granuloma and glottal insufficiency: an overlooked etiology? Laryngoscope. 2010;120(1):114–20.
84. Farwell DG, Belafsky PC, Rees CJ. An endoscopic grading system for vocal process granuloma. J Laryngol Otol. 2008;122(10):1092–5.
85. Karkos PD, George M, Van Der Veen J, et al. Vocal process granulomas: a systematic review of treatment. Ann Otol Rhinol Laryngol. 2014;123(5):314–20.
86. Havas TE, Priestley J, Lowinger DS. A management strategy for vocal process granulomas. Laryngoscope. 1999;109(2):301–6.
87. De Lima Pontes PA, De Biase NG, Gadelha ME. Clinical evolution of laryngeal granulomas: treatment and prognosis. Laryngoscope. 1999;109(2):289–94.
88. Wani MK, Woodson GE. Laryngeal contact granuloma. Laryngoscope. 1999;109(10):1589–93.
89. Bloch CS, Gould WJ, Hirano M. Effect of voice therapy on contact granuloma of the vocal fold. Ann Otol Rhinol Laryngol. 1981;90(1):48–52.
90. Wang CT, Lai MS, Lo WC, Liao LJ, Cheng PW. Intralesional steroid injection: an alternative treatment option for vocal process granuloma in ten patients. Clin Otolaryngol. 2013;38(1):77–81.
91. Ylitalo R, Lindestad PÅ. A retrospective study of contact granuloma. Laryngoscope. 1999;109(3):433–6.
92. Hirano S, Tateya I, Kojima H, Ito J. Fiberoptic laryngeal surgery for vocal process granuloma. Ann Otol Rhinol Laryngol. 2002;111(9):789–93.
93. Dominguez LM, Brown RJ, Simpson CB. Treatment outcomes of in-office KTP ablation of vocal fold granulomas. Ann Otol Rhinol Laryngol. 2017;126(12):829–34.

94. Nasri S, Sercarz JA, Mcalpin T, Berke GS. Treatment of vocal fold granuloma using botulinum toxin type A. Laryngoscope. 1995;105(6):585–8.
95. Green DC, Ward PH, Berke GS, Gerratt BR. Point-touch technique of botulinum toxin injection for the treatment of spasmodic dysphonia. Ann Otol Rhinol Laryngol. 1992;101(11):883–7.
96. Orloff LA, Goldman SN. Vocal fold granuloma: successful treatment with botulinum toxin. Otolaryngol Head Neck Surg. 1999;121(4):410–3.
97. Pham J, Yin S, Morgan M, Stucker F, Nathan CA. Botulinum toxin: helpful adjunct to early resolution of laryngeal granulomas. J Laryngol Otol. 2004;118(10):781–5.
98. Damrose EJ, Damrose JF. Botulinum toxin as adjunctive therapy in refractory laryngeal granuloma. J Laryngol Otol. 2008;122(8):824–8.
99. Fink DS, Achkar J, Franco RA, Song PC. Interarytenoid botulinum toxin injection for recalcitrant vocal process granuloma. Laryngoscope. 2013;123(12):3084–7.
100. Yılmaz T, Kayahan B, Günaydın RÖ, Kuşçu O, Sözen T. Botulinum toxin A for treatment of contact granuloma. J Voice. 2016;30(6):741–3.
101. Lee SW, Hong HJ, Choi SH, et al. Comparison of treatment modalities for contact granuloma: a nationwide multicenter study. Laryngoscope. 2014;124(5):1187–91.
102. Pham Q, Campbell R, Mattioni J, Sataloff R. Botulinum toxin injections into the lateral cricoarytenoid muscles for vocal process granuloma. J Voice. 2018;32(3):363–6.
103. Hamdan AL, Khalifee E, Jaffal H, Ghanem A. Interarytenoid botulinum toxin A injection for the treatment of vocal process granuloma. J Laryngol Otol. 2019;133(12):1041–5.
104. Newman KB, Mason UG 3rd, Schmaling KB. Clinical features of vocal cord dysfunction. Am J Respir Crit Care Med. 1995;152(4):1382–6.
105. Patterson RO, Schatz M, Horton M. Munchausen's stridor: non-organic laryngeal obstruction. Clin Allergy. 1974;4(3):307–10.
106. Christensen PM, Heimdal JH, Christopher KL, et al. ERS/ELS/ACCP 2013 international consensus conference nomenclature on inducible laryngeal obstructions. Eur Respir Rev. 2015;24(137):445–50.
107. Morris MJ, Christopher KL. Diagnostic criteria for the classification of vocal cord dysfunction. Chest. 2010;138(5):1213–23.
108. Chiang T, Marcinow AM, de Silva BW, Ence BN, Lindsey SE, Forrest LA. Exercise-induced paradoxical vocal fold motion disorder: diagnosis and management. Laryngoscope. 2013;123(3):727–31.
109. Marcinow AM, Thompson J, Chiang T, Forrest LA, de Silva BW. Paradoxical vocal fold motion disorder in the elite athlete: experience at a large division I university. Laryngoscope. 2014;124(6):1425–30.
110. Al-Alwan A, Kaminsky D. Vocal cord dysfunction in athletes: clinical presentation and review of the literature. Phys Sports Med. 2012;40(2):22–7.
111. Powell DM, Karanfilov BI, Beechler KB, Treole K, Trudeau MD, Forrest LA. Paradoxical vocal cord dysfunction in juveniles. Arch Otolaryngol Head Neck Surg. 2000;126(1):29–34.
112. Heimdal JH, Roksund OD, Halvorsen T, Skadberg BT, Olofsson J. Continuous laryngoscopy exercise test: a method for visualizing laryngeal dysfunction during exercise. Laryngoscope. 2006;116(1):52–7.
113. Morris MJ, Grbach VX, Deal LE, Boyd SY, Morgan JA, Johnson JE. Evaluation of exertional dyspnea in the active duty patient: the diagnostic approach and the utility of clinical testing. Mil Med. 2002;167(4):281–8.
114. Morris MJ, Deal LE, Bean DR, Grbach VX, Morgan JA. Vocal cord dysfunction in patients with exertional dyspnea. Chest. 1999;116(6):1676–82.
115. Sataloff RT, Mandel S, Heman-Ackah YD, Abaza M. Laryngeal Electromygrapgy. 3rd ed. San Diego, CA: Plural Publishing; 2017, p. 1–181.
116. Wysocki J, Kielska E, Orszulak P, Reymond J. Measurements of pre-and postpubertal human larynx: a cadaver study. Surg Radiol Anat. 2008;30(3):191–9.
117. Hočevar-Boltežar I, Krivec U, Šereg-Bahar M. Laryngeal sensitivity testing in youth with exercise-inducible laryngeal obstruction. Int J Rehabil Res. 2017;40(2):146–51.

118. Famokunwa B, Walsted ES, Hull JH. Assessing laryngeal function and hypersensitivity. Pulm Pharmacol Ther. 2019;56:108–15.
119. Benninger C, Parsons JP, Mastronarde JG. Vocal cord dysfunction and asthma. Curr Opin Pulm Med. 2011;17(1):45–9.
120. Vertigan AE, Bone SL, Gibson PG. Laryngeal sensory dysfunction in laryngeal hypersensitivity syndrome. Respirology. 2013;18(6):948–56.
121. Powell SA, Nguyen CT, Gaziano J, Lewis V, Lockey RF, Padhya TA. Mass psychogenic illness presenting as acute stridor in an adolescent female cohort. Ann Otol Rhinol Laryngol. 2007;116(7):525–31.
122. Forrest LA, Husein T, Husein O. Paradoxical vocal cord motion: classification and treatment. Laryngoscope. 2012;122(4):844–53.
123. Grillone GA, Annino DJ Jr, Blitzer A, Brin MF, Saint-Hilaire MH. Treatment of adductor laryngeal breathing dystonia with botulinum toxin type A. Laryngoscope. 1994;104(1):30–2.
124. Altman KW, Mirza N, Ruiz C, Sataloff RT. Paradoxical vocal fold motion: presentation and treatment options. J Voice. 2000;14(1):99–103.
125. Maillard I, Schweizer V, Broccard A, Duscher A, Liaudet L, Schaller MD. Use of botulinum toxin type A to avoid tracheal intubation or tracheostomy in severe paradoxical vocal cord movement. Chest. 2000;118(3):874–6.
126. Baxter M, Uddin N, Raghav S, et al. Abnormal vocal cord movement treated with botulinum toxin in patients with asthma resistant to optimised management. Respirology. 2014;19(4):531–7.
127. Montojo J, González R, Hernández E, Zafra M, Plaza G. Office-based laryngeal injection of botulinum toxin for paradoxical vocal fold motion in a child. Int J Pediatr Otorhinolaryngol. 2015;79(7):1161–3.
128. DeSilva B, Crenshaw D, Matrka L, Forrest LA. Vocal fold botulinum toxin injection for refractory paradoxical vocal fold motion disorder. Laryngoscope. 2019;129(4):808–11.
129. Vance D, Heyd C, Pier M, Alnouri G, Sataloff RT. Paradoxical vocal fold movement: a retrospective analysis. J Voice. 2020;S0892-1997(20):30128–4.
130. Van Houtte E, Van Lierde K, Claeys S. Pathophysiology and treatment of muscle tension dysphonia: a review of the current knowledge. J Voice. 2011;25(2):202–7.
131. Altman KW, Atkinson C, Lazarus C. Current and emerging concepts in muscle tension dysphonia: a 30-month review. J Voice. 2005;19(2):261–7.
132. Belafsky PC, Postma GN, Reulbach TR, Holland BW, Koufman JA. Muscle tension dysphonia as a sign of underlying glottal insufficiency. Otolaryngol Head Neck Surg. 2002;127(5):448–51.
133. Rosen CA, Murry T. Botox for hyperadduction of the false vocal folds: a case report. J Voice. 1999;13(2):234–9.
134. Pacheco PC, Karatayli-Ozgursoy S, Best S, Hillel A, Akst L. False vocal cord botulinum toxin injection for refractory muscle tension dysphonia: our experience with seven patients. Clin Otolaryngol. 2015;40(1):60–4.
135. Salloway S, Stewart CF, Israeli L, et al. Botulinum toxin for refractory vocal tics. Mov Disord. 1996;11(6):746–8.
136. Porta M, Maggioni G, Ottaviani F, Schindler A. Treatment of phonic tics in patients with Tourette's syndrome using botulinum toxin type A. Neurol Sci. 2004;24(6):420–3.
137. Vincent DA Jr. Botulinum toxin in the management of laryngeal tics. J Voice. 2008;22(2):251–6.
138. Kholi N, Blitzer A. Botulinum toxin for the treatment of Motor and phonetic TCS. Ann Otol Rhinol Laryngol. 2020;129(6):625–7.
139. Pandey S, Srivanitchapoom P, Kirubakaran R, Berman BD. Botulinum toxin for motor and phonic tics in Tourette's syndrome. Cochrane Database Syst Rev. 2018;1(1):CD012285.
140. Stelzig Y, Hochhaus W, Gall V, et al. Laryngeal manifestations in patients with Parkinson disease. Laryngorhinootologie. 1999;78:544–51.

141. Jiang J, Lin E, Wang J, Hanson DG. Glottographic measures before and after levodopa treatment in Parkinson's disease. Laryngoscope. 1999;109(8):1287–94.
142. Berke GS, Gerratt B, Kreiman J, Jackson K. Treatment of Parkinson hypophonia with percutaneous collagen augmentation. Laryngoscope. 1999;109(8):1295–9.
143. Surgical Treatment of Parkinson's Disease. Parkinson's Disease Clinic and Research Center. Univ of CA at San Francisco. http://pdcenter.neurology.ucsf.edu/professionals-guide/surgical-treatment. Accessed 27 Dec 2016.
144. Weaver FM, Follett K, Stern M, et al. Bilateral deep brain stimulation vs. best medical therapy for patients with advanced Parkinson disease: a randomized controlled trial. JAMA. 2009;301(1):63–73.
145. Sachdev A, Costello D, Madge S. Botulinum toxin-B injection into the lacrimal gland and posterior cricoarytenoid muscle for the treatment of epiphora and abductor spasmodic dysphonia secondary to Parkinson's disease. Orbit. 2019;38(3):248–51.

Chapter 10
Office-Based Laryngeal Laser Therapy

10.1 Introduction

The history of laser in laryngology dates back to the 1960s. Strong and Jako were the first to report the use of the CO2 laser in the treatment of benign and malignant lesions of the larynx [1]. The CO2 laser is a diode laser with a wavelength of 10.6 micrometers that is absorbed preferentially by water. Its limited depth of penetration and scattering allows precise excision of mucosal and submucosal lesions [2]. Because of its cutting and hemostatic properties, the CO2 laser became the laser of choice for many otolaryngologists. The advances in instrumentation and the invention of the micromanipulator enhanced its widespread use in endoscopic resection of laryngeal masses [3–11]. In a retrospective analysis of 49 patients with T1a glottic cancer treated with CO2 laser, Schrijvers et al. reported a local control rate similar to that of patients treated with radiation therapy [6]. Similarly, in a randomized, prospective study of 37 patients with exudative lesions of the vocal folds, Benninger et al. showed identical results in those treated with cold steel microdissection and those treated with the CO2 laser. Significant improvement was noted in perceptual voice analysis in the laser group on long-term follow-up compared with nonsignificant improvement in the microdissection group [7].

The use of CO2 laser in laryngology practice came at a cost. Inadvertent injury to the superficial, intermediate and deep layers of the lamina propria secondary to excessive tissue heating and necrosis often led to scar formation with detrimental effects on voice [12–15]. In a review of 244 patients with recurrent respiratory papillomatosis who underwent CO2 laser treatment, Dedo and Yu reported web formation in 27% of the cases [13]. Similarly, in a study of 59 patients with benign lesions of the larynx treated with CO2 laser, Shapshay et al. reported residual disease and/or hoarseness in 23 patients and worsening of voice quality in two [14]. The authors

Supplementary Information The online version contains supplementary material available at [https://doi.org/10.1007/978-3-030-91936-8_10].

A.-l. Hamdan et al., *Office-Based Laryngeal Surgery*,
https://doi.org/10.1007/978-3-030-91936-8_10

advocated the use of a pulse mode and a low-power setting. In another review of 235 patients who had undergone laser surgery, Geyer et al. reported irregular vocal folds edges and incomplete glottic closure postoperatively in 5.2% and 3.5% of the cases, respectively [15]. In their review of CO2 laser in laryngeal surgery, Sataloff et al. stressed the hazards of thermal injury and scar formation in addition to tissue loss secondary to vaporization, which often preclude histologic examination of the surgical margins. The authors also stressed the use of the super-pulse mode and the smallest spot size available (0.15 mm or less) in order to avoid injury to the underlying structures [12].

In view of the above limitations of the CO2 laser, other lasers with a wavelength range near to the absorbance peak of oxyhemoglobin were advocated. The most commonly used were the pulse dye laser (PDL) with 585 nm wavelength and the potassium titanyl phosphate (KTP) laser with a wavelength of 532 nm, both of which are no longer manufactured. Their minimal depth of penetration (less than 2 mm) and their selective absorption by hemoglobin allow treatment of submucosal lesions, especially vascular lesions, with minimal injury to the overlying mucosa [2]. For years, the use of photoangiolytic lasers was limited to the operating room with high success [16–19]. McMillan et al. investigated the efficacy of PDL in the treatment of recurrent respiratory papillomatosis (RRP) involving the larynx and reported complete regression of disease with preservation of the overlying mucosa [16]. Valdez et al. reported the use of PDL in 10 patients with RRP who underwent 13 procedures and showed complete regression in 7 patients and partial regression in two [17]. Franco et al., in their review of 41 patients with RRP treated with PDL, stressed the enhanced effect of laser therapy in facilitating dissection and in providing good hemostasis. Notably, 90% of their patients had bilateral lesions, and 63% had involvement of the anterior commissure [18]. Similarly, Burns et al. reported their experience with KTP laser in the treatment of 37 patients with laryngeal papillomatosis in the operating room and showed 90% disease regression in nearly 80% of those who were assessed postoperatively. Partial regression (50–74%) was achieved in 9% of the cases [19].

Despite the high success rate of photoangiolytic lasers in the operating room, patients in need of frequent surgical intervention may benefit from another option that spares them the risk of repeated general anesthesia and the known complications of suspension microlaryngoscopy [20–25]. Technical advances, such as development of distal chip flexible endoscopes with a working channel and the ability to deliver lasers using glass fibers, led to changes in laryngology practice towards office-based surgery [26]. Office-based laser therapy offers patients fast recovery and decreased morbidity, in addition to other advantages such as improved time efficiency and reduced cost [27–29]. The PDL was the first photoangiolytic laser to be used in an office setting [30]. Although it has been shown to be efficacious in treating laryngeal mucosal and submucosal lesions, its use had some shortcomings and limitations. Its short pulse-width was associated with a high risk of bleeding which obscured the surgical bed and decreased the efficacy of therapy, as the laser energy is absorbed by blood at the surface. This diminished selectivity, as reported by Zeitels et al., reduced effective intravascular coagulation of the PDL and predisposed to bleeding and coughing during surgery in many cases [30]. Other technical limitations of PDL included the large size of the glass fiber and frequent mechanical failures of the laser. All the above shortcomings limited its adoption in the office and paved the way for KTP laser as an alternative. The extended pulse-width of KTP laser (1.5 ms) in comparison to the PDL prolongs intravascular coagulation time and reduces the risk of bleeding. Additional technical advantages include the smaller fiber size, reduced cost, and increased hardware reliability [31]. Other lasers that also emerged for office-based therapy included are the CO2 laser and the thulium laser [32–34]. In 2006, Jacobson et al. reported their experience with flexible CO2 laser in a 74-year-old woman diagnosed with extensive laryngeal amyloidosis that extended to the trachea. Using the laser waveguide though a malleable suction (photonic band-gap assembly, developed by Omni Guide. Inc, Cambridge, MA), the authors were able to ablate the lesion in areas that had been inaccessible previously [33]. Zeitels et al. introduced thulium laser for management of benign and malignant laryngeal masses. Thulium laser is a diode laser with a wavelength of 2013 nm and a greater affinity for water than PDL and KTP lasers. Its main advantage in addition to its fiber delivery that allows its use in the office is superior hemostasis [34].

The blue laser (445 nm) is the successor to the KTP laser. It was approved by the FDA for use in the United States in March 2020 but has been used longer in Europe and elsewhere. Its use is similar to use of KTP laser, but the blue laser has specific differences with which the surgeon should be familiar. The laser energy can be delivered through a 300 micron or 400 micron fibers. For varicosities and ectasias, the author (RTS) favors settings of 2–4 watts (usually starting at 3 watts) 30 msec on time (pulse duration) and with single pulse for ectasias or 300 msec off time (pulse pause) for larger varicosities. The 300 msec off setting allows use that stimulates continuous laser application allowing the laser to be moved down or up the length of the vessel but with enough off time to allow the surgeon to take his/her foot off the pedal to stop the laser between pulses. It also provides tissue relaxation between pulses that is not available with continuous mode and that may help minimize adjacent tissue injury. The non-touch technique is the same as that for the KTP laser; but the blue laser also can be used as a contact laser. At low-power densities, this allows excellent precision. As an added feature, the blue laser also functions quite effective in cutting mode for small or moderate mass lesions and for subglottic or posterior laryngeal stenosis. For cutting, typical settings are 6–10 watts, 40–60 msec on time, and 150 msec. off time.

This chapter reviews the clinical application of office-based laser in the treatment of benign, premalignant, and early malignant lesions of the larynx. The limitations and complications of office-based laser therapy are discussed thoroughly. This information is invaluable to otolaryngologists who elect to treat patients with various laryngeal diseases in the office. As is with any surgery, patients for whom in-office laser surgery is planned should be prepared and informed fully. In addition to preparation and consent discussions reviewed elsewhere in this book, the preoperative conversation should include issues specific to the laser and laser safety. .

10.2 Review of the Clinical Application of Laser Therapy in an Office Setting

10.2.1 Office-Based Laser Therapy in Patients with Laryngeal RRP

Recurrent respiratory papillomatosis (RRP) is a disease of the respiratory epithelium caused by the human papilloma virus usually types 6 and 11. It has a bimodal age distribution affecting children and adults in their third/fourth decade of life [35–38]. Laryngeal RRP is one of the most common benign tumors of the upper aerodigestive tract and is treated traditionally in the operating room using cold steel instruments and/or lasers (diode/photoangiolytic lasers). The main goal of therapy is to maintain airway patency while preserving voice quality. Keeping the balance between phonation and breathing is important in the long-term management of patients who need frequent surgical intervention, particularly in the pediatric population. Based on a review of the US national registry of juvenile-onset RRP, a child needs on average 4.4 procedures a year, with surgical intervention every 1 to 2 months [39]. In view of the frequent need for surgical intervention, the treatment of laryngeal RRP has witnessed a marked shift over the last two decades from the operating room to the office (Video 10.1). This change has spared patients the risk of general anesthesia and the morbidity of suspension microlaryngoscopy without jeopardizing surgical outcome. In 2004, Zeitels et al. reported the successful use of office-based PDL therapy in 51 patients, among whom 30 had laryngeal papillomatosis. The authors reported 50% disease regression in 88% of the cases and improvement in self-reported voice quality in 34 patients [30]. In 2006, the same authors conducted a prospective study of 20 patients with laryngeal papillomatosis who had undergone 36 office-based KTP laser therapy. They reported success in all the cases, although disease regression was not assessed routinely on follow-up. Patients came for surgical intervention only when they had recurrence of their symptoms. The authors stressed the hemostatic property of KTP laser in the management of these patients [31]. In 2007, Koufman et al. reported 59 patients with RRP who underwent 212 office-based laser procedures using the PDL. Only 15% of their study group needed surgical intervention under general anesthesia, and none of the patients had complications during office procedures [40]. Mouadeb and Belafsky reviewed their experience with office-based PDL in the treatment of 47 patients, 60% of whom had RRP. The authors reported successful outcome in 89% of the cases [41]. In another study, Halum and Moberly reported complete disease regression in two of five patients with RRP who were treated with CO2 laser and PDL. The patients were assessed 1 month following surgery [42]. Kuet and Pitman investigated the surgical outcome of 21 patients with RRP who underwent 81 office-based laser procedures using PDL ($n = 2$) and KTP laser ($n = 19$) [43]. The authors reported improvement in the VHI-10 score (24.5 preoperatively vs. 15.9 postoperatively), GRBAS score (8.9 preoperatively vs. 4.9 postoperatively), and Derkay score (6.1

preoperatively vs. 3.0 postoperatively) [44]. In a retrospective review of 33 patients, 8 of whom had RRP, Centric et al. reported the need for hybrid treatment, such as office-based and surgical intervention in the operating room, in order to achieve complete disease control [45]. Similarly, in a review of 255 patients who underwent office-based angiolytic laser surgery, 13% of whom had RRP, Del Signore et al. reported complete disease regression in 50% of the cases [46].

In summary, office-based laser therapy is an effective and safe treatment of laryngeal RRP that spares the patient the need for general anesthesia and suspension direct laryngoscopy. In selected cases, hybrid treatment may be necessary to achieve disease control. Both diode lasers and photoangiolytic lasers are used, and the success of surgery is gauged by disease regression and improvement in voice quality. Maintaining a balance between breathing and phonation is advocated.

10.2.2 Office-Based Laser Therapy in Patients with Benign Vocal Fold Lesions

Benign lesions of the vocal folds consist primarily of polyps, nodules, cysts, pseudocysts, Reinke's edema, fibrous masses, and nonspecific lesions. The taxonomy of these lesions is still evolving with more rigorous diagnostic criteria being used to differentiate one entity from the other [47]. Phonotrauma, laryngopharyngeal reflux, and smoking are the primary risk factors eliciting a cascade of inflammatory reactions leading to mucosal and submucosal injury [48–50]. Inflammatory markers [51–52] and dysregulation in apoptosis are linked significantly to the formation of many of these lesions [53]. Affected patients usually are advised to undergo voice therapy for the purpose of enhancing vocal hygiene while also reducing laryngeal hyperfunction and mechanical stress and trauma during phonation. In patients with vocal fold scar or fibrous masses, treatment also aims to improve the pliability of the vocal fold cover. Failure to respond to conservative therapy, particularly in cases of symptomatic vocal fold polyps and cysts that have not improved with voice therapy, is an indication for microsurgical resection.

With the trend in laryngology toward office-based surgery, several treatment options are offered including laser therapy. The advances in laser technology and mode of delivery have allowed office-based laser therapy to gain significant popularity as a safe and successful alternative to laser surgery under general anesthesia. In 2006, Zeitels et al. reported five cases of benign vocal fold pathology (three cases of vocal fold edema and two cases of granuloma) who were treated successfully using thulium laser in an office setting. The authors highlighted the ablating, hemostatic, and cutting properties of the thulium laser when used in a noncontact and contact mode (Videos 10.2 and 10.3). The authors also stressed the adverse thermal effect of thulium laser on neighboring tissues and the need for selective application of this laser [34]. In 2007, in their review of office-based laser therapy, Koufman et al. reported complete regression with voice improvement in 10 of 12 patients with

Reinke's edema whose follow-up was available [40]. Similarly, Mouadeb and Belafsky reported the successful use of office-based PDL laser therapy in 104 of 117 procedures. Their study group included 16 cases of Reinke's edema, 8 cases of polyps, and 8 cases of granuloma. Only 20% of patients with Reinke's edema and 28.6% of patients with polyp required surgery in the operating room. The authors advocated the use of PDL as a "promising tool" in the management of patients with laryngeal diseases [41]. In 2013, in their review of patients treated with office-based PDL, Centric et al. reported complete regression in six of ten patients with vocal fold vascular lesions [45]. In 2015, Del Signore et al. investigated the long-term outcomes of photoangiolytic laser therapy in 255 patients, 57% of whom had polyps and/or varices, and reported the need for subsequent intervention in only 11% of the cases [46]. Similarly, in 2020, Hamdan et al. investigated the subjective and objective voice outcome of 20 patients with vocal fold polyps who were treated with thulium laser in the office and reported complete regression of the lesion in 16 and partial regression in 4. The mean score of VHI-10 decreased from 15.6 preoperatively to 4.6 postoperatively. Moreover, there was an improvement in glottic closure and mucosal wave in the majority of the patients [54]. The same authors also reported three cases of vocal fold mucus retention cysts that were treated successfully in the office using thulium laser. Follow-up at 1 year showed complete regression of the lesion in all three cases with no recurrence. The authors (ALH) advocated office-based laser therapy in patients with vocal fold cysts who are at high risk for general anesthesia and/or not willing to undergo microlaryngeal surgery [55]. Office-based laser treatment also has emerged as an option in the management of patients with vocal fold scar. Mortensen et al. reported subjective improvement in voice in 10 of 11 patients with vocal fold scar who were treated using PDL at 3-month intervals. In parallel with the significant decrease in VHI-10 score (48.44 preoperatively vs. 35.55 postoperatively), there was a decrease in perturbation parameters (jitter and shimmer) and a significant increase in mean phonatory flow [56]. Based on animal studies, the therapeutic effect of photoangiolytic lasers is mediated via upregulation of extracellular matrix components and modulation of metalloproteinase gene expression and other inflammatory genes. Another suggested mechanism is cleavage of the sub-basement membrane [57, 58].

Office-based laser treatment also has been shown to be useful in pitch modulation. Abitbol was the first to describe the use of laser in the operating room to raise the vocal pitch in selected cases. By creating an incision lateral to the vocal ligament and removing part of the thyroarytenoid muscle, the author reported an increase in vocal pitch [2]. The increase was ascribed to the inverse relationship between mass and fundamental frequency. The same principle has been applied in patients with Reinke's edema. In 2015, Koszewski et al. reported the voice changes of 19 patients with Reinke's edema who were treated with photoangiolytic lasers and showed an increase in the highest and lowest fundamental frequency (290 Hz vs. 482 Hz and 110 Hz vs. 119 Hz, respectively), a decrease in percent jitter (4.05 vs. 1.66), and an increase in maximum phonation time (8.77 seconds vs. 9.29 seconds) postoperatively. The improvement in acoustic and aerodynamic measures was accompanied by a significant decrease in VHI score and an increase in Dysphonia

Severity Index. The energy delivery during the procedure was tailored individually, and blanching of the lesion was the cut point in ending the treatment session [59]. Similarly, Hamdan et al. reported their experience with 12 patients with Reinke's edema treated with thulium laser in an office setting. There was an increase in the mean habitual pitch from 125. 11 Hz to 155.86 Hz (133.14 Hz to 170.21 Hz in females ($n - 8$) and 103.66 Hz to 117.57 Hz in males ($n = 3$)), with significant decrease in the perturbation parameters. In parallel with the improvement in the acoustic parameters, there was significant improvement in the mean VHI-10 score (15.0 preoperatively vs. 3.07, postoperatively), associated with regression (complete or partial) of the lesions in 11 of 12 patients [60].

In summary, most benign lesions of the vocal folds can be treated by laser in an office setting. Diode and photoangiolytic lasers can be used depending on the type of lesion. When hemostasis is a concern, as in patients with hemorrhagic lesions, photoangiolytic lasers usually are advocated. The success of the procedure is gaged by disease regression and improvement in voice quality.

10.2.3 Office-Based Laser Therapy in Patients with Dysplasia/Carcinoma In Situ

Laryngeal dysplasia is a challenging condition given its unpredictable rate of malignant transformation and high risk of recurrence. It is stratified into four categories: mild, moderate, severe, and carcinoma in situ, based on the degree of histologic changes. Many authors consider and treat severe dysplasia as carcinoma in view of the fine line of demarcation and subjective readings of the histologic features of these lesions. The morphologic appearance of the lesion varies and is not always predictive of its true nature or future behavior. Smoking, laryngopharyngeal reflux, and high alcohol consumption are the main risk factors for leukoplakia which may be dysplasia or carcinoma [61–63]. The treatment of laryngeal dysplasia is daunting and several treatment methods have been suggested. Traditionally, the lesion is excised in the operating room using cold steel instruments and/or lasers. With the introduction of the working channel laryngoscopes and laser glass fibers, office-based laser therapy has become another standard therapeutic modality (Video 10.4). In a review of 52 cases of laryngeal dysplasia treated with PDL, Zeitels et al. reported 50% disease involution in 88% of the cases with improvement in voice quality. The disease regression was ascribed to selective photo-angiolysis and denaturing of the basement membrane binding proteins [30]. In 2006, the same authors reported their experience with office-based KTP laser therapy in 48 patients (72 cases), 36 of whom had recurrent dysplasia. Of the 29 patients who had follow-up for 4–8 weeks after surgery, 18 had 75% disease regression, 7 had 50–75% disease regression, and 4 had less than 50% disease regression [31]. In another study using thulium laser, Zeitels et al. also described six cases of microinvasive laryngeal carcinoma that were treated successfully in an office setting. The laser was delivered using a glass fiber 0.365 mm in diameter at a power setting of 4–7 watts [34]. In

2007, Koufman et al. reported the surgical outcome of 79 patients treated with PDL, 25 of whom had glottal leukoplakia/dysplasia. With a mean follow-up of 16 months, 20 patients had been treated successfully, and only 5 required surgical treatment in the operating room [40]. In 2009, Halum and Moberly, in their study on patient tolerance of the flexible CO2 laser, reported complete regression in one patient with leukoplakia and residual disease in another [42].

In summary, office-based laser therapy may be used for treatment of patients with vocal fold dysplasia and/or carcinoma in situ. The application of photoangiolytic lasers results in selective angiolysis of the feeding vessels and denaturing of the basement membrane proteins leading to disease regression. The predictive value of the morphology of the lesion and its grade in regard to treatment and long-term control needs further investigation.

10.2.4 Rare Application of Office-Based Laser Therapy

One rare application of office-based laser therapy is vocal fold lateralization in patients with bilateral vocal fold paralysis. Hamdan et al. described a 54-year-old woman with bilateral vocal fold paralysis who underwent office-based thulium laser partial arytenoidectomy using a flexible endoscope with a working channel that was introduced through the oral cavity. The authors used a power range 3.5 to 4.5 W, duration 70 to 300 milliseconds, repetition 2 to 4 Hz, and aiming beam at 65%. The procedure was tolerated well and the patient was decannulated 3 weeks following surgery. There was significant widening of the glottal chink commensurate with improvement in her dyspnea. Notably, the patient had worsening of her voice and an increase in her VHI-10 score, as expected following arytenoidectomy [64].

10.2.5 Office-Based Application of Blue Laser in Laryngeal Surgery

As discussed early in the introduction, the blue laser is a promising tool that is replacing the photoangiolytic PDL and KTP lasers commonly used by otolaryngologists. The blue laser is distinguished by its “hybrid” property which allows both cutting when used in the contact or near-contact mode and hemostasis when used at a distance or near contact. The amount of energy delivered varies with the fiber tip to tissue distance and with handling of the fiber during surgery, particularly the speed of movement. Other factors that affect fluence are the energy setup, duration of pulse, and time of surgery. The literature is scarce on the application of blue laser in laryngology. In a recent report, Hess et al. describes the successful use of the blue laser in patients with various laryngeal pathologies including cysts, RRP, and dilated vessels. The authors stressed the need to tailor the surgery and power setting according to the type of lesion [65]. Hamdan et al. has also described 11 cases of various vocal fold pathologies treated with blue laser in an office setting and reported partial and/or complete regression of the lesion in all cases (in press). Another rare office-based application of blue laser is subglottic stenosis. Sataloff et al. described a 57-year-old male with a subglottic polyp who was treated successfully with blue laser in an office setting. The patient's symptoms of dyspnea and stridor improved immediately following complete ablation of the polypoidal mass and restoration of the airway patency (Fig. 10.1a–c). More research on voice outcomes of blue laser in office-based laryngeal surgery is needed.

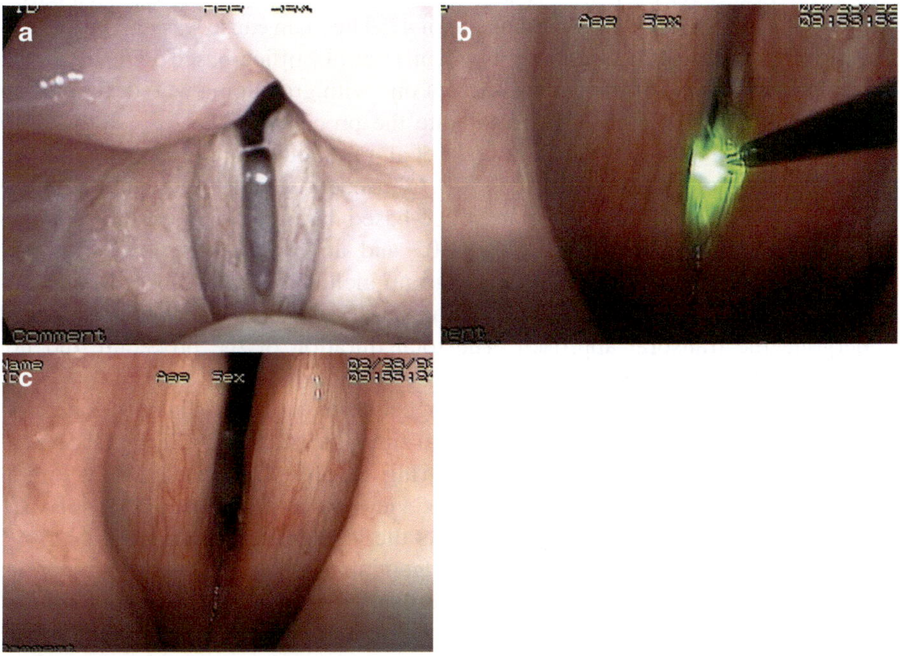

Fig. 10.1 This 57-year-old male had been intubated 1 ½ years prior to this procedure for airway compromise from Stage III lymphoma with a neck mass compressing his airway. He was extubated after 12 days and had immediate dysphonia and airway compromise. He had been followed by another physician. He presented to the author (RTS) with acutely worsening dyspnea and with stridor. (**a**) shows a polyp immediately below his vocal folds obstructing much of his airway. His vocal folds were minimally mobile due to mechanical impairment of his cricoarytenoid joints. The polyp was vaporized in the office with a blue laser (**b**). An excellent airway was established (**c**), relieving his symptoms and avoiding the need for tracheotomy

10.3 Limitations and Complications of Office-Based Laryngeal Laser Surgery

10.3.1 Limitations of Office-Based Laryngeal Laser Surgery

Office-based laser surgery has its limitations, the most important of which is patient tolerance. A low threshold for pain and/or a hyperactive gag reflex may lead to termination of the procedure. In 2004, in a review of office-based PDL treatment of 30 cases of laryngeal RRP and 52 cases of dysplasia, Zeitels et al. reported abandonment of the procedure in 5 cases. Three of the five cases were terminated because of patient discomfort and two because of insufficient visualization and/or exposure [30]. In 2007, in their review of 443 cases of office-based laryngeal laser surgery, Koufman et al. described one case of vasovagal attack that required cessation of the procedure [40]. Two years later, Mouadeb and Belafsky reported termination of 13 office-based laser therapy out of 47. The main cause was uncomfortable level of anesthesia [41]. In a study by Centric et al., office-based PDL treatment was tolerated by 97% of the patients except one with granuloma who developed an anxiety attack and was not able to tolerate the procedure [45]. In a study of 19 patients with Reinke's edema, Koszweski et al. reported stopping the procedure in 4 because of poor patient tolerance [59]. In a recent study by Hamdan et al. on patient tolerance and experience in office-based laryngeal surgery, the authors reported a tolerance score of 1.68 ± 1.05 and an overall experience score of 1.85 ± 1.13 on a scale of 1–5. The study group included 63 office-based laser procedures that were performed using the transnasal approach except for 3 who had undergone the transoral approach. The total duration of the procedure did not exceed 18.24 minutes [66].

Another limitation of office-based laryngeal laser surgery is the need for excellent dexterity. The surgeon often struggles to aim laser beam at a moving target and/or to gauge the fiber-to-tissue distance during surgery. The "line-of-sight limitation," described by Woo as the compromised view given the limited vectors of visualization, is also another challenge [67]. As the laser energy is absorbed best in a plane perpendicular to the fiber, limited tangential angles of the laser beam restrict delivery of the laser in a three dimensional plane. Moreover, the inability to retract tissue hinders visualization and limits the treatment of lesions that extend to the lower lip of the vocal folds. This limitation is further compounded by the lack of anatomic uniformity of the vocal fold that inevitably leads to uneven distribution of the laser beam energy. Any lesion that lies off the perpendicular axis of delivery is likely to receive suboptimal energy. When retraction is necessary, it can be accomplished with an indirect laryngeal suction placed transorally by an assistant.

Another technical challenge is the lack of a clear end-point as to when the surgeon should stop the surgery. Given that photoangiolytic lasers target the vessels, surgeons often rely on blanching of the lesion or blackening of a vessel, rather than complete removal in deciding when to end surgery [2, 45, 67]. Last but not least, office-based laryngeal laser surgery usually is performed without taking a specimen for histopathologic examination. This decision stems from the limited anesthesia time and/or the fear of bleeding which may decrease the efficacy of photoangiolytic lasers. Particularly, in cases in which thulium or CO2 lasers are used, part of the tissue is vaporized and the margins are usually damaged by charring and carbonization. In many cases, the lesion is vaporized completely leaving no specimen for histologic examination.

10.3.2 Complications of Office-Based Laryngeal Laser Surgery

Laser-related accidents such as cutaneous or mucosal burns and/or injury to the eyes have not been reported in office-based laryngeal surgery. This can be attributed to strict adherence to laser safety protocols and to the fact that the laser fiber is protected by the working channel of the endoscope which usually precludes inadvertent injury to the skin or to mucosal lining of the pharynx and larynx during surgery [2]. However, phonatory and airway complications have been reported and were ascribed to vocal fold hemorrhage and/or purpura, vocal fold scar, and persistent edema [40, 43, 58]. Koufman et al. reported two patients with Reinke's edema who developed vocal fold hemorrhage following laser treatment and one patient with subglottic granuloma who had the tip of the glass fiber break off during treatment [40]. Similarly, Mouadeb and Belafsky described a patient with Reinke's edema who developed stridor after office-based laser therapy, which necessitated admission and observation. The study included 47 patients who had undergone117 procedures [41]. In another study of 19 patients with Reinke's edema who underwent office-based laser therapy, Koszweski et al. reported worsening of the MPT in 3 patients and an increase in airway resistance in 1 patient. Six patients had to undergo several procedures [59]. In the study by Del Signore et al., unwanted prolonged edema and hyperemia occurred in 2.5% of the cases [46].

In summary, unsedated office-based laser therapy is a viable treatment option in patients with vocal fold pathology. Despite the advances in technology, there are still many limitations to this procedure, the most important of which is patient tolerance and restricted angle of vision while aiming with the laser beam. Complications are infrequent. These include primarily vocal fold hemorrhage, scar, and persistent edema which may lead to airway obstruction. Residual disease after a single intervention often requires multiple treatment sessions, and patients should be advised of this common scenario during the surgical consent discussion.

References

1. Strong MS, Jako GI. Laser surgery in the larynx. Early clinical experience with continuous CO2 laser. Ann Otol Rhinol Laryngol. 1972;81:791–8.
2. Abitbol J, Sataloff RT. Laryngeal laser surgery. In: Sataloff RT, editor. Professional voice: the science and art of clinical care. 4th ed. San Diego: Plural Publishing; 2017. p. 1501–21.
3. Remacle M, Hassan F, Cohen D, Lawson G, Delos M. New computer-guided scanner for improving CO 2 laser-assisted microincision. Eur Arch Otorhinolaryngol. 2005;262(2):113–9.

4. Motta G, Esposito E, Testa D, Iovine R, Motta S. Longitudinal voice outcomes following advanced CO2 laser cordectomy for glottic cancer. J Voice. 2015;29(6):772–5.
5. Sesterhenn AM, Dünne AA, Werner JA. Complications after CO2 laser surgery of laryngeal cancer in the elderly. Acta Otolaryngol. 2006;126(5):530–5.
6. Schrijvers ML, Van Riel EL, Langendijk JA, et al. Higher laryngeal preservation rate after CO2 laser surgery compared with radiotherapy in T1a glottic laryngeal carcinoma. Head Neck. 2009;31(6):759–64.
7. Benninger MS. Microdissection or microspot CO2 laser for limited vocal fold benign lesions: a prospective randomized trial. Laryngoscope. 2000;110(2 Pt 2 Suppl 92):1–17.
8. Benninger MS. Laser surgery for nodules and other benign laryngeal lesions. Curr Opin Otolaryngol Head Neck Surg. 2009;17(6):440–4.
9. Ekbom DC, Bayan SL, Goates AJ, Kasperbauer JL. Endoscopic Wedge excisions with CO2 laser for subglottic stenosis. Laryngoscope. 2020; https://doi.org/10.1002/lary.29013.
10. Incandela F, Missale F, Mora F, et al. Transoral management of adult benign laryngeal stenosis. Eur Arch Otorhinolaryngol. 2021;278(1):149–58.
11. Arias ÀM, Remacle M, Lawson G. Treatment of vocal fold scar by carbon dioxide laser and collagen injection: retrospective study on 12 patients. Eur Arch Otorhinolaryngol. 2010;267(9):1409–14.
12. Sataloff RT, Spiegel JR, Hawkshaw M, Jones A. Laser surgery of the larynx: the case for caution. Ear Nose Throat J. 1992;71(11):593–5.
13. Dedo HH, Yu KC. CO2 laser treatment in 244 patients with respiratory papillomas. Laryngoscope. 2001;111(9):1639–44.
14. Shapshay SM, Rebeiz EE, Bohigian RK, Hybels RL. Benign lesions of the larynx: should the laser be used? Laryngoscope. 1990;100(9):953–7.
15. Geyer M, Ledda GP, Tan N, Brennan PA, Puxeddu R. Carbon dioxide laser-assisted phonosurgery for benign glottic lesions. Eur Arch Otorhinolaryngol. 2010;267(1):87–93.
16. McMillan K, Shapshay SM, McGilligan JA, Wang Z, Rebeiz EE. A 585-nanometer pulsed dye laser treatment of laryngeal papillomas: preliminary report. Laryngoscope. 1998;108(7):968–72.
17. Valdez TA, McMillan K, Shapshay SM. A new laser treatment for vocal cord papilloma—585-nm pulsed dye. Otolaryngol Head Neck Surg. 2001;124(4):421–5.
18. Franco RA Jr, Farinelli WA, Zeitels SM, Anderson RR. 585-nm pulsed dye laser treatment of glottal papillomatosis. Ann Otol Rhinol Laryngol. 2002;111(6):486–92.
19. Burns JA, Zeitels SM, Akst LM, Broadhurst MS, Hillman RE, Anderson R. 532 nm pulsed potassium-titanyl-phosphate laser treatment of laryngeal papillomatosis under general anesthesia. Laryngoscope. 2007;117(8):1500–4.
20. Moore JE, Sataloff RT. Vocal fold scar. In: Sataloff RT, editor. Professional voice: the science and art of clinical care. 4th ed. San Diego: Plural Publishing; 2017. p. 1611–28.
21. Larner SP, Fornelli RA, Griffith SD. Consistent technique limits suspension laryngoscopy complications. Int Arch Otorhinolaryngol. 2019;23(3):305–10.
22. Feng AL, Song PC. Laryngeal force sensor: quantifying extralaryngeal complications after suspension microlaryngoscopy. Otolaryngol Head Neck Surg. 2018;159(2):328–34.
23. Lindemann TL, Kamrava B, Sarcu D, Soliman AM. Tongue symptoms, suspension force and duration during operative laryngoscopy. Am J Otolaryngol. 2020;41(3):102402.
24. Lafferty D, Tami A, Valentino WL, Sataloff RT. Tongue edema secondary to suspension laryngoscopy. J Voice. 2019; https://doi.org/10.1016/j.j.voice.2019.09.014.
25. Sataloff RT. Voice surgery. In: Sataloff RT, editor. Professional voice: the science and art of clinical care. 4th ed. San Diego: Plural Publishing; 2017. p. 1371–9.
26. Woo P. Office-based laryngeal procedures. Otolaryngol Clin N Am. 2006;39(1):111–33.
27. Rees CJ, Halum SL, Wijewickrama RC, Koufman JA, Postma GN. Patient tolerance of in-office pulsed dye laser treatments to the upper aerodigestive tract. Otolaryngol Head Neck Surg. 2006;134(6):1023–7.

28. Kuo CY, Halum SL. Office-based laser surgery of the larynx: cost-effective treatment at the office's expense. Otolaryngol Head Neck Surg. 2012;146(5):769–73.
29. Rees CJ, Postma GN, Koufman JA. Cost savings of unsedated office-based laser surgery for laryngeal papillomas. Ann Otol Rhinol Laryngol. 2007;116(1):45–8.
30. Zeitels SM, Franco RA Jr, Dailey AH, Burns JA, Hillman RE, Anderson RR. Office-based treatment of glottal dysplasia and papillomatosis with the 585-nm pulsed dye laser and local anesthesia. Ann Otol Rhinol Laryngol. 2004;113(4):265–76.
31. Zeitels SM, Akst LM, Burns JA, Hillman RE, Broadhurst MS, Anderson RR. Office-based 532-nm pulsed KTP laser treatment of glottal papillomatosis and dysplasia. Ann Otol Rhinol Laryngol. 2006;115(9):679–85.
32. Wang Z, Devaiah AK, Feng L, et al. Fiber-guided CO2 laser surgery in an animal model. Photomed Laser Surg. 2006;24(5):646–50.
33. Jacobson AS, Woo P, Shapshay SM. Emerging technology: flexible CO2 laser WaveGuide. Otolaryngol Head Neck Surg. 2006;135(3):469–70.
34. Zeitels SM, Burns JA, Akst LM, Hillman RE, Broadhurst MS, Anderson RR. Office-based and microlaryngeal applications of a fiber-based thulium laser. Ann Otol Rhinol Laryngol. 2006;115(12):891–6.
35. Shykhon M, Kuo M, Pearman K. Recurrent respiratory papillomatosis. Clin Otolaryngol Allied Sci. 2002;27(4):237–43.
36. Derkay CS. Task force on recurrent respiratory papillomas: a preliminary report. Arch Otolaryngol Head Neck Surg. 1995;121(12):1386–91.
37. Derkay CS, Bluher AE. Update on recurrent respiratory papillomatosis. Otolaryngol Clin N Am. 2019;52(4):669–79.
38. Fortes HR, Von Ranke FM, Escuissato DL, et al. Recurrent respiratory papillomatosis: a state-of-the-art review. Respir Med. 2017;126:116–21.
39. Armstrong LR, Derkay CS, Reeves WC. Initial results from the national registry for juvenile-onset recurrent respiratory papillomatosis. Arch Otolaryngol Head Neck Surg. 1999;125(7):743–8.
40. Koufman JA, Rees CJ, Frazier WD, et al. Office-based laryngeal laser surgery: a review of 443 cases using three wavelengths. Otolaryngol Head Neck Surg. 2007;137(1):146–51.
41. Mouadeb DA, Belafsky PC. In-office laryngeal surgery with the 585nm pulsed dye laser (PDL). Otolaryngol Head Neck Surg. 2007;137(3):477–81.
42. Halum SL, Moberly AC. Patient tolerance of the flexible CO2 laser for office-based laryngeal surgery. J Voice. 2010;24(6):750–4.
43. Kuet ML, Pitman MJ. Photoangiolytic laser treatment of recurrent respiratory papillomatosis: a scaled assessment. J Voice. 2013;27(1):124–8.
44. Derkay CS, Hester RP, Burke B, Carron J, Lawson L. Analysis of a staging assessment system for prediction of surgical interval in recurrent respiratory papillomatosis. Int J Pediatr Otorhinolaryngol. 2004;68(12):1493–8.
45. Centric A, Hu A, Heman-Ackah YD, Divi V, Sataloff RT. Office-based pulsed-dye laser surgery for laryngeal lesions: a retrospective review. J Voice. 2014;28(2):262.e9–262.e12.
46. Del Signore AG, Shah RN, Gupta N, Altman KW, Woo P. Complications and failures of office-based endoscopic angiolytic laser surgery treatment. J Voice. 2016;30(6):744–50.
47. Naunheim MR, Carroll TL. Benign vocal fold lesions: update on nomenclature, cause, diagnosis, and treatment. Curr Opin Otolaryngol Head Neck Surg. 2017;25(6):453–8.
48. Won SJ, Kim RB, Kim JP, Park JJ, Kwon MS, Woo SH. The prevalence and factors associated with vocal nodules in general population: cross-sectional epidemiological study. Medicine. 2016;95(39):e4971.
49. Czerwonka L, Jiang JJ, Tao C. Vocal nodules and edema may be due to vibration-induced rises in capillary pressure. Laryngoscope. 2008;118(4):748–52.
50. Tao C, Jiang JJ. Mechanical stress during phonation in a self-oscillating finite-element vocal fold model. J Biomech. 2007;40(10):2191–8.

51. Gu J, Huang Y. β-Defensin-2 is overexpressed in human vocal cord polyps. Eur Arch Otorhinolaryngol. 2017;274(2):901–7.
52. Zhang HP, Zhang R. Correlations between serum apolipoprotein AI and formation of vocal cord polyp. J Voice. 2017;31(3):380.e1–6.
53. Novaleski CK, Carter BD, Sivasankar MP, Ridner SH, Dietrich MS, Rousseau B. Apoptosis and vocal fold disease: clinically relevant implications of epithelial cell death. J Speech Lang Hear Res. 2017;60(5):1264–72.
54. Hamdan AL, Khalifee E, Ghanem A. Application of thulium laser as office-based procedure in patients with vocal fold polyps. J Voice. 2020;34(1):140–4.
55. Hamdan AL, Rizk SA. Unsedated office-based thulium laser therapy in patients with vocal fold cysts. Ear Nose Throat J. 2021;100(1):NP39.
56. Mortensen MM, Woo P, Ivey C, Thompson C, Carroll L, Altman K. The use of the pulse dye laser in the treatment of vocal fold scar: a preliminary study. Laryngoscope. 2008;118(10):1884–8.
57. Prufer N, Woo P, Altman K. Pulse dye and other laser treatments for vocal scar. Curr Opin Otolaryngol Head Neck Surg. 2010;18(6):492–7.
58. Sheu M, Sridharan S, Paul B, et al. The utility of the potassium titanyl phosphate laser in modulating vocal fold scar in a rat model. Laryngoscope. 2013 Sep;123(9):2189–94.
59. Koszewski IJ, Hoffman MR, Young WG, Lai YT, Dailey SH. Office-based photoangiolytic laser treatment of Reinke's edema: safety and voice outcomes. Otolaryngol Head Neck Surg. 2015;152(6):1075–81.
60. Hamdan AL, Ghanem A, Abi Akl PR, El Hage A. Unsedated office-based thulium laser therapy in patients with reinke's edema. J Voice. 2020;S0892-1997(20):30109–0.
61. Isenberg JS, Crozier DL, Dailey SH. Institutional and comprehensive review of laryngeal leukoplakia. Ann Otol Rhinol Laryngol. 2008;117(1):74–9.
62. Lee DH, Yoon TM, Lee JK, Lim SC. Predictive factors of recurrence and malignant transformation in vocal cord leukoplakia. Eur Arch Otorhinolaryngol. 2015;272(7):1719–24.
63. Van Hulst AM, Kroon W, van der Linden ES, et al. Grade of dysplasia and malignant transformation in adults with premalignant laryngeal lesions. Head Neck. 2016;38(1):E2284–90.
64. Hamdan AL, Khalifee E, Jaffal H, Abi Akl PR. Laser partial arytenoidectomy as an office procedure. Ear Nose Throat J. 2019;98(4):217–9.
65. Hess M, Fleischer S, Ernstberger M. New 445 nm blue laser for laryngeal surgery combines photoangiolytic and cutting properties. Eur Arch Otorhinolaryngol. 2018;275(6):1557–67.
66. Hamdan AL, Jabbour C, Khalifee E, Ghanem A, El Hage A. Tolerance of patients using different approaches in laryngeal office-based procedures. J Voice. 2021;S0892-1997(20):30456–2.
67. Woo P. Office-based laryngeal procedures. Rev Otolaryngol Clin North Am. 2006;39(1):111–33.

Chapter 11
Office-Based Laryngeal Injections of Steroids and Other Pharmaceutical Agents

11.1 Office-Based Laryngeal Steroid Injections

Glucocorticoids are molecules that are present naturally in our body. Their endogenous secretion is regulated by the hypothalamic-pituitary-adrenal axis. Glucocorticoids play a regulatory role in physiologic and pathophysiologic conditions such as metabolic disorders and immune diseases. Their effect is modulated via genomic and nongenomic pathways. By acting on membrane-associated receptors in various cells such as macrophages, monocytes, and lymphocytes, glucocorticoids can induce inhibition of inflammatory mediators. Similarly, their transcriptive and transactive genomic effects modulate the inflammatory response to various stimuli leading to a decrease in vasodilation and edema [1, 2].

Glucocorticoids are used commonly in laryngology in the treatment of acute and chronic inflammatory disorders. In a meta-analysis on the effect of steroid administration (intramuscularly, orally, and subcutaneously) in laryngotracheitis, Kairys et al. reported significant benefit within 12–24 h [3]. The authors noted that the response was dose-dependent [3]. Similarly, in a systematic review of 19 studies on the diagnosis and management of croup, Johnson stressed the effectiveness of oral, systemic, and nebulized (budesonide) corticosteroids as adjuncts to racemic epinephrine and humidification in the treatment of acute respiratory symptoms [4]. Ossoff et al., in their case series of 15 patients with acute epiglottitis, advocated the use of steroids, particularly when combined with antibiotics and humidified oxygen [5]. Steroids also are used in the management of chronic inflammatory and autoimmune diseases that affect the larynx [6–9]. Bower et al. highlighted the role of systemic steroids in the treatment of life-threatening laryngeal manifestations of sarcoidosis [6]. Similarly, Korbet et al. described a case of inactive systemic lupus erythematosus (SLE) diagnosed with arytenoiditis who was treated successfully

Supplementary Information The online version contains supplementary material available at [https://doi.org/10.1007/978-3-030-91936-8_11].

A.-l. Hamdan et al., *Office-Based Laryngeal Surgery*,
https://doi.org/10.1007/978-3-030-91936-8_11

with steroids. The symptoms of dyspnea and airway obstruction improved markedly following therapy [7]. Solans-Laqué et al. reported six cases of Wegner's granulomatosis (now called granulomatosis with polyangiitis) and subglottic stenosis, four of whom were controlled with systemic steroids and cyclophosphamide, and one was treated successfully with intralesional steroid injection and tracheal dilation [9]. The authors stressed the disparity between the clinical stage of the disease and laryngeal involvement.

Despite the efficacy of steroids in the treatment of laryngeal inflammatory disorders, their systemic side effects remain a major concern. These include aggravation of hypertension, diabetes, gastroesophageal reflux disease, glaucoma, and osteoporosis among other metabolic disorders [2, 10]. To circumvent many of these above effects, intralesional steroid injection (ILSI) has been advocated as an alternative to systemic therapy. Its main advantage is the high regional drug concentration associated minimal adverse systemic effects. Traditionally, ILSI was performed in the operating room following laryngeal microsurgery and as adjuvant therapy in patients with chronic inflammatory diseases [11–15]. With the advances in technology and successful application of topical anesthesia to the upper airway, laryngeal steroid injections are now performed safely in an office setting. Common indications include vocal fold benign lesions, vocal fold scar, and subglottic stenosis. A review of office-based steroid injections in the management of these conditions is presented below. The surgical outcomes and complications of ILSI also are reviewed. This information is invaluable to otolaryngologists who need to counsel patients regarding success rate and failure of office-based steroid injections.

11.2 Office-Based Steroid Injections in Laryngotracheal Stenosis

Laryngotracheal stenosis is characterized by narrowing of the upper airway leading to impairment in breathing. The most common causes are prolonged intubation, laryngopharyngeal reflux, autoimmune diseases, and neoplasms. The clinical presentation of laryngotracheal stenosis varies with the extent of the disease. Patients with mild obstruction may be asymptomatic or present with decrease in exercise tolerance, whereas patients with severe obstruction often complain of shortness of breath and stridor [16–18]. Laryngotracheal stenosis is treated endoscopically and/or using open surgical techniques. The management strategy depends on the etiology of the stenosis, its severity, and the presence of associated comorbidities. Endoscopic treatment consists primarily of dilatation, radial incisions using cold steel instruments or laser, and endoscopic removal of fibrotic scar using mucosal flaps. Open surgery may involve segmental tracheal resection, cricotracheal resection, and/or laryngotracheoplasty [18, 19].

Steroid injection has been recommended as an adjunct treatment for many cases. The effect is mediated via a decrease in fibroblast activity and hence collagen deposition [20, 21]. Several studies have shown that ILSI is beneficial in reducing recurrence of scar formation and in prolonging surgery-free intervals [22–25]. In a review of 45 patients with subglottic stenosis treated with serial dilatation and submucosal corticosteroid injections, Wierzbicka et al. reported improvement in 56–75% of the cases. The mean follow-up was 76 months [22]. Similarly, Wolter et al. reported successful treatment with corticosteroid injection and dilatation of 12 patients with subglottic stenosis. All patients except one were decannulated with no long-term phonatory sequelae [23]. In another study of 21 patients with Wegner's granulomatosis and subglottic stenosis, Hoffman et al. advocated steroid injection prior to microsurgery. Each patient underwent 2.4–4.1 ILSIs depending on the extent of the disease [24]. Similarly, Feinstein et al. reported steroid injection as an adjunct procedure in the management of patients with subglottic stenosis in 42.5% of cases [25].

Given the success of steroid injections as adjunct therapy to surgery in the operating room, surgeons are treating patients in the office, as well. Several studies showed that steroid injections in patients with laryngeal and proximal tracheal stenosis can be performed safely in an office setting while the patient is awake. In 2017, Hoffman et al. reported a series of 19 patients with idiopathic subglottic stenosis who underwent serial office-based steroid injections and reported a decrease in stenosis to 20–25% as the number of injections increased. Office-based steroid injections obviated the need for intervention in the operating room in 14 of 17 patients who had more than 3 injections [26]. In 2018, Bertelsen et al. studied the efficacy of in-office repeated ILSI in 24 patients with subglottic and proximal tracheal stenosis and reported extension of surgery-free intervals in those who underwent at least 2 procedures (10.1 months preinjection vs. 22.6 months postinjection) [27]. Similarly, in 2018, Franco et al. reviewed 13 patients with idiopathic subglottic stenosis who underwent repeated ILSI (4–6 rounds) and reported improvement in per cent peak expiratory flow by 23.1%. The clinical improvement in breathing was comparable to those treated in the operating room [28]. In 2019, in a study of 13 patients with subglottic stenosis who underwent endoscopic dilatation and adjuvant office-based steroid injection, Pan et al. reported prolongation of surgery-free interval from 288 to 545 days. The number of injections per patient on average was 4.2 [29]. In 2020, Hoffman et al. reported 16 patients with idiopathic subglottic stenosis (20–50% stenosis) who underwent office-based steroid injections using the transnasal route. The results showed improvement in the dyspnea index, a validated ten-item questionnaire on upper airway dyspnea [30]. There was improvement in the stenotic segment in 12 of the 16 patients. One patient had worsening of his breathing, and three had no change. In one case, there was worsening of the VHI score, highlighting the rare but possible, impact of steroid injection on airflow dynamics and possibly phonation [31].

In summary, steroid injections can be used as adjunct therapy in patients with laryngotracheal stenosis. The procedure can be performed safely in the office while the patient is awake. Repeated injections can lead to an increase in severe symptom free intervals and improvement in the severity of stenosis. Dyspnea and airway symptoms may worsen immediately following injection but improve in the long term. Dysphonia may be a transient side effect to ILSI and rarely may be permanent.

11.3 Office-Based Vocal Fold Steroid Injection

11.3.1 Office-Based Steroid Injection in Vocal Fold Scar

Vocal fold scar occurs as a result of trauma or disease affecting the vocal folds. Following a three-phase response that starts with migration of neutrophils and inflammatory mediators, there is remodeling of the lamina propria layered structure associated with a change in the cellular and extracellular matrix (ECM) landscape. In a histologic study of vocal fold scar in rabbit larynges, Thibeault et al. showed a decrease in collagen formation, an increase in procollagen, and a decrease in elastin 6 days following injury. These histologic changes were associated with an increase in shear modulus elasticity and dynamic viscosity [32]. In another study by Tateya et al. on acute histologic changes following injury to the vocal folds, the authors reported changes in extracellular components, namely, collagen, fibronectin, and hyaluronic acid, mostly at the 3–5th day. Collagen type 1 production peaked at day 5 and then decreased, whereas collagen type 3 kept increasing until day 14 [33]. The late proliferative phase following injury is characterized by neo-angiogenesis and migration of fibroblasts, with subsequent overproduction of collagen and decrease in elastin formation. Rousseau et al. investigated the histologic and rheologic properties of scarred vocal folds during the chronic phase of wound repair 6 months after injury, and they noted an increase in collagen deposition in thick bundles and fragmentation of elastin fibers [34]. The study was conducted on a rabbit model in which the vocal fold lamina propria was stripped surgically down to the muscle [34]. Similar results were reported in another study by the same authors on a canine model. At 6 months following surgery, there was a decrease in elastin and an increase in collagen formation. The elastin fibers were broken and tangled at 2 months post-injury [35]. As a result of the aforementioned histologic changes in the ECM constituents, the viscoelastic shear properties of the vocal fold are affected. Remodeling in the lamina propria structures leads to marked alteration in the vibratory behavior of the layers of the vocal fold [36]. Strobovideolaryngoscopy often reveals decreased pliability of the vocal folds with a decrease in mucosal waves amplitude attributed to tethering of the vocal fold cover to the underlying structures. In severe cases, incomplete closure of the vocal folds may be observed with signs of glottic insufficiency Aerodynamic measures show a decrease in maximum phonation time, an increase in mean flow rate, and a decrease in glottal resistance. Acoustically, there is an increase in the perturbation parameters, noise-to-harmonic ratio, and voice turbulence index, all confirming to disturbances in the vocal signal [20, 37].

Patients with vocal fold scar are offered various options. These include vocal fold microflap surgery with insertion of fat or fascia [38–40], laryngeal framework surgery [41], injection laryngoplasty [42], and laser therapy [43]. Recently, fibroblast growth factors and stem cell therapy have been described with successful results [44–46]. There is also extensive literature on the use of steroid injection either as an adjunct or primary treatment option in patients with vocal fold scars

[47–49]. In 2006, Mortensen and Woo investigated the outcome of 34 patients who underwent office-based steroid injection and reported significant improvement in dysphonia and mucosal wave amplitude on laryngeal videostroboscopic examination [47]. Twelve patients of their study group had vocal fold scar. In 2016, Young et al. investigated the effect of dexamethasone injection in 25 patients with vocal fold scar who had undergone an average of 3.5 sessions each and reported decrease in VHI score, decrease in the grade of dysphonia using GRBAS, decrease in phonatory threshold pressure, and an increase in fundamental frequency. The patients also had voice therapy [49].

The improvement in the clinical and aerodynamic measures following glucocorticoid steroid injection in vocal fold scars can be ascribed to changes in extracellular matrix constituents secondary to alteration in fibroblast activity. The concentration and distribution of hyaluronic acid, fibronectin, decorin, and collagen concentration are affected. Campagnolo et al. reported a significant decrease in collagen deposition (mean total area of collagen 86.23 μm^2 vs. 273.67 μm^2 in the control group) on the 3rd and 7th day following injection of 0.1 ml dexamethasone sodium phosphate within the vocal fold. The study was conducted on the vocal folds of rabbits; and one side was incised and injected with steroids, whereas the opposite side was only incised and served as s a control [50]. Similarly, Coleman et al. investigated the histomorphometric changes associated with corticosteroid injection following vocal fold microflap surgery in 15 dogs and showed a 3-week delay in neovascularization and a 12-day delay in the inflammatory response [51]. Although there was a delay in healing, there were no significant changes in any of the laryngeal stroboscopic parameters, namely, extent and pliability of mucosal waves and malleability. In another investigation on human vocal fold fibroblasts, Zhou et al. showed that glucocorticoid injection not only downregulated the inflammatory response but also decreased fibroblast proliferation and extracellular matrix metabolism [52]. See Video 11.1 illustrating vocal fold steroid injection using the transnasal approach and Videos 11.2 and 11.3 using the transoral approach in awake patients.

In summary, steroid injection is an alternative treatment to endoscopic vocal fold surgery and/or laryngeal framework surgery in the management of vocal fold scars. The procedure can be performed safely in an office setting while the patient is fully awake. Vocal fold steroid injections have shown to restore vocal fold pliability and glottic closure in some cases. The effect is mediated via remodeling of the lamina propria layered structure.

11.3.2 Office-Based Steroid Injection in Benign Lesions of the Vocal Folds

Benign lesions of the vocal folds are common causes of dysphonia. A nomenclature paradigm by Rosen et al. stratified these lesions into nodules, polyps, cysts, pseudocysts, fibrous masses, and reactive and nonspecific lesions [53]. The histopathologic spectrum includes thickening of the mucosal basement membrane, submucosal fibrin deposits, hyalinization, hemorrhage, neovascularization, edema, and inflammatory infiltrates [54]. Affected patients usually are treated with voice therapy that aims at reducing voice abuse/misuse and laryngeal hyperfunction. Voice therapy consists primarily of patient education on voice hygiene, vocal function exercises/training, and use of voice amplification and many other techniques [55, 56]. Failure to respond to voice therapy is often an indication for surgical intervention. Patients with masses usually undergo microflap or minimicroflap vocal fold surgery which allows dissection and removal of the lesion while preserving the overlying mucosal lining [15, 57, 58]. The rational is to reduce injury to the deep layers of the lamina propria and hence scar formation [20, 59].

Vocal fold steroid injection is used frequently as an adjunct therapy in patients undergoing phonomicrosurgery. The injection is administered at the site of the lesion and/or in the surgical bed following excision. Steroids act by decreasing paracellular permeability and by regulating extracellular matrix metabolism and collagen formation [37, 60]. In a study on the efficacy of adjunct steroid injection following microsurgical resection of benign lesions of the vocal folds, Cho et al. reported a lower rate of recurrence in those who underwent steroid injection vs. those who did not. Adjunct steroid injection was associated with a 0.3-fold lower risk of persistent dysphonia following surgery. The study was conducted on 221 patients (136 polyps, 49 nodules, and 30 cysts) who were divided into two groups, those who had steroid injection and those who did not [11]. Steroid injection also has been described as a primary treatment modality of benign lesions of vocal folds under direct laryngoscopy. Ramavat et al. reported the efficacy of steroid injection in a randomized controlled study of 29 patients with benign vocal fold lesions, 15 of whom were treated with ILSI alone. The results showed a reduction in the size of the lesions and a decrease in VHI and GRBAS scores 12 weeks following treatment. Similarly, there was increase in fundamental frequency and maximum phonation time MPT ($n = 15$). Notably, the decrease in shimmer and jitter was more significant in those who underwent phonomicrosurgery ($n = 14$) in comparison to those who had steroid injection alone [61]. With the trend in laryngology practice toward office-based surgery, steroid injections in patients with benign vocal fold lesions are now performed using indirect laryngoscopy. In 1962, Yanagihara et al. was the first to report vocal fold steroid injection in the treatment of vocal fold nodules using a laryngeal mirror. The authors reported effectiveness in 62–79% of the cases [62]. Because of lack of precision and other factors, vocal fold steroid injection in an office setting was not adopted widely until refinements in optic technology and instrumentation evolved. The introduction of flexible endoscopy followed later by an endoscope with a working channel and distal chip camera allowed sophistication of this procedure. In 1993, Nonomura et al. reported satisfactory results in 21 patients (9 with nodules and 12 with chronic inflammation) who underwent vocal fold steroid injection using "fiberoptic laryngosurgery technique." In view of the high success rate, the authors advocated intracordal steroid injection as an effective treatment alternative in patients with mild vocal fold inflammatory disorders who are refractory to conservative therapy [63]. In 2003, Tateya et al. reported their experience with ILSI in 44 patients with mild Reinke's edema using triamcinolone acetonide. The authors found significant improvement or remission following injection in almost all cases. There was a significant increase in the mean fundamental frequency by 13 Hz (168 Hz preinjection vs. 181 Hz postinjection) and an increase in maximum phonation time (9.0 s preinjection vs. 11.4 s postinjection). The procedure was performed thru the transoral approach under fiberoptic guidance [64]. In another study of 27 patients with vocal fold nodules who underwent triamcinolone acetonide injections in the superficial layer of the lamina propria, the same authors reported complete regression of the lesion in 17 patients and partial regression in 10. The regression in the size of the lesion was accompanied by subjective improvement or recovery of voice symptoms, as well as improvement in mean MPT (10.9–13.9 s, respectively) and mean flow rate (236–166 ml/s, respectively) [65]. In 2006, Mortensen and Woo described their experience in office-based steroid injections in 34 patients and reported an overall success rate of 82%. Eleven of the 18 patients with vocal fold polyps or nodules had significant improvement in voice quality. The patients were evaluated subjectively using the GRBAS perceptual rating and laryngeal videostroboscopy. No complications were reported [47]. In 2009, Hsu et al. investigated the outcome of percutaneous steroid injection in 24 patients with vocal fold polyps and reported complete remission in 12 of the 22 who completed surgery. There was improvement in laryngeal videostroboscopic findings and in acoustic and aerodynamic measures. The authors emphasized on the safety of this procedure and its efficacy in the management of patients with vocal fold polyps [66]. In 2011, Lee et al. reviewed their experience with 80 patients with vocal fold nodules who underwent steroid injection via the cricothyroid membrane. There was partial decrease in the size of the nodules in 49% and complete regression in 44% of cases. Moreover, there was a decrease in perturbation parameters and an increase in MPT [67]. The same year, Woo et al. investigated the efficacy of percutaneous steroid injections in patients with benign vocal fold lesions and reported an overall success rate of 84%. Forty of 115 patients had complete remission, and 57 had partial remission. The authors reported statistically significant improvement in both objective and subjective outcome measures at 1 and 3 months following surgery [68]. In 2013, Wang et al. investigated the effect of transnasal endoscopic steroid injection in 30 patients with vocal fold nodules and polyps and reported regression or complete disappearance of the lesion in 29 cases at 3 months follow-up. There was a decrease in VHI-10 scores (22.5 vs. 14.5), perceptual rating of dysphonia, and a decrease in the perturbation parameters. However, there was an increase in the mean MPT by 2.2 seconds. Notably, there was no significant difference in the outcome measures between patients with vocal fold nodules and patients with vocal fold polyps [69]. In 2014, in a study of 176 patients with vocal fold nodules and polyps, 92 of whom had received vocal fold steroid injection using the transoral or transnasal approach, Wang et al. reported regression in the size of the lesion in 39% of the cases at 1–2 months. The regression in the size of the lesion was associated with a significant decrease in VHI-10 score by 9.5 points (24.4 preinjection vs.14.9 postinjection) [70]. The authors used a quantitative method described by Mallur et al. for assessment of the size of the vocal fold lesion [71]. Wang et al. found that patients with vocal fold nodules had earlier regression in the size of the lesion following steroid injection in comparison to those treated with vocal hygiene education alone. Similarly, patients with vocal fold polyps had significant reduction in the size of the lesion in comparison to those who had vocal hygiene education alone. Those with nonhemorrhagic polyps had better outcome than those with hemorrhagic polyps (48% vs. 34%, respectively). However, although patients who had undergone steroid injection did better than those who had vocal hygiene education, still 11% of the former group needed surgical intervention using either KTP laser or laryngo-microsurgery [70]. In 2015, Wang et al. performed a comprehensive review of 126 patients with benign lesions of the vocal folds who underwent ILSI and reported improvement in symptoms and decrease in the size of the lesion size in more than 80% of cases. The authors also found a negative correlation between duration of symptoms, voice demand, VHI score, and perceptual voice evaluation. Patients with vocal fold nodules and high occupational vocal load were less likely to improve than those with no or low vocal demand. Similarly, patients with long-standing duration of polyps and/or history of laryngopharyngeal reflux did not improve as much as those with recent history of polyps and no history of laryngopharyngeal reflux. Interestingly, although there was a significant improvement in the mean MPT at 1 month follow-up, the increase at 2 months was not significant for all three categories, nodules, polyps, and cysts [72]. In 2016, Lee and Park reviewed long-term efficacy in 84 patients with benign vocal fold lesions who had undergone percutaneous steroid injection and reported complete and partial remission in 44% and 26.2% of the cases, respectively. The improvement was stable up to 2 years following treatment [73]. In 2017, Wang et al. investigated the long-term effect of ILSI in patients with benign lesions of the vocal folds and reported improvement in 74% of the cases at 1 month but only 50% in the long term. Patients with vocal fold polyps had better outcomes than patients with vocal fold nodules (54% vs. 49%) [74].

In summary, patients with benign lesions of the vocal folds may benefit from steroid injections in an office setting. The patient should be notified that repeated injections are often needed, and surgery remains an option for those who do not improve. It is also important to note that the underlying predisposing factors for the development and progression of these lesions are not addressed by injection or surgery. Bad phonatory behavior and poor vocal hygiene may jeopardize the outcome and lead to recurrence, and voice therapy prior to injection or surgery is recommended.

11.3.3 Office-Based Steroid Injection in Vocal Fold Bamboo Nodes

Bamboo nodes were described initially by Hosako et al. in 1993 as yellowish, transverse, submucosal lesions of the vocal folds [75]. Histologically, these lesions are fusiform in shape and characterized by central necrosis surrounded by inflammatory cells and macrophages. Affected patients may have impairment in vocal fold vibration and change in voice quality. Several treatment options are available. These include treatment of the underlying disease, systemic steroids, voice therapy, and/or surgery. Microsurgical excision under direct laryngoscopy is advocated usually only in cases who are refractory to conservative management [76]. Oker et al. reviewed the clinical course of 15 patients with bamboo nodes and reported successful treatment with voice therapy in 53% of the cases. They also noted spontaneous improvement in three patients [77]. Intralesional steroid injection is an alternative treatment. Todic et al. reviewed ten cases of bamboo nodes, six of whom were treated with systemic steroids and one with ILSI. The authors stressed the association of bamboo nodes with autoimmune diseases and the benefit of combined voice therapy and steroids [78]. Schwemmle et al. reported a 43-year-old woman with bamboo nodes who was treated with repeated steroid injections but with little success. The patients needed surgical removal of the lesion which ultimately led to improvement in voice quality [79]. With the recent advances in technology, ILSI are now being performed in the office. Imaizumi et al. reported a 30-year-old woman who was treated successfully with steroid injection in an outpatient setting. The authors advocated the use of steroid injection in patients with bamboo nodes who fail conservative therapy [80]. With the wider spread of office-based laryngeal surgery, the use of ILSI in the treatment of the laryngeal manifestations of autoimmune diseases is expected to increase. See Video 11.4 illustrating steroid injection using the percutaneous approach in a patient with vocal folds bamboo nodes.

11.3.4 Complications of Office-Based Vocal Fold Steroid Injection

Although office-based laryngeal steroid injection has advantages in terms of achieving high intralesional drug concentration with minimal systemic effects, complications may occur in up to one third of patients. High vocal demand, persistent voice abuse, smoking, and laryngopharyngeal reflux are significant predisposing factors. The most commonly reported complications are vocal fold hematoma and deposition of crystals in the superficial layer of the lamina propria, particularly with the use of triamcinolone solutions [67, 69, 72, 81]. Affected patients often report worsening of the voice associated with a decrease in mucosal wave amplitude on stroboscopic examination. In a study by Wang et al. of 30 patients with vocal fold polyps and nodules, the authors reported vocal fold hematoma in three cases, all of whom improved spontaneously with no need for surgical intervention [69]. In a review by the same authors in 2015, 34 of 126 patients who underwent ILSI for benign lesions of the vocal folds developed vocal fold hematoma. Additionally, 4% of their study population developed triamcinolone deposits, which resolved spontaneously 2 months after the injection [72]. Similarly, Lee et al. reported two cases of triamcinolone deposits within the vocal folds following steroid injection in patients with vocal fold nodules. The deposits dissolved without the need for surgery [67]. Because of this problem, the authors stopped using suspensions such as triamcinolone for routine vocal fold injection many years age in favor of dexamethasone, a solution safe for intravenous use. This eliminates the problem of the white plaques and stiffness from triamcinolone that can persist for up to 8 months. Another rare complication of ILSI is vocal fold atrophy that often presents with breathiness and glottic insufficiency on laryngeal examination. In a review of 80 cases of ILSI via the cricothyroid membrane, Lee et al. reported four cases of vocal fold atrophy that resolved within 2 months [67]. In another study by Wang et al. of 126 patients with benign vocal fold lesions who had undergone office-based ILSI, 1 patient developed vocal fold atrophy [72].

Recurrence is another significant concern in patients undergoing office-based ILSI. In an investigation on the long-term results of ILSI, Wang et al. reported an increase in cumulative failure rate from 12% at 6 months to 32% at 2 years. Cumulative failure rate was defined as recurrence of symptoms and/or need for surgical intervention. Patients with vocal fold polyps had better outcomes than patients with vocal fold nodules. The authors attributed the high recurrence rate to persistence of phonotraumatic behavior in patients with benign lesions of the vocal folds [74]. In another study by Tateya et al. of 28 patients with vocal fold nodules, recurrence was noted in 8 patients. The follow-up period ranged between 2 and 37 months [65]. In a systematic review by Wang et al. in 2013 that included 321 patients with benign vocal fold disorders who underwent steroid injection, the authors reported a recurrence rate between 4% and 31% [81]. Lee et al. reported six patients who had recurrence even at 4 weeks following steroid injections in vocal fold nodules [67]. In another review by the same authors of 84 patients who received ILSI, the average recurrence time interval was 8.5 months and ranged between 3 and 36 months. Important predisposing factors were history of voice abuse and being a professional voice user [73].

In summary, office based steroid injections can cause complications despite the advantages of delivering high intralesional drug concentration. These include vocal fold hematoma, deposition of crystals within the superficial layer of the lamina propria if a suspension rather than a solution is used, and rarely vocal fold atrophy. Most of these complications resolve spontaneously without the need for surgical intervention.

11.4 Office-Based Laryngeal Intra-articular Steroid Injections in Patients with Autoimmune Diseases

Laryngeal manifestations of autoimmune diseases are common. In rheumatoid arthritis (RA), the prevalence can reach 88%, with dysphonia being reported in two thirds of the cases [82–84]. Patients may present with a plethora of symptoms and signs depending on the stage of the disease and site of involvement. In the acute phase, complaints of change in voice quality, sore throat, difficulty in swallowing, and referred otalgia are reported often. In the chronic stage, patients may present with persistent dysphonia, respiratory distress, and stridor [84]. Many of the phonatory and airway symptoms stem from acute and chronic changes in the cricoarytenoid and/or cricothyroid joints. These changes include edema, fibrosis, destruction of the articular surfaces, and/or deposition of rheumatoid nodules in close relation to the joint. The rate of involvement varies with the degree of physician's awareness and the use of radiologic imaging in the assessment of these patients [84]. In many cases, the clinical presentation is masked by comorbid diseases.

Based on numerous studies, the management of laryngeal articular involvement relies on adequate control of the underlying disease using systemic steroids, methotrexate, or other medications to suppress the immune system. With the advances in technology, corticosteroids are delivered via injections into the articular surface of the affected joint, thus sparing the patient the adverse effect of systemic steroids. In 1977, Habib reported a case of rheumatoid arthritis who presented with stridor secondary to involvement of the cricoarytenoid joints. The patient was managed successfully with intra-articular steroid injection [85]. Simpson et al. described six cases of RA who had substantial improvement following periarticular steroid injections. The authors emphasized the added value of steroid injections if performed by a well-trained physician [86]. Similarly, in a study of five patients with RA treated with intra-articular steroid injections and systemic therapy, Dockery et al. reported improvement in phonatory and respiratory symptoms [87]. In all the above cases, the injections were performed in the operating room under general anesthesia. With the increase in the landscape of office-based laryngeal surgery, intra-articular steroid injections can be performed in an awake setting. The author (RTS) designed a right-angle injection needle to facilitate intra-articular injection. The needle is disposable, and injection handles for the needles are available for direct and for peroral indirect injection (Integra Lifesciences, Princeton, NJ).

11.5 Office-Based Laryngeal Injections of Cidofovir

Recurrent respiratory papillomatosis RRP is a disease of the respiratory epithelium characterized by papillomatous growth caused usually by human papilloma virus (HPV) types 6 and 11. It affects all age groups and can lead to symptoms such as dyspnea, dysphonia, stridor, and chronic cough. RRP has been treated traditionally with surgery. The high recurrence rate of this disease and the need for frequent surgical intervention have prompted the use of adjunct treatment such as immunotherapy and antiviral therapy [88]. Cidofovir is a potent antiviral medication used in the treatment of many viruses including HPV. It is a cytosine nucleotide analogue, a prodrug that undergoes phosphorylation to become an active metabolite that leads to decrease in cell proliferation and enhanced apoptosis [89, 90]. Traditionally, cidofovir injections have been used for the treatment of *Cytomegalovirus* (CMV) retinitis. Its success in the treatment of CMV led to its widespread use in patients with RRP who undergo frequent surgical interventions. The purpose of treatment is to reduce the frequency of surgical intervention which often leads to scar and worsening of voice quality [91].

Cidofovir injections usually are performed under general anesthesia following debulking of the laryngeal RRP using cold steel instruments and/or lasers. In 1997, Wellens et al. were the first to describe intralesional cidofovir injection in the larynx [92]. A follow-up in 1998 by the same authors described cidofovir in 17 patients with laryngeal papillomatosis. The authors reported successful results in 16 of 17 cases [93]. Similarly, Wilson et al. reported three cases of laryngeal papillomatosis treated successfully with intralesional cidofovir injection [94]. Pransky et al. reported the efficacy of cidofovir injection in ten patients and reported complete or partial regression all. The authors advocated the use of cidofovir as an adjunct treatment following surgical excision [95]. Galletti et al. described a protocol that consists of debulking the lesion under microdirect suspension laryngoscopy followed by intralesional or perilesional cidofovir injection and the use of indole-3-carbinol orally. The objective of this protocol is to control the disease and reduce the frequency of surgical intervention often associated with scar formation [96]. In 2003, Naiman et al. investigated the efficacy of cidofovir intralesional injections at monthly intervals in 26 patients with RRP. One third of the study group had complete remission, and two thirds had minimal residual disease that necessitated surgical intervention. The overall response rate was better in those with supraglottic and/or glottic lesions in comparison to those with subglottic lesions. The treatment was performed under direct laryngoscopy and general anesthesia [97]. In 2003, Lee and Rosen investigated the efficacy of cidofovir injection combined with surgery in 13 patients with RRP and reported remission in 76.9% of the cases. Each patient underwent 3.5 injections on average using a concentration that varied between 2.5 and 5 mg/cc [98]. Dikkers reported the successful use of cidofovir injection in combination with microsurgical excision in seven patients with glottic lesions. The injections were repeated every 6 weeks, and each patient received a cumulative dose that varied between 10.5 and 128 mg [99]. In 2015, Kim and Baizhumanova supported the efficacy of combining surgery with adjuvant therapy using cidofovir or pulsed dye laser in a group of 29 patients who were followed up for more than 2 years. The authors reported improvement in voice quality, a decrease in VHI score, subglottic pressure, noise-to-harmonic ration, and degree of subharmonic component. The authors advocated removal of submucosal glands in order to reduce the frequency of recurrence [100]. In 2019, Jackwoska et al. reported their experience with 42 patients with RRP who were treated with CO2 laser and intralesional cidofovir injections and reported improvement in voice quality in all patients, with a decrease in VHI scores. Moreover, there was a decrease in jitter and shimmer with improvement in spectrographic analysis after treatment [101].

Cidofovir injections are not performed in an office setting commonly (Video 11.5). There are only two case studies on office-based cidofovir injections in the treatment of laryngeal RRP. Co and Woo reported their experience with five patients with RRP who underwent serial office-based laryngeal injections following CO2 laser therapy in the operating room. The authors reported improvement in voice quality associated with partial remission of the disease on laryngeal examination. Moreover, there was prolongation in the time needed for microsurgical intervention [102]. Chhetri et al. reported their experience with five patients with RRP who had undergone repeated cidofovir injections using the percutaneous technique. The authors reported a marked decrease in the size of the lesion in all patients after a mean treatment duration of 12 months. Notably, all patients had laser therapy prior to the percutaneous injections. In conclusion, they advocated office-based cidofovir injection as an adjunct to laser therapy in patients traditionally treated under direct laryngoscopy and general anesthesia. The authors also noted the limitation of this technique in patients with supraglottic and or subglottic lesions [103].

In summary, cidofovir injection can be used as adjunct therapy in patients with RRP. The main reasons for the high recurrence of laryngeal RRP are hidden areas (often microscopic) not resected under direct laryngoscopy and the conservative surgery often performed to minimize phonatory complications. Given the propensity of RRP to recur in the upper airway, frequent injections are needed in many cases. Patients should be informed that office-based cidofovir injections may prolong the time interval between for surgical intervention but do not eliminate the need for surgery in many cases.

11.6 Office-Based Laryngeal Injection of 5-Fluorouracil

5-Flurorouracil is a drug that is used primarily in the treatment of patients with cancer. It is a pyrimidine analog that is converted intracellularly into active metabolites that disrupt RNA synthesis and decrease production of thymidine, hence DNA replication [104]. Recent reports indicate that it is also useful in the treatment of patients with hypertrophic scars. In a systematic review of evidence-based therapy in hypertrophic scars, Nischwitz et al. reported intralesional injection of 5-FU as a therapeutic modality that reduces scar formation and enhances its pliability. The authors stressed the need for future studies to optimize its mode of delivery and tissue permeability [105]. In another review, Jiang et al. found that combining 5-FU with triamcinolone acetonide (TAC) improves the efficacy of keloid treatment and is superior to TAC treatment in isolation [106]. 5-FU also has gained popularity as a therapeutic drug in patients with laryngotracheal stenosis. In 2009, Baptistella et al. investigated the rate of collagen fiber deposition in the vocal folds of pigs following partial excision using carbon dioxide laser. The study group was divided into three subgroups, control ($n = 6$), 5-FU ($n = 6$), and the mitomycin ($n = 6$) subgroup. After 1 month, histologic examination showed a lower concentration of collagen fiber deposition in the 5-FU and mitomycin subgroups in comparison to the control subgroup (2269.19 μm and 2196.36 μm, respectively, vs. 3428.66 μm) [107]. In 2015, Gu et al. investigated fibrous scar formation in a rabbit model following treatment with ethosomes (lipid vesicles) containing 5-FU. Using hematoxylin and eosin (HE) staining and fluorescence microscopy, the authors showed decrease and dispersion of fibroblast and collagen fibers, leading to a decrease in laryngotracheal stenosis. Ethosomes with small diameter had better permeability and hence drug delivery than ethosomes with large diameters [108]. In a similar study in which tracheal scar was induced by scraping the mucosal surface, Mao et al. showed a decrease in airway stenosis 21 days following administration of ethosomes containing 5-fluorouracil. The authors stressed the potential benefit of 5-FU in treating patients with laryngotracheal stenosis [109]. The results of these animal studies have been supported by the author (RTS) in his treatment of patients with posterior glottis stenosis, subglottic stenosis, and true vocal fold scar. Intralesional 5-FU injections have helped improve vocal fold mucosal wave and appear to reduce recurrence of laryngeal stenosis [110].

In view of the above, laryngeal injection of 5-FU in patients with laryngeal stenosis and or vocal fold scar is a promising therapeutic modality. The easy access to the laryngeal inlet via the transnasal or perioral route in an awake patient should foster 5-FU injections in an office setting.

11.7 Office-Based Laryngeal Injection of Growth Factors

Other pharmaceutical agents that are used increasingly in the treatment of aging/scared vocal folds are growth factors. Advances in regenerative medicine and tissue engineering have paved the way for clinical use of growth factors in managing age-induced histologic changes such as decrease in hyaluronic acid and increase collagen deposition. Numerous studies over the last two decades suggest that growth factors, particularly basic fibroblast growth factor (b-FGF), may have a therapeutic effect on the aged and scared vocal fold by promoting wound healing and angiogenesis and by stimulating the proliferative function of the aged fibroblasts [111–115]. Hirano et al. investigated the effect of growth factors (hepatocyte growth factor and b-FGF) cultured with aged fibroblasts and reported a significant increase in hyaluronic acid production. The increase was dose-dependent for the hepatocyte growth factor and not dose-dependent for the b-FGF [111]. These results were substantiated by Suehiro et al. who also proved that treating vocal fold fibroblasts with b-FGF leads to upregulated expression of hyaluronic acid synthase and fibronectin and downregulated expression of procollagen type 1. The authors used quantitative polymerase chain reaction for the assessment of extracellular matrix constituents and gene expression [112]. In an animal study in which scar fibroblasts and normal fibroblasts were cultured with hepatocyte growth factor, Graupp et al. showed that the response to growth factor stimulation was present only in the fibroblasts extracted from young rats and not aged ones. The authors stressed the age-dependent response and the need to consider age in clinical trials [113]. Basic fibroblast growth factors also improve or slow down vocal fold atrophy. In a study in which b-FGF was injected into denervated thyroarytenoid muscles (TA), Kaneko et al. showed an increase in the number of neuromuscular junctions and a decrease in muscle atrophy. The denervated TA cross-sectional area was larger in those treated with b-FGF in comparison to those not treated [114]. In 2016, Satoshi et al. conducted the first human study on the effect of b-FGF on the fibroblasts and extracellular matrix of the lamina propria in six elderly. Ten micrograms of b-FGF were injected in the superficial layer of the lamina propria using a curved needle that was introduced perorally under local anesthesia. The authors reported an improvement in VHI-10, perceptual evaluation, as well as acoustic and aerodynamic measures 6 months after treatment [115]. The author (RTS) has been using growth factors available commercially as AmnioFix (MiMedx, Marietta, GA), a dehydrated amnion/chorion membrane allograft available as a particulate that can be rehydrated for injection into vocal fold scar. Preliminary results have been encouraging.

In summary, the use of fibroblast growth factors is a promising therapeutic modality in patients with vocal fold aging and or scarring. The effect is mediated via an increase in hyaluronic acid concentration and a decrease in collagen production. With the trend toward office based laryngeal surgery fibroblast growth factors can be injected in an awake patient. Future reports on a larger number of patients are needed to assert the long-term efficacy of this treatment.

References

1. Sibilia J. Corticosteroids and inflammation. Rev Prat. 2003;53(5):495–501.
2. Barnes PJ. Corticosteroids: the drugs to beat. Eur J Pharmacol. 2006;533(1–3):2–14.
3. Kairys W, Olmstead M, O'Connor T. Steroid treatment of laryngotracheitis: a meta-analysis of the evidence from randomized trials. Pediatrics. 1989;83(5):683–93.
4. Johnson W. Croup. BMJ Clin Evid. 2014;2014:0321.
5. Ossoff H, Wolff P, Ballenger J. Acute epiglottitis in adults: experience with fifteen cases. Laryngoscope. 1980;90(7 Pt 1):1155–61.
6. Bower S, Belen E, Weg G, Dantzker R. Manifestations and treatment of laryngeal sarcoidosis. Am Rev Respir Dis. 1980;122(2):325–32.
7. Korbet M, Block J, Lewis J. Laryngeal complications in a patient with inactive systemic lupus erythematosus. Arch Intern Med. 1984;144(9):1867–8.
8. Teitel D, MacKenzie R, Stern R, Paget A. Laryngeal involvement in systemic lupus erythematosus. Semin Arthritis Rheum. 1992;22(3):203–14.
9. Solans-Laqué R, Bosch-Gil JA, Canela M, Lorente J, Pallisa E, Vilardell-Tarres M. Clinical features and therapeutic management of subglottic stenosis in patients with Wegener's granulomatosis. Lupus. 2008;17(9):832–6.
10. Caplan A, Fett N, Rosenbach M, Werth VP, Micheletti RG. Prevention and management of glucocorticoid-induced side effects: a comprehensive review: a review of glucocorticoid pharmacology and bone health. J Am Acad Dermatol. 2017;76(1):1–9.
11. Cho JH, Kim SY, Joo YH, Park YH, Hwang WS, Sun DI. Efficacy and safety of adjunctive steroid injection after microsurgical removal of benign vocal fold lesions. J Voice. 2017;31(5):615–20.
12. Campagnolo AM, Tsuji DH, Sennes LU, Imamura R. Steroid injection in chronic inflammatory vocal fold disorders, literature review. Braz J Otorhinolaryngol. 2008;74(6):926–32.
13. Krespi YP, Husain S, Mitrani M, Husain S, Meltzer CJ. Treatment of laryngeal sarcoidosis with intralesional steroid injection. Ann Otol Rhinol Laryngol. 1987;96(6):713–5.
14. Remacle M, Frederickx Y, Pigeolet Y, Bertrand B. Laryngeal manifestations of sarcoidosis. Acta Otorhinolaryngol Belg. 1986;40(6):889–906.

15. Bouchayer M, Cornut G. Microsurgery for benign lesions of the vocal fold. Ear Nose Throat J. 1998;67(6):446–66.
16. Heman-Ackah YD, Sataloff RT. Laryngotracheal trauma. In: Sataloff RT, editor. Professional voice: the science and art of clinical care. 4th ed. San Diego: Plural Publishing; 2017. p. 1611–28.
17. Spiegel JT, Sataloff RT. Posterior glottic stenosis. In: Sataloff RT, editor. Professional voice: the science and art of clinical care. 4th ed. San Diego: Plural Publishing; 2017. p. 1641–8.
18. Gelbard A, Francis DO, Sandulache VC, Simmons JC, Donovan DT, Ongkasuwan J. Causes and consequences of adult laryngotracheal stenosis. Laryngoscope. 2015;125(5):1137–43.
19. Lano CF Jr, Duncavage JA, Reinisch L, Ossoff RH, Courey MS, Netterville JL. Laryngotracheal reconstruction in the adult: a ten year experience. Ann Otol Rhinol Laryngol. 1998;107(2):92–7.
20. Moore JE, Sataloff RT. Vocal fold scar. In: Sataloff RT, editor. Professional voice: the science and art of clinical care. 4th ed. San Diego: Plural Publishing; 2017. p. 1605–10.
21. Carroll A, Hanasono M, Mikulec A, Kita M, Koch J. Triamcinolone stimulates bFGF production and inhibits TGF-β1 production by human dermal fibroblasts. Dermatol Surg. 2002;28(8):704–9.
22. Wierzbicka M, Tokarski M, Puszczewicz M, Szyfter W. The efficacy of submucosal corticosteroid injection and dilatation in subglottic stenosis of different aetiology. J Laryngol Otol. 2016;130(7):674–9.
23. Wolter E, Ooi H, Witterick J. Intralesional corticosteroid injection and dilatation provides effective management of subglottic stenosis in Wegener's granulomatosis. Laryngoscope. 2010;120(12):2452–5.
24. Hoffman S, Thomas-Golbanov K, Chan J, Akst M, Eliachar I. Treatment of subglottic stenosis, due to Wegener's granulomatosis, with intralesional corticosteroids and dilation. J Rheumatol. 2003;30(5):1017–21.
25. Feinstein J, Goel A, Raghavan G, et al. Endoscopic management of subglottic stenosis. JAMA Otolaryngol Head Neck Surg. 2017;143(5):500–5.
26. Hoffman R, Coughlin R, Dailey H. Serial office-based steroid injections for treatment of idiopathic subglottic stenosis. Laryngoscope. 2017;127(11):2475–81.
27. Bertelsen C, Shoffel-Havakuk H, O'Dell K, Johns MM 3rd, Reder LS. Serial in-office intralesional steroid injections in airway stenosis. JAMA Otolaryngol Head Neck Surg. 2018;144(3):203–10.
28. Franco A Jr, Husain I, Reder L, Paddle P. Awake serial intralesional steroid injections without surgery as a novel targeted treatment for idiopathic subglottic stenosis. Laryngoscope. 2018;128(3):610–7.
29. Pan R, Rosow E. Office-based corticosteroid injections as adjuvant therapy for subglottic stenosis. Laryngoscope Investig Otolaryngol. 2019;4(4):414–9.
30. Hoffman R, Francis O, Mai P, Dailey H. Office-based steroid injections for idiopathic subglottic stenosis: patient-reported outcomes, effect on stenosis, and side effects. Ann Otol Rhinol Laryngol. 2020;129(4):361–8.
31. Gartner-Schmidt L, Shembel C, Zullo G, Rosen A. Development and validation of the Dyspnea Index (DI): a severity index for upper airway-related dyspnea. J Voice. 2014;28(6):775–82.
32. Thibeault L, Gray D, Bless M, Chan W, Ford N. Histologic and rheologic characterization of vocal fold scarring. J Voice. 2002;16(1):96–104.
33. Tateya T, Tateya I, Sohn JH, Bless DM. Histological study of acute vocal fold injury in a rat model. Ann Otol Rhinol Laryngol. 2006;115(4):285–92.
34. Rousseau B, Hirano S, Chan RW, et al. Characterization of chronic vocal fold scarring in a rabbit model. J Voice. 2004;18(1):116–24.
35. Rousseau B, Hirano S, Scheidt TD, et al. Characterization of vocal fold scarring in a canine model. Laryngoscope. 2003;113(4):620–7.
36. Hansen K, Thibeault L. Current understanding and review of the literature: vocal fold scarring. J Voice. 2006;20(1):110–20.

37. Woo P, Casper J, Colton R, Brewer D. Diagnosis and treatment of persistent dysphonia after laryngeal surgery: a retrospective analysis of 62 patients. Laryngoscope. 1994;104(9):1084–91.
38. DeFatta A, DeFatta J, Sataloff RT. Laryngeal lipotransfer: review of a 14-year experience. J Voice. 2013;27(4):512–5.
39. Kishimoto Y, Hirano S, Kojima T, Kanemaru SI, Ito J. Implantation of an atelocollagen sheet for the treatment of vocal fold scarring and sulcus vocalis. Ann Otol Rhinol Laryngol. 2009;118(9):613–20.
40. Neuenschwander MC, Sataloff RT, Abaza MM, Hawkshaw MJ, Reiter D, Spiegel JR. Management of vocal fold scar with autologous fat implantation: perceptual results. J Voice. 2001;15(2):295–304.
41. van den Broek M, Heijnen J, Hendriksma M, et al. Bilateral medialization thyroplasty in patients with vocal fold atrophy with or without sulcus. Eur Arch Otorhinolaryngol. 2020;277(7):2023–9.
42. Lahav Y, Malka-Yosef L, Shapira-Galitz Y, Cohen O, Halperin D, Shoffel-Havakuk H. Vocal fold fat augmentation for atrophy, scarring, and unilateral paralysis: long-term functional outcomes. Otolaryngol Head Neck Surg. 2021;164(3):631–8.
43. Prufer N, Woo P, Altman KW. Pulse dye and other laser treatments for vocal scar. Curr Opin Otolaryngol Head Neck Surg. 2010;18(6):492–7.
44. Hirano S, Sugiyama Y, Kaneko M, Mukudai S, Fuse S, Hashimoto K. Intracordal injection of basic fibroblast growth factor in 100 cases of vocal fold atrophy and scar. Laryngoscope. 2020. https://doi.org/10.1002/lary.29200.
45. Mattei A, Magalon J, Bertrand B, Philandrianos C, Veran J, Giovanni A. Cell therapy and vocal fold scarring. Eur Ann Otorhinolaryngol Head Neck Dis. 2017;134(5):339–45.
46. Hertegård S, Cedervall J, Svensson B, et al. Viscoelastic and histologic properties in scarred rabbit vocal folds after mesenchymal stem cell injection. Laryngoscope. 2006;116(7):1248–54.
47. Mortensen M, Woo P. Office steroid injections of the larynx. Laryngoscope. 2006;116(10):1735–9.
48. Mortensen M. Laryngeal steroid injection for vocal fold scar. Curr Opin Otolaryngol Head Neck Surg. 2010;18(6):487–91.
49. Young G, Hoffman R, Koszewski J, Whited W, Ruel N, Dailey H. Voice outcomes following a single office-based steroid injection for vocal fold scar. Otolaryngol Head Neck Surg. 2016;155(5):820–8.
50. Campagnolo M, Tsuji H, Sennes U, Imamura R, Saldiva H. Histologic study of acute vocal fold wound healing after corticosteroid injection in a rabbit model. Ann Otol Rhinol Laryngol. 2010;119(2):133–9.
51. Coleman R, Smith S, Ossoff P, et al. Histomorphometric and laryngeal videostroboscopic analysis of the effects of corticosteroids on microflap healing in the dog larynx. Ann Otol Rhinol Laryngol. 1999;108(2):119–27.
52. Zhou H, Sivasankar M, Kraus H, Sandulache C, Amin M, Branski C. Glucocorticoids regulate extracellular matrix metabolism in human vocal fold fibroblasts. Laryngoscope. 2011;121(9):1915–9.
53. Rosen A, Gartner-Schmidt J, Hathaway B, et al. A nomenclature paradigm for benign midmembranous vocal fold lesions. Laryngoscope. 2012;122(6):1335–41.
54. Cipriani A, Martin E, Corey P, et al. The clinicopathologic spectrum of benign mass lesions of the vocal fold due to vocal abuse. Int J Surg Pathol. 2011;19(5):583–7.
55. Behlau M, Oliveira G. Vocal hygiene for the voice professional. Curr Opin Otolaryngol Head Neck Surg. 2009;17(3):149–54.
56. Rose B, Horman M, Sataloff RT. Voice therapy. In: Sataloff RT, editor. Professional voice: the science and art of clinical care. 4th ed. San Diego: Plural Publishing; 2017. p. 1171–93.
57. Courey S, Stone E, Gardner M, Ossoff H. Endoscopic vocal fold microflap: a three-year experience. Ann Otol Rhinol Laryngol. 1995;104(4):267–73.

58. Sataloff RT, Spiegel JR, Heuer RJ, et al. Laryngeal mini-microflap: a new technique and reassessment of the microflap saga. J Voice. 1995;9(2):198–204.
59. Rosen CA. Vocal fold scar: evaluation and treatment. Otolaryngol Clin N Am. 2000;33(5):1081–6.
60. Zettl KS, Sjaastad MD, Riskin PM, Ratty G, Machen TE, Firestone GL. Glucocorticoid-induced formation of tight junctions in mouse mammary epithelial cells in vitro. Proc Natl Acad Sci U S A. 1992;89(19):9069–73.
61. Ramavat S, Tiwana H, Banumathy N, Bakshi J, Panda N, Goel A. Efficacy of intralesional steroid injection in small benign vocal fold lesions. J Voice. 2019;33(5):767–72.
62. Yanagihara N, Azuma F, Koike Y, Honjo I, Imanishi Y. Intracordal injection of dexamethasone. Pract Otorhinolaryngol (Basel). 1964;57:496–500.
63. Nonomura M, Kojima H, Omori K, Kanaji M. Fiberscopic intracordal steroid injection. Koutou (Larynx Jpn). 1993;5(1):59–61.
64. Tateya I, Omori K, Kojima H, et al. Steroid injection for Reinke's edema using fiberoptic laryngeal surgery. Acta Otolaryngol. 2003;123(3):417–20.
65. Tateya I, Omori K, Kojima H, Hirano S, Kaneko K, Ito J. Steroid injection to vocal nodules using fiberoptic laryngeal surgery under topical anesthesia. Eur Arch Otorhinolaryngol. 2004;261(9):489–92.
66. Hsu B, Lan C, Chang Y. Percutaneous corticosteroid injection for vocal fold polyp. Arch Otolaryngol Head Neck Surg. 2009;135(8):776–80.
67. Lee H, Yeo O, Choi I, et al. Local steroid injection via the cricothyroid membrane in patients with a vocal nodule. Arch Otolaryngol Head Neck Surg. 2011;137(10):1011–6.
68. Woo JH, Kim DY, Kim JW, Oh EA, Lee SW. Efficacy of percutaneous vocal fold injections for benign laryngeal lesions: prospective multicenter study. Acta Otolaryngol. 2011;131(12):1326–32.
69. Wang T, Lai S, Liao J, Lo C, Cheng W. Transnasal endoscopic steroid injection: a practical and effective alternative treatment for benign vocal fold disorders. Laryngoscope. 2013;123(6):1464–8.
70. Wang T, Liao J, Lai S, Cheng W. Comparison of benign lesion regression following vocal fold steroid injection and vocal hygiene education. Laryngoscope. 2014;124(2):510–5.
71. Mallur S, Tajudeen A, Aaronson N, Branski C, Amin R. Quantification of benign lesion regression as a function of 532-nm pulsed potassium titanyl phosphate laser parameter selection. Laryngoscope. 2011;121(3):590–5.
72. Wang T, Lai S, Hsiao Y. Comprehensive outcome researches of intralesional steroid injection on benign vocal fold lesions. J Voice. 2015;29(5):578–87.
73. Lee W, Park N. Long-term efficacy of percutaneous steroid injection for treating benign vocal fold lesions: a prospective study. Laryngoscope. 2016;126(10):2315–9.
74. Wang T, Lai S, Cheng W. Long-term surveillance following intralesional steroid injection for benign vocal fold lesions. JAMA Otolaryngol Head Neck Surg. 2017;143(6):589–94.
75. Hosako Y, Nakamura M, Tayama N, et al. Laryngeal involvement in systemic lupus erythematosus: a case report. Koutou (Larynx Jpn). 1993;5:171–5.
76. Hilgert E, Toleti B, Kruger K, Nejedlo I. Hoarseness due to bamboo nodes in patients with autoimmune diseases: a review of literature. J Voice. 2008;22(3):343–50.
77. Oker N, Julien-Laferrière A, Herman P, Chevaillier G. Bamboo nodes on a series of 15 patients: vocal fold lesion as a sign of autoimmune disease and microphonotrauma. J Voice. 2019;33(3):357–62.
78. Todic J, Schweizer V, Leuchter I. Bamboo nodes of vocal folds: a description of 10 cases and review of the literature. Folia Phoniatr Logop. 2018;70(1):1–7.
79. Schwemmle C, Kreipe HH, Witte T, Ptok M. Bamboo nodes associated with mixed connective tissue disease as a cause of hoarseness. Rheumatol Int. 2013;33(3):777–81.
80. Imaizumi M, Tada Y, Okano W, Tani A, Omori K. Effectiveness of steroid injections for bamboo nodules: a case report. Ear Nose Throat J. 2016;95(4–5):E21–3.

81. Wang CT, Liao LJ, Cheng PW, et al. Intralesional steroid injection for benign vocal fold disorders: a systematic review and meta-analysis. Laryngoscope. 2013;123(1):197–203.
82. Voulgari V, Papazisi D, Bai M, Zagorianakou P, Assimakopoulos D, Drosos A. Laryngeal involvement in rheumatoid arthritis. Rheumatol Int. 2005;25(5):321–5.
83. Abe K, Mitsuka T, Yamaoka A, et al. Sudden glottic stenosis caused by cricoarytenoid joint involvement due to rheumatoid arthritis. Intern Med. 2013;52(21):2469–72.
84. Hamdan A, El-Khatib MO, Dagher W, Othman I. Laryngeal involvement in rheumatoid arthritis. Middle East J Anesthesiol. 2007;19(2):335.
85. Habib MA. Intra-articular steroid injection in acute rheumatoid arthritis of the larynx. J Laryngol Otol. 1977;91(10):909–10.
86. Simpson GT, Javaheri A, Janfaza P. Acute cricoarytenoid arthritis: local periarticular steroid injection. Ann Otol Rhinol Laryngol. 1980;89(6):558–62.
87. Dockery KM, Sismanis AR, Abedi ES. Rheumatoid arthritis of the larynx: the importance of early diagnosis and corticosteroid therapy. South Med J. 1991;84(1):95–6.
88. Taliercio S, Cespedes M, Born H, et al. Adult-onset recurrent respiratory papillomatosis: a review of disease pathogenesis and implications for patient counseling. JAMA Otolaryngol Head Neck Surg. 2015;141(1):78–83.
89. Anderi G, Snoeck R, Piette J, Delvenne P, De Clerq E. Antiproliferative effects of acyclic nucleoside phosphatases on human papillomavirus (HPV)-harboring cell-lines compared with HPV-negative cell lines. Oncol Res. 1998;10(10):523–31.
90. Snoeck R, Andrei G, De Clercq E. Cidofovir in the treatment of HPV-associated lesions. Verh K Acad Geneeskd Belg. 2001;63(2):93–120.
91. Jackowska J, Wojnowski W, Hashimoto A, et al. Voice improvement in patients with recurrent respiratory papillomatosis after combined treatment with cidofovir and CO 2 laser surgery. Lasers Med Sci. 2019;34(7):1433–40.
92. Wellens W, Snoeck R, Desloovere C, et al. Treatment of severe laryngeal papillomatosis with intralesional injections of cidofovir [(S)-1-(3-hydroxy-phosphonyl-methoxypropyl) cytosine, HPMPC, Vistide]. In: Proceedings of the XVI World Congress of Otorhinolaryngology-Head and Neck Surgery. Bolona: Monduzzi Editore; 1997. p. 455–9.
93. Snoeck R, Wellens W, Desloovere C, et al. Treatment of severe laryngeal papillomatosis with intralesional injections of cidofovir [(S)-1-(3-hydroxy-2-phosphonylmethoxypropyl) cytosine]. J Med Virol. 1998;54(3):219–25.
94. Wilson WR, Hashemiyoon R, Hawrych A. Intralesional cidofovir for recurrent laryngeal papillomas: preliminary report. Ear Nose Throat J. 2000;79(4):236–8, 240.
95. Pransky SM, Albright JT, Magit AE. Long-term follow-up of pediatric recurrent respiratory papillomatosis managed with intralesional cidofovir. Laryngoscope. 2003;113(9):1583–7.
96. Galletti F, Freni F, Gazia F, Gallo A. Vocal cord surgery and pharmacological treatment of a patient with HPV and recurrent respiratory papillomatosis. BMJ Case Rep. 2019;12:e231117.
97. Naiman AN, Ceruse P, Coulombeau B, Froehlich P. Intralesional cidofovir and surgical excision for laryngeal papillomatosis. Laryngoscope. 2003;113(12):2174–81.
98. Lee AS, Rosen CA. Efficacy of cidofovir injection for the treatment of recurrent respiratory papillomatosis. J Voice. 2004;18(4):551–6.
99. Dikkers FG. Treatment of recurrent respiratory papillomatosis with microsurgery in combination with intralesional cidofovir--a prospective study. Eur Arch Otorhinolaryngol. 2006;263(5):440–3.
100. Kim HT, Baizhumanova AS. Is recurrent respiratory papillomas a manageable or curable disease? Laryngoscope. 2016;126(6):1359–64.
101. Jackowska J, Wojnowski W, Hashimoto A, et al. Voice improvement in patients with recurrent respiratory papillomatosis after combined treatment with cidofovir and CO2 laser surgery. Lasers Med Sci. 2019;34(7):1433–40.
102. Co J, Woo P. Serial office-based intralesional injection of cidofovir in adult-onset recurrent respiratory papillomatosis. Ann Otol Rhinol Laryngol. 2004;113(11):859–62.

103. Chhetri DK, Blumin JH, Shapiro NL, Berke GS. Office-based treatment of laryngeal papillomatosis with percutaneous injection of cidofovir. Otolaryngol Head Neck Surg. 2002;126(6):642–8.
104. Longley DB, Harkin DP, Johnston PG. 5-fluorouracil: mechanisms of action and clinical strategies. Nat Rev Cancer. 2003;3(5):330–8.
105. Nischwitz S, Rauch K, Luze H, Hofmann E, Draschl A, Kotzbeck P, Kamolz LP. Evidence-based therapy in hypertrophic scars: an update of a systematic review. Wound Repair Regen. 2020;28(5):656–65.
106. Jiang ZY, Liao XC, Liu MZ, Fu ZH, Min DH, Yu XT, Guo GH. Efficacy and safety of intralesional triamcinolone versus combination of triamcinolone with 5-fluorouracil in the treatment of keloids and hypertrophic scars: a systematic review and meta-analysis. Aesthet Plast Surg. 2020;44(5):1859–68.
107. Baptistella E, Malafia O, Czeczko N, Filo J, Nassif P, do Nascimento M, Pachnicki J. Comparative study in swines' vocal cords healing after excision of fragment with CO2 laser with mitomycin and 5-fluorouracil postoperative topical application. Acta Cir Bras. 2009;24(1):13–8.
108. Gu J, Mao X, Li C, Ao H, Yang X. A novel therapy for laryngotracheal stenosis: treatment with ethosomes containing 5-fluorouracil. Ann Otol Rhinol Laryngol. 2015;124(7):561–6.
109. Mao X, Cheng X, Zhang Z, Wang Z, Wang Z. The therapy with ethosomes containing 5-fluorouracil for laryngotracheal stenosis in rabbit models. Eur Arch Otorhinolaryngol. 2017;274(4):1919–24.
110. Moore JA, Sataloff RT, Hawkshaw M. Vocal fold scar: current concepts and management. Oxford: Compton; 2016. p. 59–60.
111. Hirano S, Bless M, Muñoz del Río A, Connor P, Ford N. Therapeutic potential of growth factors for aging voice. Laryngoscope. 2004;114(12):2161–7.
112. Suehiro A, Hirano S, Kishimoto Y, Tateya I, Rousseau B, Ito J. Effects of basic fibroblast growth factor on rat vocal fold fibroblasts. Ann Otol Rhinol Laryngol. 2010;119(10):690–6.
113. Graupp M, Kiesler K, Friedrich G, Ainödhofer H, Gruber HJ, Kieslinger P, Saxena A, Hirano S, Gugatschka M. Vocal fold fibroblast response to growth factor treatment is age dependent: results from an in vitro study. J Voice. 2014;28(4):420–3.
114. Kaneko M, Tsuji T, Kishimoto Y, Sugiyama Y, Nakamura T, Hirano S. Regenerative effects of basic fibroblast growth factor on restoration of thyroarytenoid muscle atrophy caused by recurrent laryngeal nerve transection. J Voice. 2018;32(6):645–51.
115. Ohno S, Hirano S, Yasumoto A, Ikeda H, Takebayashi S, Miura M. Outcome of regenerative therapy for age-related vocal fold atrophy with basic fibroblast growth factor. Laryngoscope. 2016;126(8):1844–8.

Chapter 12
Office-Based Laryngeal Biopsy, Excision of Masses, and Dilation

Abdul-latif Hamdan, Robert Thayer Sataloff, Ghiath Alnouri, and Mary J. Hawkshaw

12.1 Introduction

Laryngeal biopsy and excision of vocal fold masses traditionally are performed under general anesthesia. Microscopic suspension laryngoscopy was first introduced in 1960 by Scalco and quickly became the standard approach for endolaryngeal microsurgery [1]. The main advantages are the stability of the surgical field and the ability of the surgeon to use both hands while performing surgery. The magnified image using the microscope is also an advantage because it allows precision and avoidance of injury to the intermediate and deep layer of the lamina propria which may result in scar formation [2–4]. Major limitations of direct laryngeal surgery are the use of general anesthesia in most of cases (although suspension microlaryngoscopy can be performed under local/regional anesthesia with the patient awake), distorted glottic configuration because of laryngeal suspension, and limited exposure in

Supplementary Information The online version contains supplementary material available at [https://doi.org/10.1007/978-3-030-91936-8_12].

A.-l. Hamdan (✉)
Otolaryngology, Head & Neck Surgery, American University of Beirut Medical Center, Beirut, Lebanon

Department of Otolaryngology Head and Neck Surgery, Drexel University College of Medicine, Philadelphia, PA, USA
e-mail: ah77@aub.edu.lb

R. T. Sataloff · M. J. Hawkshaw
Otolaryngology – Head and Neck Surgery, Drexel University, Philadelphia, PA, USA
e-mail: rtsataloff@phillyent.com

G. Alnouri
Department of Otolaryngology – Head and Neck Surgery, Drexel University College of Medicine, Philadelphia, PA, USA
e-mail: galnouri@phillyent.com

A.-l. Hamdan et al., *Office-Based Laryngeal Surgery*,
https://doi.org/10.1007/978-3-030-91936-8_12

patients with cervical spine disease and/or anatomic variations from normal or with neck motion limitations. To attempt to circumvent many of these limitations, particularly in patients at high risk for general anesthesia, indirect laryngeal surgery was recognized as a safe alternative after its inception in the early 1900s [5]. The indirect approach in an awake patient permits functional monitoring of the voice with the larynx in neutral position. Another advantage is cost containment. In-office laryngeal surgery is far less expensive than use of an operating room (OR). However, limited precision while operating, limited manipulation of tissues such as retraction or palpation, and the need for patient cooperation can be major limitations [6–9].

This chapter reviews the current literature on indirect laryngeal brush biopsy, biopsy, excision of vocal fold masses, and laryngeal dilation. The clinical indications, benefits, and limitations using the indirect approach are discussed.

12.2 Office-Based Laryngeal Brush Biopsy

Office-based laryngeal brush biopsy is a diagnostic test used commonly in patients with suspicious laryngeal/pharyngeal lesions. It is indicated when frequent sampling is needed, particularly when the morphologic appearance of the lesion is nonspecific and requires frequent monitoring. The rational is to obtain a specimen representative of the pathologic changes, whether they are inflammatory, infectious, or neoplastic. Office-based laryngeal brush biopsy offers a safe alternative to direct and indirect laryngeal biopsy in some cases. It provides a transepithelial sample that can go as deep as the basement membrane reaching the small capillaries underneath it, without jeopardizing the vocal ligament and hence compromising voice. When done in the office, the patient is spared the risk of general anesthesia and the morbidity associated with laryngeal suspension. The technique is simple and familiar to many otolaryngologists who perform office-based laryngeal surgery. After having applied topical anesthesia to the larynx and pharynx, the laryngeal brush is introduced either through the working channel of a flexible endoscope or perorally under guidance using a flexible or rigid telescope. The details of the perioral and transnasal approaches in office-based laryngeal surgery are discussed in Chap. 7 of this book. The surgeon should ensure that the lesion is brushed rigorously in all directions in order to acquire an adequate sample [6]. The specimen is examined histologically using traditional techniques. A negative brush biopsy is reassuring although not definitive, and the patient often can be observed closely (unless there is high suspicion of malignancy), whereas a positive brush biopsy is an indication for a full-thickness biopsy. Based on a review of 24 cases, Woo reported a positive predictive value of a brush biopsy of 87% in comparison to a standard biopsy [6]. In a study by Afrogheh et al. on the effectiveness of liquid-based, transepithelial, flexible brush cytology in patients with high-grade laryngeal mucosal lesions, the authors reported a 97% sensitivity and 100% specificity in comparison with the results of biopsies taken in the operating room under general anesthesia. The authors stressed the ease of performing this procedure in an office setting while the patient is awake [10].

12.3 Office-Based Laryngeal Biopsy

Office-based laryngeal biopsy, similar to office-based brush biopsy, is a safe alternative to direct laryngeal biopsy under general anesthesia. The surgical technique differs slightly from office-based brush biopsy in that a full-thickness specimen of the lesion is obtained which allows better assessment of deep tissue invasion. Using a 3-mm cup forceps introduced via the working channel of the flexible endoscope or a cup forceps or scissors perorally usually under flexible laryngoscopic guidance, the lesion is biopsied or excised fully. See Fig. 12.1 illustrating the perioral approach and Fig. 12.2 illustrating the transnasal approach. Because it is a full-thickness biopsy, blood is invariably seen at the site of the biopsy [6–10]. See Video 12.1 showing a transnasal endoscopic laryngeal biopsy. Depending on the depth and location of the biopsy, dysphonia may ensue as a result of injury to the intermediate and deep layer of the lamina propria. Patients should be alerted to the possible changes in voice during preoperative counselling. Common indications for office-based laryngeal biopsy are laryngeal papilloma, granuloma, erythroplakia, leukoplakia, and suspected neoplasms, with the latter two being the most alarming. Similar to oral leukoplakia, laryngeal leukoplakia may be precancerous in up to 40% of the cases. In a review by Isenberg et al. which included 2188 laryngeal biopsies, the prevalence of mild/moderate dysplasia and squamous cell carcinoma was 33.5% and 15.2%, respectively. Close to half (53%) had no dysplasia [11]. In that same review, the rate of malignant transformation increased with the degree of dysplasia. Lesions with moderate to severe dysplasia were more likely to transform into carcinoma than lesions with mild dysplasia. Only 3.7% of patients with no dysplasia in their initial biopsy developed carcinoma on follow-up in comparison to 10.1% of those with mild to moderate dysplasia and 18.1% in those with severe dysplasia/carcinoma in situ [11].

The risk of malignant transformation even in the absence of dysplasia on initial histologic examination suggests the need for diligent follow-up and repeated biopsies when indicated. Surgeons should be familiar with the current literature on the diagnostic yield of office-based laryngeal biopsy in patients with vocal fold leukoplakia.

12.3.1 Diagnostic Yield of Office-Based Laryngeal Biopsy in Patients with Vocal Fold Leukoplakia

The high rate of neoplastic transformation in vocal fold leukoplakia makes these lesions worrisome. Although the predictive value role of the morphologic appearance of these lesions using laryngeal videostroboscopic examination, with or without narrow band imaging, has been investigated thoroughly by numerous authors [12–16], tissue biopsy remains the core diagnostic test. With the trend in laryngology practice toward office-based surgery, indirect laryngeal biopsy in an office

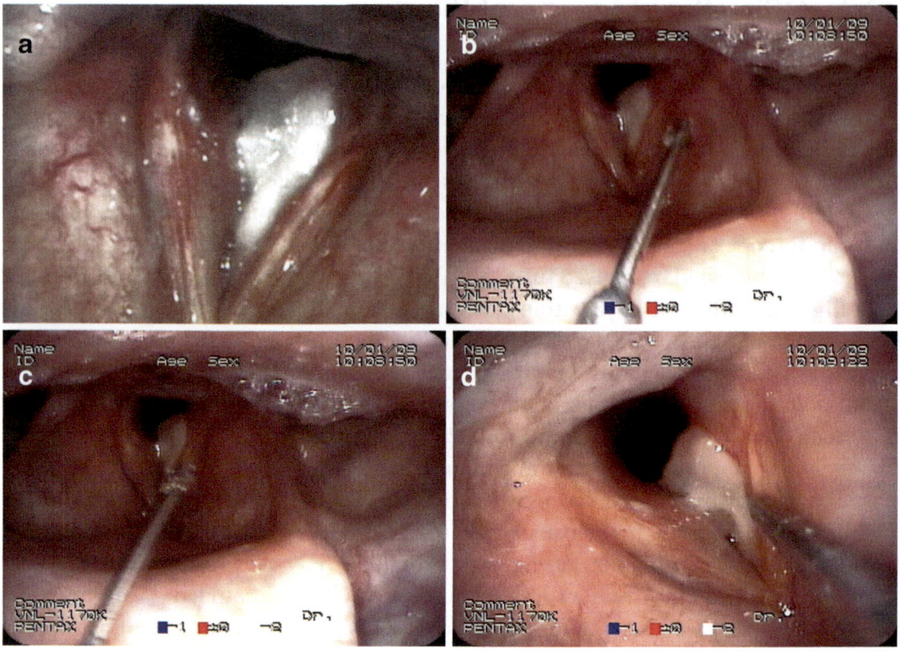

Fig. 12.1 (**a**) Rigid strobovideolaryngoscopy reveals a large granuloma extending along the musculomembranous left true vocal fold. The granuloma contacts the right true vocal fold; the vibratory function of the vocal fold, as seen on stroboscopic examination, suggests a second lesion that is hidden from view by the large, easily visible granuloma. (**b**) A transnasal flexible laryngoscopy is performed to visualize the larynx. The laryngoscope is placed initially just beyond the soft palate, at the level of the oropharynx, to allow for ease of transoral placement of indirect laryngoscopy needle, and then the laryngoscope is advanced. (**c**) Four percent lidocaine is applied topically through the indirect laryngoscopy needle under flexible laryngoscopic guidance and is placed directly onto the vocal folds. (**d**) Once the desired anesthetic effect has been established, a subepithelial injection of 1% lidocaine with 1:100,000 epinephrine is injected into the base of the lesion, at the junction of normal and abnormal tissue, for hydrodissection to help separate the mass from normal tissue. ((**a–d**) Republished with permission. Sataloff et al. [35], p. 19). (**e**) In this case, this inflammatory lesion was removed easily after hydrodissection with straight microcup forceps. However, for more delicate lesions without preexisting stiffness at the base, heart-shaped forceps, scissors, and delicate dissection instruments are available and preferable. (**f**) A second, similar granuloma is removed from the right true vocal fold. In this case, Sataloff left-angled cup forceps provided easy, precise resection of the lesion at its base, without the need for excessive traction and without tearing the surrounding normal mucosa. This was possible because this was a small, friable inflammatory lesion. Heart-shaped forceps and scissors are preferable in some cases. The position of these granulomas on the musculomembranous portion of the vocal folds was unusual. ((**e**, **f**) Republished with permission. Sataloff et al. [35], p. 20). (**g**) Using a 25-gauge Sataloff Indirect Laryngeal Needle, steroid (Decadron 10 mg/ml) is injected into the vocal fold at the site of the base of resection of the granuloma

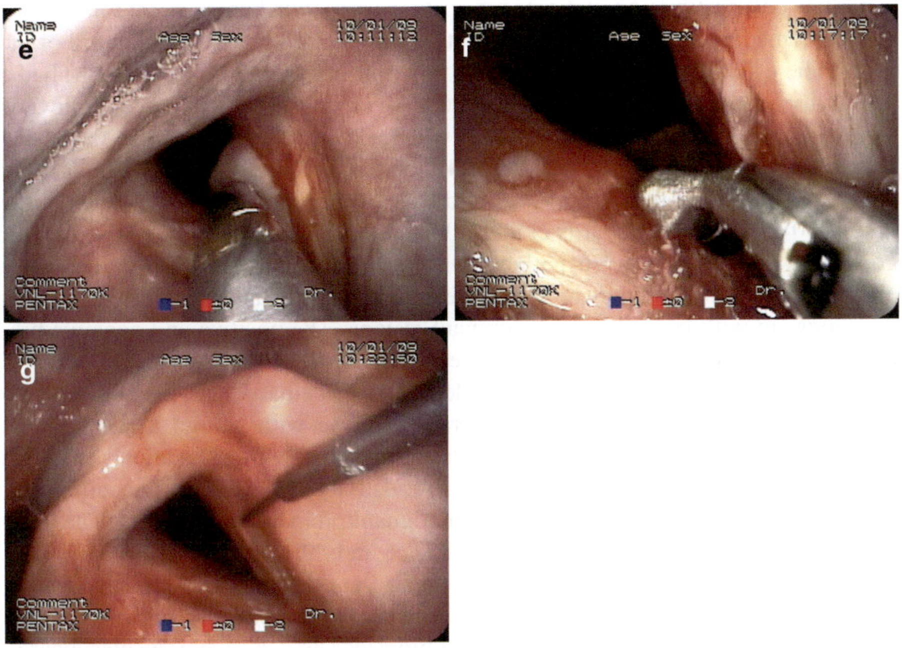

Fig. 12.1 (continued)

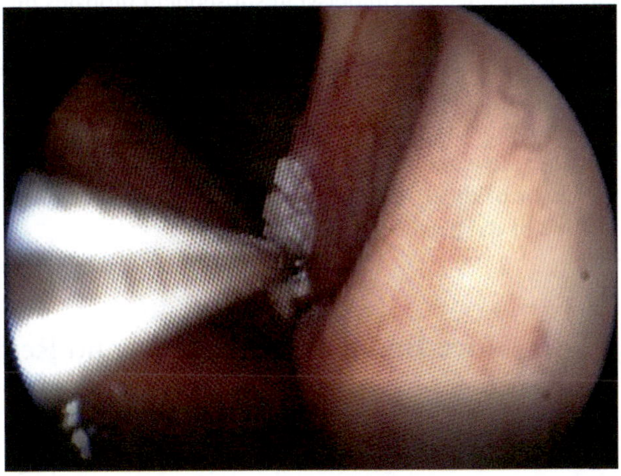

Fig. 12.2 A 62-year-old male, smoker, presenting with a history of dysphonia. On laryngeal examination, the patient had left vocal fold leukoplakia. This figure shows biopsy of the left vocal fold lesion using cup forceps introduced through the working channel of a nasopharyngoscope. (Republished with permission. Sataloff et al. [35], p. 20)

setting has become the first choice for many patients. Although the procedure is tolerated well by many patients with minimal or no complications [17, 18], main concerns include diagnostic yield and the depth of tissue resected. Cohen et al. compared the pathology results of office-based biopsies vs. biopsies taken under direct laryngoscopy in 96 patients with suspicious laryngeal lesions. The results trended toward an underestimation of disease severity in those with benign vocal fold lesions or carcinoma in situ. False negative results were reported in almost one third of the cases. The office-based laryngeal biopsy (via transnasal fiberoptic approach) had a sensitivity and specificity of 69.2% and 96.1%, respectively [19]. In another review by Zalvan et al. that included 26 patients who had undergone both office-based and operating room-based laryngopharyngeal biopsies, the authors found similarity in the results in 81% of the cases. Vocal fold lesions accounted for 69% of their study group [20]. Similarly, Richards et al. evaluated the accuracy of office-based laryngopharyngeal biopsies in 76 patients who also had biopsies taken under direct microlaryngoscopy, and they reported a sensitivity of 60% and specificity of 87% in the subgroup with premalignant/malignant lesions. The positive and negative predictive values were 78% and 74%, respectively. However, false negative rate was almost 33% [21]. The authors concluded that office-based laryngeal biopsy in patients with leukoplakia is most accurate in those with benign and malignant lesions and less so in patients with dysplasia. In a review of 581 patients who had office-based biopsy, Cha et al. reported a sensitivity of 88.2% and specificity of 86.7% in the subgroup of patients with malignant/premalignant lesions. The positive and negative predictive values were 85.7% and 89.1%, respectively. The false negative rate was higher in patients with small (less than 1 cm) and nonfungating lesions. The authors advocated operative re-biopsy in patients with suspicious lesions and in those in whom office-based biopsies showed severe dysplasia/carcinoma in situ [22]. In another study on the diagnostic yield of office-based laryngeal biopsy in vocal fold leukoplakia, Hamdan et al. reported change in diagnosis in four of five patients who underwent subsequent biopsies under direct laryngoscopy [23].

In summary, office-based biopsy of vocal fold lesions is a reliable and safe alternative to direct laryngeal biopsy in an OR. Its diagnostic yield is high in patients with benign and malignant lesions. In cases of mild to moderate dysplasia, biopsy under direct laryngoscopy is recommended. Close monitoring of patients with biopsies negative for malignancy is advocated strongly in view of the unpredictable behavior of these lesions. The risk of malignant transformation correlates with the degree of dysplasia.

12.4 Office-Based Laryngoscopy and Removal of Lesions

Office-based indirect laryngeal intervention has gained popularity as an alternative to direct laryngoscopy for treatment of various laryngeal conditions. The operative image is provided using a mirror, rigid telescope, or flexible endoscope with or without stroboscopic light, while the surgery is performed using curved devices that are introduced perorally [24] or using flexible surgical instruments introduced via the working channel of a flexible endoscope. In 1975, Saito et al. reported stroboscopic microsurgery while patients were under neuroleptanalgesia [25]. Mahieu et al. in 1992 and Dikkers in 1994 introduced indirect microlaryngostroboscopic surgery using a rigid 90-degree telescope or laryngeal mirror. Their approach was met with resistance because of patient discomfort and technical difficulties [26, 27]. In 1998,

Tai et al. described the use of flexible laryngovideostroboscopy during surgery. The authors used this approach successfully in 150 of 157 patients, with a mean operating time of 5 min. The most commonly performed surgeries were injection laryngoplasty ($n = 87$) and laryngeal biopsies ($n = 48$). The authors also stressed the poor of precision of this approach, particularly in broad-based or submucosal lesions of the vocal folds [28]. In 2000, Omori et al. introduced video-endoscope-assisted laryngeal surgery using a charge-coupled device (CCD) chip built into the tip of the endoscope. While the scope was introduced transnasally for visualization, the surgery was performed via the transoral approach using fine-tipped forceps and scalpels. The study group included 114 patients with various laryngeal pathologies, the most common of which were polyps ($n = 34$) and epithelial hyperplasia ($n = 36$). The authors stressed the high level of image resolution that the CCT technology provided in comparison with the fiberoptic endoscope [29]. In 2002, Hirano et al. reported their experience using fiberoptic laryngeal surgery in 27 patients with vocal process granuloma. While the fiberoptic endoscope coupled to a CCD camera system is introduced transnasally, fine-tipped forceps are used transorally for removal of the lesion. In cases of incomplete removal and/or the presence of remaining tags, steroid injection or laser vaporization may be used as adjunct therapy. The recurrence rate was high in patients with contact granuloma (10 of 27), which necessitated repeated intervention [30]. Similarly, in 2010, Lan et al. reported their experience in 20 patients with vocal fold polyps who underwent office-based flexible laryngovideostroboscopic surgery. The authors found significant improvement in the overall grade of dysphonia, aerodynamic measure (MPT), and stroboscopic parameters, including closure, mucosal wave, and phase symmetry. With a follow-up that extended up to 6 months, no complications such as vocal fold scar, aspiration, or major bleeding were encountered [31]. In 2015, Wang et al. compared transnasal vocal fold polypectomy with conventional microlaryngeal surgery under suspension laryngoscopy and reported similar long-term results with the two approaches. The lesions were first cauterized using KTP laser and then excised using flexible, blunt-bended grasping forceps. There were significantly worse self-reported voice outcomes in the short term (2 weeks) in the group who underwent suspension microlaryngoscopy vs. the group who underwent flexible transnasal surgery (visual analogue scale (VAS) 7.7 ± 1.4 VS. 5.9 ± 2.0, respectively). The authors speculated that the higher score in the former group was due to the discomfort associated with intubation and laryngeal suspension [32]. In 2020, Shahshahan et al. described the removal of a pedunculated vocal fold polyp in an 84-year-old woman who presented with dysphonia and incomplete closure of the vocal folds on laryngeal examination. The lesion was excised under local anesthesia using a side-biting cup forceps introduced orally. Follow-up after 6 months revealed no recurrence of the lesion [33].

Microdissection including microflap and mini-microflap surgery can be performed in an office setting using indirect instruments designed to permit precise in-office surgery (Fig. 5.1). However, vocal fold movement from respiration and other factors makes it impossible to achieve consistently precision as good and predictable as can be obtained in a paralyzed, anesthetized patient in an operating room. Nevertheless, when the clinical situation warrants indirect excision even from the vibratory margin, good results usually can be achieved.

In summary, in-office resection of vocal fold masses is a viable option to patients at high risk of general anesthesia. The success of the surgery is contingent on adequate topical anesthesia to the upper airway and patient collaboration. The surgery may be performed perorally using curved surgical instruments or transnasally using flexible devices introduced through the working channel of the operating endoscope. It is important to note that office-based removal of vocal fold masses does not preclude suspension microlaryngeal surgery in patients with residual disease or recurrence.

12.5 Office-Based Laryngeal Dilation

Laryngeal stenosis is challenging and can be hazardous, especially in patients who do not have a tracheotomy. Some patients require repeated dilation, particularly patients with stenosis related to radiation therapy received previously for head and neck carcinoma. Traditionally, such patients have been dilated in an OR. However, that approach always raises concerns, and the surgical team must always be prepared to perform an urgent tracheotomy. Frequently, the airway is too narrow to permit intubation. So, anesthesia is induced, and rapid dilation is performed in an effort to create enough space to permit intubation with a small endotracheal tube. Then, the tube is removed and replaced, often repeatedly, as the procedure is continued. Often, jet ventilation must be avoided because the stenosis limits egress and may predispose to rupture of pulmonary blebs and creation of pneumothorax. Making matters more difficult, sometimes patients do not present to the otolaryngologist's office until the airway is substantially compromised. This scenario is disturbingly common especially in older head and neck cancer survivors; and it may necessitate emergent tracheotomy in the OR, or even in the office.

The author (RTS) developed an alternative, in-office approach in the 1980s. It has not achieved wide popularity and remains generally unknown. The Sataloff laryngeal dilator is a strongly built indirect instrument that is similar in many ways to a Jackson dilator, but it is shorter (Fig. 12.3). It can be introduced into the larynx through the mouth, using flexible endoscopic visual guidance. Its introduction is preceded by cautious application of topical laryngeal anesthesia, with caution

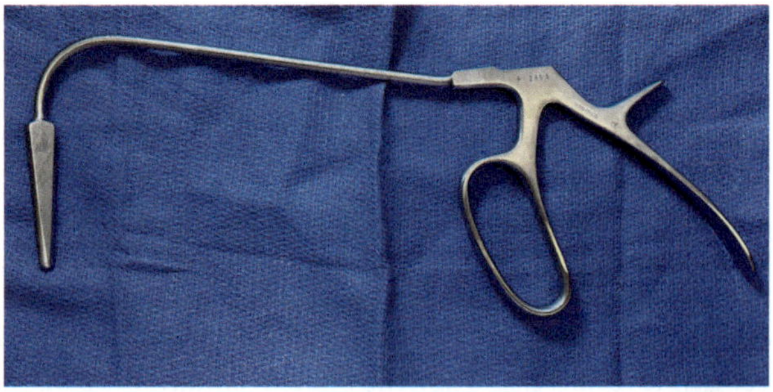

Fig. 12.3 Sataloff Indirect Laryngeal Dilator. (Integra LifeSciences, Princeton, NJ, USA)

stressed because irritation of a compromised airway could precipitate obstruction. In some cases, superior laryngeal nerve block can be used instead of, or as an adjunct to, topical anesthesia. Interestingly, radiated patients often have little or no laryngeal sensation, especially those who have undergone multiple laryngeal dilations; and such patients may require no anesthesia for this procedure. Introduction and withdrawal of the dilator require a substantial (bordering on somewhat frightening) amount of force (Video 12.2). However, the procedure is extremely fast, generally taking only a few seconds. Although performing it in patients who have a tracheotomy is always more comfortable for the surgeon, it usually can be performed safely in patients without a tracheotomy; but the surgeon should always be prepared to establish an airway emergently. The author (RTS) has never had to do so in the office.

12.6 Other Office-Based Endolaryngeal Procedures

Most procedures that can be performed in the operating room can be performed in the office, if necessary. Even procedures that require considerable force such as reduction of a dislocated arytenoid cartilage can be performed in an office setting rather than the operating room, as described previously (Figs. 12.4 and 12.5) [34]. When clinical circumstances warrant efforts to avoid taking a patient to the OR, it is reasonable for surgeons to consider seriously performing almost any endolaryngeal procedure in an office setting.

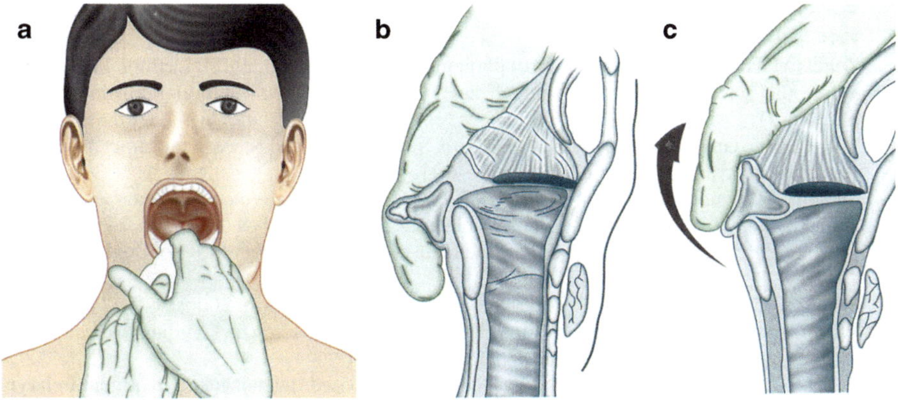

Fig. 12.4 Digital reduction of a dislocated arytenoid can be accomplished in the office occasionally, especially for patients who are edentulous and who have had recent posterior dislocation or redislocation following recent arytenoid reduction. The patient's tongue is retracted by the patient or an assistant, leaving the surgeon's other hand free for external counterpressure (**a**). The surgeon's index or middle finger is placed in the pyriform sinus, engaging the dislocated arytenoid (**b**). The surgeon's other hand applies external counterpressure and the arytenoid is reduced digitally (**c**). (Republished with permission. Sataloff et al. [35], p. 257)

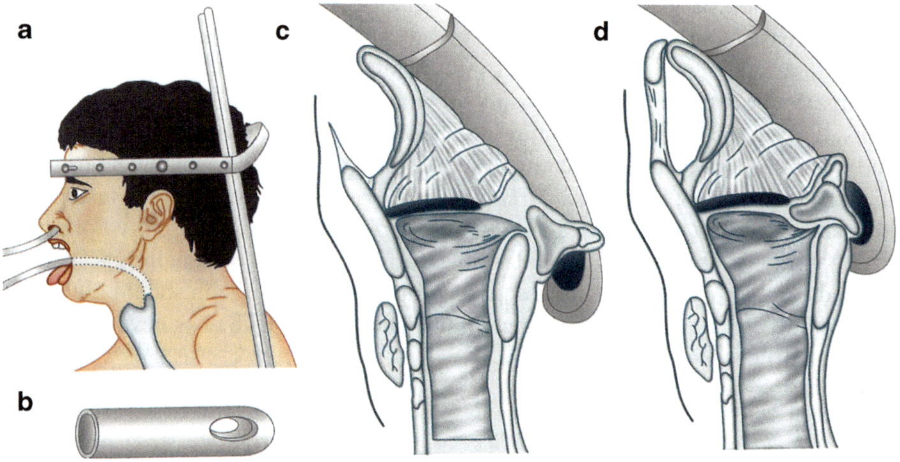

Fig. 12.5 This procedure can be used in the office for patients with posterior arytenoid dislocation and difficult anatomical constraints, such as this patient in a halo. (**a**) A flexible laryngoscope is placed in the nostril to observe the larynx. A right-angle instrument, such as a laryngeal bayonet forceps, is covered with a shortened red rubber catheter. The hole in the red rubber catheter (**b**) assists in making stable contact with the dislocated arytenoid. The posterior inferior aspect of the dislocated arytenoid is engaged (**c**) and drawn superiorly, and anteromedially, to reduce the dislocated cartilage (**d**). (Republished with permission. Sataloff et al. [35], p. 258)

References

1. Scalco AN, Shipman WF, Tabb HG. Microscopic suspension laryngoscopy. Ann Otol Rhinol Laryngol. 1960;69(4):1134–8.
2. Zeitels M. History and development of phonomicrosurgery. In: Sataloff RT, editor. Professional voice: the science and art of clinical care. 4th ed. San Diego: Plural Publishing; 2017. p. 1347–71.
3. Thibeault L, Gray D, Bless M, Chan W, Ford N. Histologic and rheologic characterization of vocal fold scarring. J Voice. 2002;16(1):96–104.
4. Sataloff RT. Voice surgery. In: Sataloff RT, editor. Professional voice: the science and art of clinical care. 4th ed. San Diego: Plural Publishing; 2017. p. 1371–8.
5. Bruning W. Uber eine neue Behanlungsmethode der Rekurrenslahmung. Ver Deutsch Laryng. 1911;18:23.
6. Woo P. Office-based laryngeal procedures. Otolaryngol Clin N Am. 2006;39(1):111–33.
7. Wellenstein J, Schutte W, Takes P, et al. Office-based procedures for the diagnosis and treatment of laryngeal pathology. J Voice. 2018;32(4):502–13.
8. Rosen A, Amin R, Sulica L, et al. Advances in office-based diagnosis and treatment in laryngology. Laryngoscope. 2009;119(S2):S185–212.
9. Shoffel-Havakuk H, Sadoughi B, Sulica L, Johns MM 3rd. In-office procedures for the treatment of benign vocal fold lesions in the awake patient: a contemporary review. Laryngoscope. 2019;129(9):2131–8.
10. Afrogheh A, Pelser A, Hille J, Attwood R, Loock J, Schubert PT. Application of liquid-based transepithelial flexible brush cytology in the detection of high-grade laryngeal mucosal lesions. Diagn Cytopathol. 2015;43(1):21–7.

11. Isenberg S, Crozier L, Dailey H. Institutional and comprehensive review of laryngeal leukoplakia. Ann Otol Rhinol Laryngol. 2008;117(1):74–9.
12. Chen M, Li C, Yang Y, Cheng L, Wu H. A morphological classification for vocal fold leukoplakia. Braz J Otorhinolaryngol. 2019;85(5):588–96.
13. Fang J, Lin N, Lee L, et al. Classification of vocal fold leukoplakia by clinical scoring. Head Neck. 2016;38(1):E1998–2003.
14. Rzepakowska A, Sielska-Badurek E, Osuch-Wójcikiewicz E, Sobol M, Niemczyk K. The predictive value of videostroboscopy in the assessment of premalignant lesions and early glottis cancers. Otolaryngol Pol. 2017;71(4):14–8.
15. Li J, Xu W, Cheng LY. Application of stroboscopy and narrow band imaging endoscopy in the diagnosis of vocal cord leukoplakia. Zhonghua Er Bi Yan Hou Tou Jing Wai Ke Za Zhi. 2017;52(11):806–11.
16. Ni G, Zhu Q, Zhang Q, Zhang G, Wang Q. Diagnosis of vocal cord leukoplakia: the role of a novel narrow band imaging endoscopic classification. Laryngoscope. 2019;129(2):429–34.
17. Lippert D, Hoffman R, Dang P, McCulloch M, Hartig K, Dailey H. In-office biopsy of upper airway lesions: safety, tolerance, and effect on time to treatment. Laryngoscope. 2015;125(4):919–23.
18. Hamdan AL, Jabbour C, Khalifee E, Ghanem A, El Hage A. Tolerance of patients using different approaches in laryngeal office-based procedures. J Voice. 2021. https://doi.org/10.1016/j.voice.2020.12.009.
19. Cohen JT, Safadi A, Fliss DM, Gil Z, Horowitz G. Reliability of a transnasal flexible fiberoptic in-office laryngeal biopsy. JAMA Otolaryngol Head Neck Surg. 2013;139(4):341–5.
20. Zalvan H, Brown J, Oiseth J, Roark M. Comparison of trans-nasal laryngoscopic office based biopsy of laryngopharyngeal lesions with traditional operative biopsy. Eur Arch Otorhinolaryngol. 2013;270(9):2509–13.
21. Richards L, Sugumaran M, Aviv E, Woo P, Altman W. The utility of office-based biopsy for laryngopharyngeal lesions: comparison with surgical evaluation. Laryngoscope. 2015;125(4):909–12.
22. Cha W, Yoon W, Jang Y, et al. Office-based biopsies for laryngeal lesions: analysis of consecutive 581 cases. Laryngoscope. 2016;126(11):2513–9.
23. Hamdan AL, Ghanem A, El Natout T, Khalifee E. Diagnostic yield of office-based laryngeal biopsy in patients with leukoplakia; a case study with review of the literature. J Voice. 2021 Jan 27;S0892-1997(20)30446-X.
24. Sataloff Indirect Laryngeal Instrument Set. Integra LifeSciences. https://www.integrafile.com/file/general/1461595462.pdf. Published 2016. Accessed 31 Mar 2021.
25. Saito S, Fukuda H, Kitahara S. Stroboscopic microsurgery of the larynx. Arch Otolaryngol. 1975;101(3):196–201.
26. Mahieu F, Dikkers G. Indirect microlaryngostroboscopic surgery. Arch Otolaryngol Head Neck Surg. 1992;118(1):21–4.
27. Dikkers G, Sulter M. Suspension microlaryngoscopic surgery and indirect microlaryngostroboscopic surgery for benign lesions of the vocal folds. J Laryngol Otol. 1994;108(12):1064–7.
28. Tai K, Chu Y, Chang Y. Transoral laryngeal surgery under flexible laryngovideostroboscopy. J Voice. 1998;12(2):233–8.
29. Omori K, Shinohara K, Tsuji T, Kojima H. Videoendoscopic laryngeal surgery. Ann Otol Rhinol Laryngol. 2000;109(2):149–55.
30. Hirano S, Kojima H, Tateya I, Ito J. Fiberoptic laryngeal surgery for vocal process granuloma. Ann Otol Rhinol Laryngol. 2002;111(9):789–93.
31. Lan C, Hsu B, Chang Y, et al. Office-based treatment of vocal fold polyp with flexible laryngosvideostroboscopic surgery. J Otolaryngol Head Neck Surg. 2010;39(1):90–5.
32. Wang T, Liao J, Huang W, Lo C, Cheng W. Comparison of treatment outcomes of transnasal vocal fold polypectomy versus microlaryngoscopic surgery. Laryngoscope. 2015; 125(5):1155–60.

33. Shahshahan N, Panossian H, Sataloff RT. In-office resection of vocal fold polyp. Ear Nose Throat J. 2020;99(3):NP33–4.
34. Sataloff RT. Cricoarytenoid and cricothyroid joint fixation and injury: evaluation and treatment. In: Sataloff RT, Chowdhury F, Portnoy JE, Hawkshaw MJ, Joglekar S, editors. Surgical techniques in otolaryngology-head and neck surgery; laryngeal surgery. New Delhi: Jaypee Brothers; 2014. p. 251–63.
35. Sataloff RT, Chowdhury F, Portnoy JE, Hawkshaw MJ, Joglekar S. Laryngeal surgery. New Delhi: Jaypee Brothers; 2014.

Index

A.-l. Hamdan et al., *Office-Based Laryngeal Surgery*,
https://doi.org/10.1007/978-3-030-91936-8

GPSR Compliance

The European Union's (EU) General Product Safety Regulation (GPSR) is a set of rules that requires consumer products to be safe and our obligations to ensure this.

If you have any concerns about our products, you can contact us on ProductSafety@springernature.com

In case Publisher is established outside the EU, the EU authorized representative is:

Springer Nature Customer Service Center GmbH
Europaplatz 3
69115 Heidelberg, Germany

Batch number: 10732090

Printed by Printforce, the Netherlands